Instructor's Resou

for

Barlow and Durand's

Abnormal Psychology

Fourth Edition

John P. Forsyth
University at Albany, State University of New York

Megan M. Kelly
University at Albany, State University of New York

Tiffany Fuse
University at Albany, State University of New York

Velma Barrios
University at Albany, State University of New York

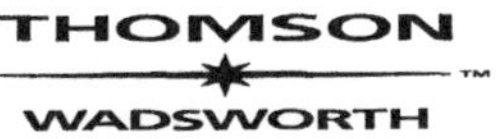

Australia • Canada • Mexico • Singapore • Spain • United Kingdom • United States

Printed in the United States of America
1 2 3 4 5 6 7 08 07 06 05 04

Printer: West Group

0-534-63367-6

For more information about our products, contact us at:
Thomson Learning Academic Resource Center
1-800-423-0563

For permission to use material from this text or product, submit a request online at **http://www.thomsonrights.com.**
Any additional questions about permissions can be submitted by email to **thomsonrights@thomson.com.**

Thomson Wadsworth
10 Davis Drive
Belmont, CA 94002-3098
USA

Asia
Thomson Learning
5 Shenton Way #01-01
UIC Building
Singapore 068808

Australia/New Zealand
Thomson Learning
102 Dodds Street
Southbank, Victoria 3006
Australia

Canada
Nelson
1120 Birchmount Road
Toronto, Ontario M1K 5G4
Canada

Europe/Middle East/South Africa
Thomson Learning
High Holborn House
50/51 Bedford Row
London WC1R 4LR
United Kingdom

Latin America
Thomson Learning
Seneca, 53
Colonia Polanco
11560 Mexico D.F.
Mexico

Spain/Portugal
Paraninfo
Calle/Magallanes, 25
28015 Madrid, Spain

TABLE OF CONTENTS

Preface

Welcome to the revised Instructor's Manual for the textbook *Abnormal Psychology: An Integrative Approach, 4th Edition* by David H. Barlow and V. Mark Durand. The main textbook represents a comprehensive and highly integrative approach to the nature of abnormal psychology and human suffering. In the same spirit, this Instructor's Manual is designed to help facilitate an integrative approach to the teaching of abnormal psychology. To help achieve this aim, this manual begins with a series of resource integration guides that outline and integrate teaching materials (e.g., test bank, video, teaching activities) and resources (i.e., supplemental reading, web resources) with the content of each chapter. What follows next is a chapter devoted to an overview of the science and art of teaching, including more specific points that are somewhat unique to the teaching of abnormal psychology. The remaining chapters provide the content and resources to help you bring *Abnormal Psychology: An Integrative Approach, 4/e* to life in the classroom, including transparency masters covering each of the DSM-IV-TR diagnostic criteria for psychological disorders. The last portion of this manual is geared for instructors making the transition from either the Carson, Butcher, and Mineka or Davison, Neale, and Kring Abnormal textbooks to Barlow and Durand's Abnormal textbook. Though many of the best teaching ideas and resources have been retained from the previous manual, many new ones have been added, and the format and content have been reorganized and updated. The material contained herein is a starting point in the process of learning and discovery; what you do with the material, including other resources, in the classroom is what really matters.

Overview and Content of Each Chapter

1. **Learning Objectives**: A list of some of the most important points covered in the chapter that you may wish to describe and expand upon with your students.

2. **Chapter Outline**: A thorough outline that provides an elaborate overview of the textbook chapter material to assist you in organizing your lectures.

3. **Overall Summary**: A short paragraph or two describing the "gist" of the chapter.

4. **Key Terms and InfoTrac Exercises**: An extensive list of psychological terms found in the chapter. Key terms and concepts from the chapter are integrated with InfoTrac College short writing and web-based exercises. One InfoTrac writing assignment is focused on a single article. The remaining writing activities include 5-10 web-based articles for each key term. A "Future Trend" topic rounds out this section and includes relevant web based links for students and instructors.

5. **Classroom Activities, Demonstrations, and Lecture Topics**: This section includes some practical suggestions for the classroom and provides some popular activities and demonstrations to enhance the learning process. Included in this section are video activities that accompany the CNN video, Inside/Out, and Deficits of Mind and Brain Videos. When applicable, such video-based activities can be used in conjunction with the text video series to facilitate learning of relevant chapter concepts or to reinforce points. Though most activities are

designed for smaller class sizes, some are included that may help facilitate learning in larger lecture sections.

6. **Supplementary Reading Material**: A list of relevant supplemental books and articles for further background reading regarding particular topics in the chapter. Sources noted with a symbol can be found on "*Infotrac, the online library*" provided by Wadsworth/Thompson Publishing. Contact your Thomson Learning representative for further details.

7. **Supplementary Video Resources**: A list of videotapes relevant to each chapter. Some of the video segments are derived from Wadsworth/Thompson sources: "Abnormal Psychology: Inside/Out," "Deficits of Mind and Brain," and "Post-Traumatic Stress Disorder: A Path to Remember." Each of these videos, and many others, can be obtained from your Thomson Learning representative. Commercial video and documentaries, some of which can be found at a local video rental store, are also listed.

8. **Internet Resources**: Each chapter contains several interesting websites for instructors and students to visit. Because web pages come and go frequently, instructors are encouraged to visit the site(s) regularly, particularly if internet resources are assigned to students.

9. **Warning Signs for Psychological Disorders and DSM-IV-TR Transparencies Masters**: Where applicable, each chapter includes transparency ideas (e.g., warning signs of psychological disorders) and transparency masters depicting all of the DSM-IV-TR diagnostic criteria for each of the disorders covered in the main text. Transparency masters can be found at the end of each chapter.

Our main goal in preparing this manual was to help instructors develop an integrative *context* for teaching the *content* of abnormal psychology. A secondary goal was to make the material useful for all abnormal psychology instructors, regardless of the college level at which the particular course in abnormal psychology is taught. Please do not hesitate to contact us with any comments or suggestions at the following address:

John P. Forsyth, Ph.D.
Associate Professor of Clinical Psychology
Faculty Director, Anxiety Disorders Research Program
University at Albany, State University of New York
Department of Psychology
Social Sciences 369
1400 Washington Avenue
Albany, NY 12222 U.S.A.
email: forsyth@albany.edu
WEB:http://www.albany.edu/~forsyth

Acknowledgments

I also would like to thank and express my deep appreciation to the textbook authors (David H. Barlow and V. Mark Durand) for this opportunity to provide material that I hope will help facilitate bringing their textbook to life in the classroom, and the tremendous support and encouragement provided by senior editor Marianne Taflinger and assistant editor Dan Moneypenny of Wadsworth Publishing. I am also grateful for the editorial assistance of several of my senior graduate students, particularly the three co-authors of this Instructor's Manual, Megan Kelly, Tiffany Fuse, and Velma Barrios, and the efforts of Carlos Finlay and Dean Acheson in helping prepare other materials related to this project. Lastly, I wish to thank my wife Celine, whose abiding support and encouragement over the years has enabled me to immerse myself in the science, practice, and teaching of abnormal psychology in ways that I never thought possible.

John P. Forsyth, Ph.D.

THE SCIENCE AND ART OF TEACHING ABNORMAL PSYCHOLOGY

There are many ways one can teach, just as there are many ways to learn. No method will fit everyone. A particular method or style of teaching that you have found to be effective for small classes, may not be workable for very large classes. The trick is coming up with an effective teaching style that you are comfortable with, and one that fits the particular needs of your students and the classroom environment. What your students likely want and need are strategies to help them learn, information that is relevant to them and made relevant for them, and instructors that are flexible in meeting these needs. In my experience teaching abnormal psychology, I have found that the simple credo *"teach unto others as you would like to be taught, not necessarily as you were taught"* goes a long way in making for a lively, positive, constructive, and enjoyable learning experience. Consistent with this theme, the following suggestions may help you as an instructor breathe new life to the presentation of the material and keep you and your students engaged in abnormal psychology for the entire semester and beyond.

THE SCIENCE OF TEACHING

I. Preparation Techniques

There are many systems of preparation. What works best for one instructor may not work well for another. What works for everyone is to develop a system and use it. Examples of such systems include:

A. *The Cookbook System.* This system is an approach that is very much like using a cookbook to prepare a meal. Instructors using this system prefer to base all lectures on the textbook chapters and related ancillaries (nothing more, nothing less); assign all chapters in the order they appear in the text; use a college generated syllabus to plan student objectives; and choose test items from course text ancillaries without modification. Though this system is time-efficient and can be effective, it is not particularly inspiring for students. Indeed, the comments you will likely hear from students (if you hear them directly at all) is that the instructor simply lectures from the book. Unless you require mandatory attendance in your classes, you will likely find that once students learn that you use the Cookbook System, they will stop coming to class.

B. *The Personalized System.* Unlike the Cookbook approach, the personalized system is flexible and tailored to instructor style, course content, and the needs of the students. The personalized system takes the textbook and related ancillaries as starting points, but not as end points. Within this system, instructors develop learning objectives based on a personalized and tailored syllabus; assign selected textbook chapters and not necessarily in the order they appear in the textbook; bring to class material and information gleaned from other sources to enhance and/or supplement the material in the textbook; develop new and different learning objectives and activities based on past experience and student feedback; and often tailor exam questions so that they correspond with what the instructor wants students to know, or at least information that they should know. The danger of this approach, particularly if taken too far, is that the course can become so personalized and idiosyncratic that students become confused as to the content and objectives of the course, have difficultly in knowing what to expect and how they will be evaluated, and may even stop reading the book if the book material becomes irrelevant to them.

C. *An Integrative Approach.* A third strategy is to integrate and combine personalization with structure. In my experience, this approach has been most effective in teaching abnormal psychology. For example, it is difficult, but not impossible, to cover each chapter in the Barlow and Durand textbook in a single semester. The same axiom is true for most abnormal textbooks on the market today. Thus, instructors often need to pick and chose what chapters to have students read, what textbook material they will cover (and at what level of detail) in the classroom, and other activities to include as a means to foster learning. Course structure in the form of a syllabus and predictable class format are important in this process, but also allow room for tailoring to fit needs and demands. It has been my experience that supplementing the textbook material in lecture with other related information, personal stories, and case material is enormously beneficial, for it helps stimulate critical thinking while enriching classroom lectures. Similarly, one could also tailor exam questions provided with the textbook to suit what you, as an instructor, want the students to know for a particular exam. Using the multimedia accompaniment to the textbook (i.e., Multimedia Manager for Abnormal Psychology 2004 A Microsoft® PowerPoint® Link Tool) also provides students with a semblance of structure and predictability in the classroom and serves as a guide for note taking. The integrated approach to teaching abnormal psychology, therefore, gives students the structure they expect, while expands upon the range of content in a unique, flexible, and dynamic fashion.

II. Student Evaluation of Techniques

Generally, students tend to prefer course structure with a balance of flexibility, creativity, and good will on the part of the instructor. It has been our experience that when you are perceived as approachable and genuinely interested in students' welfare and success, then you and your course will stand a greater likelihood of being evaluated positively. Students also want timely, accurate, and fair feedback about their performance. Such feedback benefits both the instructor and student. Taking the time to provide written or oral feedback about how you have graded student papers and other work products can foster learning, but also favorable impressions of you as an instructor who cares about students.

Several possible methods exist to provide student feedback in a manner that fosters growth and learning. You may try sprinkling short evaluative descriptors throughout a paper (e.g., "interesting point," "neat idea," "need more detail here"). Such comments send the message that you are doing more than grading a student's paper; you care about what they said, how they said it, and about the learning process more generally. You could also try summarizing your impressions and suggestions at the end of a student paper, using a standardized evaluative form you may have developed, or even sending comments to students via email. Here it is also important to covey feedback constructively in a manner that directs students to how they can improve upon their next assignment. Unless you provide prompt and constructive feedback, students will be unable to do something different the next time a similar assignment is due.

III. On Becoming a More Effective Instructor

Becoming a more effective instructor can be viewed as a concrete end point (you have it or you don't), or as a lifelong evolving process; a career goal that one strives to attain, but is not satisfied that one has ever attained it. This is very much like the act of being a good parent, a good neighbor, good spouse, friend, or being a more compassionate human being. These and other examples illustrate experiential processes that have no concrete end points. The same is true of being a good teacher.

As a process, developing one's teaching effectiveness can be enhanced in several ways (e.g., taking workshops, observing other instructors known for their outstanding teaching, talking with colleagues, having other colleagues sit in and comment on your teaching, and general practice). Yet, feedback about your perceived teaching effectiveness will likely come from another more direct source: your students. Unfortunately, much of this feedback comes at the very end of the semester when it is too late to do anything about it; though you should use this feedback in modifying your course for the next time that you teach it. Rather than waiting for institutional end-of-semester/quarter student evaluations, plan to evaluate yourself several times throughout the semester/quarter. Aside from using student performance on tests and other written work, consider some of the following examples which students can submit anonymously: (a) have students rate your success on meeting one or more teaching goals using a 5-point scale (1 = never met goal, 5 = always met goal) and do your own self-evaluation using the same standard; (b) have students comment on your teaching strengths and weaknesses at the mid point of the semester, including what they like and don't like about the course so far; and (c) ask to see student notes and assess whether students are getting what you say, what they consider important, and areas that need more emphasis or clarification. Getting feedback early on can position you to do something differently before it is too late.

ARTFUL TEACHING

Artful teaching represents a balance of course content with skill in conveying the content in an interesting and lively manner. The art of teaching is very much about learning how to teach effectively, and how to reach your target audience with your message and knowing that you have done so. Below are several points that may be of help in this regard.

A. *Get to Know Your Students*. Instructors that get to know their students often report that teaching is fun. Students, in turn, who have the opportunity to get to know their instructor find learning more enjoyable. Instructors will likely have an easier time getting to know their students when the class size is small. When class sizes are enormous, the task is more difficult, but no less important. The average size for my abnormal psychology classes never dips below 140 students and is taught in a room that looks more like an amphitheater than a classroom. Yet, I make an effort to get to know the students by name early on and I explicitly tell them from the outset that I want to get to know them. So, I encourage students to drop by my office, even if it is just to say hello. I refer to the students by name when they raise a question or respond in class. I frequently move about the classroom during lectures, greet students at the door, and linger afterwards so that students can talk with me after class. Most important, when a student makes the effort to see me, I ask them their name if I do not know it, and try to remember it for the next time. The payoff of this strategy is great, but the task is difficult and requires an ongoing commitment. Indeed, when students know you and you know them, they will often perceive you as more human, more approachable, and will be more likely to participate in classroom discussion. In the same vein, you will be more likely to see your students not simply as students, but as human beings. To help facilitate this process, you may, for instance, keep a file card on each student with their name or preferred nickname, a phone number that is acceptable to call, interests and goals, reasons for taking the course. Some instructors request that when students speak in class, they state their names before doing so, whereas others use formal seating charts. You may also try having students form study groups and then make an effort to meet personally with each group several times during the semester to discuss goals and progress in the course.

B. *Getting to Know You.* An important process that is often overlooked in teaching is personal reflection and self-assessment of your own personal, professional, affective, cognitive, and behavioral reasons and goals for teaching. Why do you teach abnormal psychology? What do you get out of teaching this course? Do you believe that you are at your peak of teaching effectiveness? Are you genuinely enthusiastic about teaching abnormal psychology? Do you have a positive relationship with your students? It is so easy to get into a teaching rut, particularly when one teaches the same course semester after semester. The easy part is to recognize the rut. The hard part is to do something about it. It may be helpful, for instance, to observe a colleague and to see whether you can extract something new to try in your own teaching. You may also set a goal to try something that is normally outside your comfort zone. For instance, how about setting a goal of lecturing from bulleted overheads or PowerPoint slides and without formal notes. Alternatively, you may try being less rule-governed when it comes to sticking to the exact pace of the material as outlined in the syllabus. Try breaking up the lecture with personal stories, and even humor. Be spontaneous if you otherwise tend not to be that way. Remember that, as an instructor, you are part of the learning process, and you too can grow in ways not previously thought. I can guarantee 100% that you will not become a different instructor if you continue to do the same thing time and time again. If you are not satisfied with your approach and style, experiment, and try something new.

C. *Providing Fair and Regular Evaluations of Student Performance.* Most students would love to hear their instructors say that they will do away with all exams and tests. Most instructors, however, would be quite reluctant to take this suggestion seriously. Yet, instructors should take quite seriously how students perceive the content validity and overall fairness of the evaluations they choose to adopt. Often, I ask students following an exam what they thought of it, and listen carefully to what they have to say. Other methods of soliciting such feedback include: (a) going over the most frequently missed items in class after the exam is returned, (b) reviewing examples of good essays or short answers in-class with the permission of the student(s) involved. Usually, students will respond favorably to exams and the like when they perceive the material as relevant to the content covered in the text and in-class lecture and discussions. One strategy that has worked in the past to enhance this process is to tailor exam questions contained in the instructor ancillaries to fit unique material covered in class. To enhance the degree of relevance, I often preface questions with statements such as "*As illustrated in class by your instructor…*," "*As discussed in class, but not in the text…*," "*As described in class and the text…*," and at times "*As described in the text…*" Prefacing exam questions in this fashion serves to create the perception that the exam material is relevant, that attending class is relevant, and that there is a correspondence between the exam questions, the textbook, and lecture/discussion. Whether such correspondence does, in fact, exist will depend on whether such statements reflect reality. Capricious use of such preface remarks in exam questions will likely backfire and is not recommended.

Finally, unless unannounced quizzes and exams are used routinely as part of the evaluation process, it is a good idea to indicate clearly in the course syllabus (a) the nature of the course evaluation process, (b) the form that the evaluations will take (e.g., quizzes, exams, multi-choice questions, fill-in-the blank, short or long essays, papers), (c) how grades will be calculated, including opportunities for remediation and extra credit (if any), and (d) the purpose of the chosen forms of evaluating student achievement. Indeed, how you evaluate your students' grasp on the material and how often you do it is important in the learning process. Usually, I cover this information from the outset and then repeat it several times throughout the semester. In so doing, I attempt to convey a message that I do care about how well students do in the course; that I want them to learn and believe that they can do so; and that doing well and learning can take several forms beyond what they earn as a final letter grade. Ultimately, instructors want their students to do well, and regular and fair evaluations can greatly facilitate the student's ability to achieve this goal. As I often tell students in my abnormal psychology course, "*you have to work hard to get an A, but you also have to work hard to earn an F.*"

D. *Establishing Classroom Policies.* The policies that you set for your Abnormal Psychology course need to support both active and motivated learning in the students as well as your goals, personality, and teaching style. Policies should be consistently applied and established immediately during the first day of class. As a general rule, you will encounter problems when you change your policies mid-stream, either by loosening your standards (e.g., dropping your attendance requirement, allowing assignments to be turned in after the due date specified on the syllabus) or by making standards more difficult (e.g., changing grading criteria, moving exams earlier than indicated on the syllabus). The most common policies addressed by instructors appear below with suggestions for how to handle them.

1. *Attendance and Punctuality.* College students are adults that come to us with varying degrees of socialization as well as cultural norms regarding attendance and punctuality. Most instructors hope that students will take their course in Abnormal Psychology seriously and make time for it, but the reality is that some students will not because they simply do not care, whereas others will not make the course a priority because they are trying to fit their education into a difficult to manage schedule (e.g., working full or part-time, raising a family, involvement in other relationships and activities). Attendance can obviously facilitate class discussion and decrease repetitious questions by students who miss previous classes. Promptness will encourage greater coverage of the material and less disruption in the learning process. Class attendance can be enhanced by using a seating chart to take attendance regularly, by having students sign in, or by having students answer concept questions at the end of lecture. The most direct, non-mechanical way to increase class attendance is to make the classroom a rewarding, fun, and intellectually stimulating environment.

2. *Handling Late Assignments and Make-Ups.* Most of the world operates on deadlines because they matter and failing to meet them can have very real negative consequences. Some instructors will refuse to accept any late work, whereas others acknowledge that even the IRS takes late returns, though often will a penalty attached.

Here the issue is one of fairness and balance. Set a policy early and stick to it. Clearly specify deadlines for assignments and exams in the syllabus and stick to it, but watch out for being capricious or overly dogmatic in your approach. Though all of us believe more or less that deadlines matter and should be adhered to, the reality is that all of us have failed to met deadlines at one time or another. Require students to provide written official documentation for missed or late assignments and exams. Alternatively, you may allow students to drop their lowest score on an exam or assignment, or inform students that make-up exams will be more difficult or require additional work. Whatever policy you choose to adopt, it is important to be consistent, fair, and human in how you apply it. Provide students with a reasonable explanation as to why you cannot bend the rules in a given case (e.g., out of fairness to the other students), and be reasonable when it comes to legitimate circumstances beyond the student's control.

3. *Extra Credit*. Though recent data suggest that 82% of faculty provide for some form of extra credit, students who earn their grade by doing the required work often resent students who earn the same grade through extra credit. Instructors will no doubt differ on whether they allow extra credit and the form that such credit will take. I have allowed extra credit in the context of my Abnormal Psychology course in the form of (a) participation in psychology department sponsored research and (b) empirical reviews of studies in the field of abnormal psychology. I know of other abnormal psychology instructors who provide opportunities for extra credit in the form of critically reviewing a movie that addresses some important domain of abnormal behavior and human suffering, and even taking pop music and showing how the lyrics relate to some form of psychopathology. Extra credit can often be quite useful as an adjunct tool to encourage new learning and to reward extra effort and motivation. If you decide to offer extra credit, you should (a) clearly state the rules about such credit in your syllabus, (b) tie the extra credit in some meaningful way to course content, (c) provide several project alternatives, (d) limit the amount of extra credit to 5% of the total points for the course, (e) keep extra credit independent of the points necessary in the determination of the final course grade (e.g., students should not need the extra credit to earn an A), and alternatively require that students must have completed all required assignments for their extra credit to count toward their final grade.

4. *Abnormal Psychology Syllabus*. Institutions will differ in their requirements for what an instructor must include in their syllabi. You should, therefore, check with your campus or department for guidelines. Some instructors prefer a short abbreviated syllabus, reasoning that it is more likely to be read. Others, however, prefer a detailed syllabus so that expectations are clearly spelled out in writing. Normally, it is safer to air on the side of being more detailed. An example of this author's syllabus is provided below. Note in this example that I was not able to reasonably cover all the material in the textbook during a regular 15 week semester, and in fact chose to spend more time on some topics and less on others. This is to be expected. Also note that extra supplies were not required for the course. If students require supplies (e.g., buying their text booklets or Scantron sheets), then you should so state. Finally, you may only have 10 weeks with which to conduct your course. In

SYLLABUS EXAMPLE

COURSE SYLLABUS FOR ABNORMAL PSYCHOLOGY
A PSY 338; Sections 3413 & 3414

Instructor:	John P. Forsyth, PhD
Office:	SS 227; Ph: 442-4862; email: forsyth@csc.albany.edu
Office Hours:	SS 227; Mon. & Fri. 4:00 - 5:00pm, or by appointment
Class Times & Room:	Mon., Wed., and Friday 10:10am - 11:05am; Lecture Center 23

Graduate Teaching Assistants: To be named.

REQUIRED TEXT

Barlow, D. H., & Durand, V. M. (2005). *Abnormal psychology: An integrative approach, (4th ed.).* Monterey, CA: Wadsworth.

RECOMMENDED SUPPLEMENTAL MATERIALS (Optional)

Santogrossi, D. A. (2005). *Study guide for abnormal psychology: An integrative approach (4th ed.).* Monterey, CA: Wadsworth.

WEB RESOURCES

The text publisher (Wadsworth/Thompson) offers an online resource center with practice multiple-choice quizzes and links to relevant sites for each chapter (http://www.wadsworth.com/psychology_d/). Followlinks via Student Resources and then the textbook.

COURSE OBJECTIVES

(a) to provide students with an integrative overview of the field of abnormal psychology and major psychological problems and disorders;
(b) to familiarize students with the multiple causes of psychopathology as viewed from a number of different theoretical perspectives;
(c) to illustrate an integrative view of research in the area of abnormal behavior;
(d) and, to discuss intervention and prevention strategies for psychological disorders.

ATTENDANCE AND SCHOLARLY CONDUCT

Formal attendance in class is required, but it will not be policed. It is your responsibility to come to class, or to otherwise obtain information presented in class from another class member. *Please note that to do well on the exams, you will need to attend class lectures as some of the material presented in lecture will not be found in your textbook.*

Students will be treated with respect and courtesy and I expect the same. In order to create an environment that is conducive to learning in a large lecture hall, it is critical that your in-class behavior contributes to a positive learning environment. Thus, behaviors that are disruptive or insulting to me or other students (such as unsolicited talking, coming late, leaving early, slamming doors, or failing to comply with my instructions) will not be tolerated. I expect that cell phones will be turned off during lectures and all exams.

EXAMS

There will be five exams. All exams will be multiple choice format and will cover material presented in lectures, in-class videos, and text readings. The first four exams will be 50 items long and will be given during class time. The final exam will be approximately 100 items and will be partly comprehensive. The **final exam is scheduled for Tuesday May 11, 10:30am-12:30pm (LC23)**. You will not be permitted to take the final exam at a different time.

MAKE-UPS

Please note that, except under extreme circumstances, no make-up exams will be given. If you miss an exam without prior authorization by Dr. Forsyth, you will receive 0 points for that particular exam. Also note that simply not showing for an exam, and then contacting the instructor afterwards will an excuse (however justified), is not good form. You should make every effort to attend all exams, and/or otherwise contact the instructor ahead of time if an emergency arises.

EXTRA CREDIT

You may earn up to 20 pts of extra credit that can be applied toward your final cumulative grade point total by doing any combination of the following:

Participating as a research subject. You may earn 2 pts of extra credit for each hour you participate as a research subject in a Department of Psychology study. Opportunities to participate in IRB approved research are posted in the basement of Social Sciences across from where grades are typically posted. To earn credit for research participation you will need to sign up (and show up!) for one or more studies. Upon completion of your participation in a research project, you will need to have the experimenter complete and sign a **RESEARCH PARTICIPATION FORM** (see attached). Completed research participation forms will be collected only on exam days as indicated on the syllabus and will be cross-checked for accuracy with the experimenter. Attempts to alter and/or plagiarize in any way the information documented on the Research Participation Form will result in an automatic grade of "F" for the course.

Writing an article summary. You may also earn extra credit by doing up to four article summaries. For each article summary, you must read a recent article (within the last 3 years; i.e., between 1999 and 2003) from one of the following journals (available in the campus science library): *Journal of Abnormal Psychology, Behaviour Research and Therapy, Journal of Behavior Therapy and Experimental Psychiatry, Behavior Therapy, Journal of Clinical Psychology, Journal of Consulting and Clinical Psychology, American Journal of Psychiatry*, and *Journal of Experimental Psychology: Applied*. The article must come from one of the above journals and it must be a data-based study (i.e., data were collected, presented, and analyzed), not a review or conceptual article (i.e., an article where no new data are presented). To receive credit for your summary, you must turn in a short, one page (double-spaced), typed summary of the article along with a copy of the full article stapled to your summary. Your summary should address your thoughts about the article (e.g., what did you think about it?, what did you learn?, how did it relate to ideas presented in the text or in class?, and did it raise other interesting questions for you?). Article summaries will be collected in-class on exam days (i.e., exams 1, 2, and 3 only) and you may turn in more than one article summary on a given day. Article summaries will not be collected at any other time, and will not be accepted for extra credit after the 3rd regular exam (4/3/03) before the final (no exceptions!). You will receive up to 5 pts for each article summary you complete up to a maximum of 20 pts of extra credit.

Thus, by doing article summaries and/or participating in research, you can earn up to an additional 20 pts (not more) toward your final grade. Please note that no other extra credit will be accepted to improve your grade.

ACADEMIC DISHONESTY

Any student caught cheating on an exam and/or altering/plagiarizing extra credit assignments will receive a grade of "F" for the course. Please refer to your student handbook for a description of what constitutes academic dishonesty.

SPECIAL NEEDS

Any students with disabilities or other special needs that may require special accommodations for this course should make this known to the instructor during the first week of the class.

COURSE GRADE

Your grade will be based on the cumulative points you earn from all exams and any extra credit earned on or before the 4th regular exam. Keep in mind that you can earn an A in the course without doing extra credit. Also keep in mind that there will be no curve in calculating grades. A = 285-300+ pts, A- = 270-284 # pts., B+ = 258-269 # pts., B = 253-257 # pts., B- = 240-252 # pts., C+ = 228-239 # pts., C = 224-227 # pts., C- = 210-223 # pts., D = 180-209 # pts., E < 180 # pts.

Use the spaces below to keep track of your cumulative points from exams and extra credit.

EXAM 1	______pts.	EXTRA CREDIT	______pts.
EXAM 2	______pts.	EXTRA CREDIT	______pts.
EXAM 3	______pts.	EXTRA CREDIT	______pts.
EXAM 4	______pts.	RESEARCH EXTRA CREDIT	______pts.
Subtotal exam pts	______/200 pts.	Subtotal extra credit pts	______/20 pts.

EXAM TOTAL POINTS	______/ 200 pts.
EXTRA CREDIT TOTAL POINTS	______/ 20 pts.
FINAL EXAM	______/ 100 pts.
TOTAL POINTS	______pts.

COURSE OUTLINE (15 Week Semester)

1/22	First Day of Class: Overview of Course
1/24, 1/26, & 1/29	chapt. 1: Abnormal Behavior in Historical Context
1/31 & 2/2	chapt. 2: An Integrative Approach to Psychopathology
2/5, 2/7, & 2/9	chapt. 3: Clinical Assessment and Diagnosis
2/12	**EXAM 1 (Article Summary/Research Extra Credit Accepted)**
2/14 & 2/16	chapt. 4: Research Methods
2/19	**NO CLASS (PRESIDENT'S DAY)**
2/21 & 2/23	chapt. 5 & 7: Anxiety and Mood Disorders
2/26, 2/28, & 3/2	**NO CLASS (SPRING BREAK)**
3/5, 3/7, & 3/9	chapt. 5 & 7: Anxiety and Mood Disorders
3/12	**EXAM 2 (Article Summary/Research Extra Credit Accepted)**
3/14, 3/16, & 3/19	chapt. 8: Eating & Sleep Disorders (MIDTERM)
3/19, 3/21, & 3/23	chapt. 6: Somatoform and Dissociative Disorders
3/26, 3/28, & 3/30	chapt. 9: Physical Disorders and Health Psychology
4/2	**EXAM 3 (Article Summary/Research Extra Credit Accepted; NOTE: Last Day That Article Summary Extra Credit Will be Accepted)**
4/4 & 4/6	chapt. 10: Sexual and Gender Identity Disorders
4/9, 4/11, 4/13, & 4/16	**NO CLASS**
4/18, 4/20, 4/23	chapt. 12: Personality Disorders
4/25	**EXAM 4 (Only Research Extra Credit Accepted)**
4/27, 4/30, & 5/2	chapt. 13: Schizophrenia and Other Psychotic Disorders
5/4 & 5/7	chapt. 16: Mental Health Services: Legal & Ethical Issues
FINAL EXAM	**Tuesday, May 11, 2002 10:30 - 12:30 LC23** (Arrive On Time!)

********HAVE A NICE SUMMER!********

RESEARCH PARTICIPATION FORM

EXTRA CREDIT

Dr. Forsyth's Abnormal Psychology 338, Spring 2004

Note to Experimenters:

Please complete all the information on this form in ink and return to the subject. **Do not complete Green Bubble Sheets for subject pool credit for this participant**. The subject will be responsible for returning this completed form to Dr. Forsyth for issuance of extra credit for Abnormal Psychology 338.

Date of Participation: ___/___/2004

Name of Experiment and Subject Pool Number:

____

Number of Hours of Participation: ______ Students ID# _____ - _____ - ______

_______________________ _______________________

Student's Name (please print) Student's Signature

_______________________ _______________________

Experimenter's Name (please print) Experimenter's Signature

TIPS AND STATEGIES FOR TEACHING ABNORMAL PSYCHOLOGY

I. Setting the Tone: Making the First Week Count

Students do not want to waste their time during the first week of classes and often resent instructors who just take the roll and dismiss them. Whether you provide a dynamic lecture, offer a fascinating preview of coming attractions, or cultivate classroom norms of interaction and learning, students will appreciate your attention to the important first week of classes for it is here that you set the tone for what is to come.

Abnormal psychology is intrinsically interesting and many students will be taking this course because they are curious about psychological disorders and human suffering more generally. Others will take the course to meet requirements. And still others will be drawn to the course because either they or someone they know has struggled with some form of abnormal behavior and psychological suffering. In fact, you can expect that a substantial portion of the students in your class will know someone close to them with a diagnosable psychological disorder. Of those that do not, they will most likely know someone with a psychological disorder before they reach the age of 50. You may also be surprised that many students taking your class have had, or currently suffer from, some form of diagnosable psychological disorder. It is partly because human suffering is so ubiquitous to the human condition that so many are drawn to this course so as to understand why this is so. A simple exercise during the first day or two of classes can help drive home this important point.

After providing a preview of the nature of the course and the range of topics that will be covered, I often move in to a discussion about the ubiquity of human suffering and how the course is, at the core, about several very real extreme forms of suffering. Most students have suffered at one point in their lives, and all have witnessed someone else suffer. Yet, students often fail to make contact with this simple fact. Getting them to think about how they have suffered can help set a context for what is to come. To drive home this point, you can ask for a show of hands in response to the questions "*how many of you have suffered at some point in your lives?,*" or "*how many of you have felt extremely lonely, anxious, depressed, isolated, confused, bothered by unwanted thoughts, emotions, felt emotional and physical pain, embarrassment, or humiliation?*" Many will raise their hands if you provide a context for doing so. You may also add a vivid case description of a person's personal account with psychological suffering, including other life problems not commonly listed as part of the diagnostic criteria for psychological disorders. I usually follow such activities with another exercise based on the known prevalence rates for several psychological conditions. I treat the class as a population, and then randomly select an approximate number of students from the class that would be representative of different rates of psychological disorders. I ask them stand up, and have others take a look around. I then move to lifetime prevalence rates, and the issue of comorbidity. Eventually, more than half of the class is standing. Many students leave the class hooked, wanting to learn more.

II. Sensitivity, Language, and Humor

Given the ubiquity of psychological suffering, you will need to be particularly sensitive in how you talk about the psychological disorders covered in the textbook. Consistent with the textbook, you should try to use "people first" language when describing disorders. This form of talk reflects the view that people are not their disorders – they are not "schizophrenics," "autistics," "alcoholics," or "social phobics" – but people who suffer from schizophrenia, autism, and the like. Using this type of language (and explain why to your students) should help establish a respectful context within which to discuss the people described in the textbook, including clinical cases that you may use to illustrate certain concepts. Invariably some students will volunteer to talk about their own experiences with psychological suffering and treatment. I let students know that this will likely happen and that such talk is not discouraged. Establishing a respectful tone in class is therefore essential to such openness, compassion, and learning.

An issue that is related to the language concern is the use of humor in connection with describing people who have psychological disorders and their symptoms. Some psychological disorders are associated with symptoms that can appear quite funny (e.g., some of the delusions associated with schizophrenia), whereas many others could be set in the context of humor. Indeed, there are several places on the world-wide web where one could find humorous quips and images associated with most of the psychological disorders covered in the text. As an instructor, I have often found humor to be quite helpful in lightening what can be a very serious subject matter and as a means to help the students learn. Yet, the kind of humor I tend to use is generic. That is, I avoid making fun of the real suffering persons experience with psychological disorders and the disorders themselves. Again, the reason I avoid making such topics the target of humor is sensitivity to the students in class who may have intimate contact with such problems. For instance, I have had students talk to me about their phobias, their experience with bi-polar disorder, panic disorder, eating disorders, including students who come by my office to get more information about available treatments because either they or someone they know is suffering. Yet, knowing this has not dissuaded me from using humor in the context of teaching abnormal psychology. In fact, I use humor quite frequently in the classroom.

For example, when discussing narcissistic personality disorder, I often put up a PowerPoint slide listing the diagnostic criteria, and then ask students if they know someone who is egotistical, self-centered, grandiose, power hungry, and who treats others as mere objects, and the like. Then, with a mouse click, a picture of me appears on the slide, and students break out in laughter. Similarly, when discussing the research base of narcolepsy, I will often point out that some dogs have it too, and then go on to act out (playing the role of a dog) how emotionality might trigger a cataplexic attack when an owner walks through the door of his house and the dog (me in this case) comes rushing excitedly to greet his master. I pant wide eyed, run as if toward the door, and then collapse on the floor of the classroom and snore loudly. The response by students is again laughter, but the intention of using humor in this fashion is to help students learn and never forget what they have learned. In fact, I have had many students approach me semesters later to say that they have not forgotten the bit I did in class, and most importantly what narcolepsy is. Other students have commented to me that using humor was a nice way to lighten what can be a very saddening subject matter. As an instructor, you will need to use your best judgment regarding how and when you will use humor in the classroom. My suggestion is to use it judiciously, and to always follow it with a more serious tone that reflects sensitivity and understanding about the very real suffering of those involved.

III. Prototypical Versus "Real" Cases: Seeing is Believing

Clinical cases presented in the textbook are there because they best illustrate the concepts, diagnostic criteria, and the pure nature of a particular disorder in question. Such cases are not in the textbook because they represent how persons with such disorders normally look. We know that diagnostic comorbidity is the rule clinically, not the exception. The textbook authors know this too and your students should be reminded of this fact. The classroom is a wonderful opportunity to use the cases described in the text as a starting point for discussion about other complex problems often encountered by persons suffering from psychological disorders. You may wish to use cases from your own clinical experience to illustrate the complexity of human suffering; provided, of course, that you take steps to safeguard the patients' identity and confidentiality. Alternatively, you may examine casebooks from other sources and use that information in the classroom. The world-wide web is also a rich source of relevant information, and several sites (some good, others not so good) contain stories and case histories from persons who have struggled with psychopathology and human suffering. Verbally illustrating clinical cases in the classroom is central to making the course content relevant to students, but often it is no substitute for seeing and hearing from actual persons manifesting the symptoms themselves.

It has been my experience that using video and movies depicting actual patients is invaluable as a teaching tool in the classroom. Wadsworth provides some nice video ancillaries of persons with a range of psychological disorders (e.g., Abnormal Psychology Inside Out/ CNN Series); however, I normally supplement this material with video segments that I have collected from other sources (e.g., dateline, discovery channel, PBS, 20/20, 48 hours, the nightly news). Students nowadays seem to respond quite favorably to visual stimulation that is dramatic and a classroom environment that is dynamic. Most news stories of persons with psychological conditions fit this bill, and many programs (not all) do a reasonable job of providing nice illustrations of what it is like to suffer from a psychological disorder. Some major Hollywood films also nicely illustrate a range of psychopathology and are included in this instructor's manual as a reference source. Using multimedia in the classroom is increasingly becoming a must, and functions to provide variety and spice to your lectures. Try having a blank tape at home that you can use to record such material for use in the classroom. Over time you will find that you will amass a nice collection of teaching material that can be used to illustrate the very real nature of psychopathology and human suffering to your students.

IV. Using Multimedia in the Classroom

At one time, multimedia in the classroom meant lecturing and using white chalk and a chalkboard to drive home a point visually. Many instructors still find comfort in this form of pedagogy, particularly as it is workable in most classroom environments. Students, however, often want more from their instructors than white chalk lectures. Colleges and universities are increasingly recognizing this fact, and a national movement is underway to retool classroom environments to bring them up to speed with current advances in technology. So, you will often hear terms such as "smart classroom" to denote a classroom environment that is equipped with several technological tools to help instructors be more effective teachers. Smart classrooms come in all shapes and sizes, but many include sophisticated computer-interfaced audio and visual capabilities and often connections to the world-wide web. Such technology can greatly enhance the classroom experience, and can even help make you a more effective teacher. Yet, technology alone is unlikely to improve your teaching effectiveness. Good instructors will see technology as a tool to help their students learn, and will use it appropriately and creatively to create a rich and dynamic learning environment in the classroom. Abnormal psychology lends itself quite nicely to a multimedia format in the classroom, and Wadsworth provides several multimedia tools that you may wish to try out (e.g., Multimedia Manager for Abnormal Psychology 2004
A Microsoft® PowerPoint® Link Tool, Inside/Out Video Segments, CNN Video Series, Transparency Acetates and Masters). Some instructors will no doubt be a bit sheepish about using technology in the classroom. This is understandable. Most colleges and universities have staff ready to assist you in making the transition to multimedia in the classroom. You may be surprised that technology is not difficult to use in the classroom and that it can make your job

quite a bit easier and more fun too. You may also find that once you start using technology in the classroom, you will put away the chalk and never look back.

V. Bringing Abnormal Psychology to Life in the Classroom

There is no substitute for being well prepared for teaching. The content and ideas expressed in this instructor's manual are here to help you in your preparation to teach and in your efforts to help students to learn about abnormal psychology. This instructor's manual should serve as a guide in this process, not as an end itself. In other words, the instructor's manual is not a cookbook for what to teach, but rather a guide to facilitate your own process or exploration and discovery as an instructor. Indeed, good preparation extends beyond the content of any instructor's manual and even the content covered in a course textbook. Taking the time to peruse material from other sources can help spark new ideas, new spins on topics, and even offer you supplemental content that you may bring into your classroom. For instance, you could elaborate on the issue of empirically supported treatments in the context of discussing any of the psychological disorders contained in the textbook. Alternatively, you may wish to discuss managed care and the role of psychology in a rapidly changing health care marketplace. When abnormal psychology makes the news, bring it into your classroom and relate it with the course material. Help students become more critical thinkers by presenting competing perspectives on a topic. Get them to use all of their senses in the classroom. When you come up with creative ways to make abnormal psychology relevant and real in the lives of the students you teach, your students will learn and be more likely to retain what they learned long after they complete your course.

VI. Helping Abnormal Psychology Stick With Your Students Through Their Lives

We know that students are more likely to learn when they actively engage in the material they are trying to learn and have some fun doing so. As an instructor, you can foster more active engagement by promoting activities that immerse students in the material whether in or outside the classroom. Such engagement may simply take the form of promoting use of the supplemental student study guide. Beyond this, you may also encourage your students to get involved in psychological research, do critical reviews of articles related to abnormal psychology, perhaps critically evaluate how a film or song depicts features of a psychological disorder, form debate teams, or perhaps do volunteer work in a mental health setting. Making lectures interesting, thought provoking, and at times entertaining, can go a long way to helping students learn.

As instructors, we tend not to think beyond the borders of our students as students. We forget that our students will someday be graduates, parents, teachers, lawyers, business people, and that some will be academics, politicians, and even psychologists. We also tend to forget that many of our students will someday be consumers of mental services, and that this particular course will be their first and last formal contact with the field of abnormal psychology. I have found this expanded view of "student" as enormously beneficial in how I approach the task of teaching in and outside the classroom. Developing critical thinking skills in students and a passion for abnormal psychology is a large part of the teaching equation. The other part of the equation is more practical: to help students to make informed and accurate decisions about the nature of mental health and its alleviation based on the best available scientific evidence. Most textbooks will avoid taking such a stand for obvious reasons, but students and the general public need to know what psychological science knows about human suffering and its successful alleviation. All treatments are not equally efficacious for psychological problems. Students need to know this as consumers of psychological science and potential consumers of mental health services. Students also need to know that our best available treatments (plural) for psychological disorders and associated problems in living will likely change as science teaches us more effective ways to alleviate an increasingly wide range of human suffering. Such changes in our state-of-the-art understanding will occur long after our students leave the classroom. Yet, our hope is that what our students learn while they are with us will carry on with them long after they graduate.

Teaching Supplements for
Abnormal Psychology: An Integrative Approach, 4/e

Below is a list of resources available to you from your Wadsworth/Thompson learning representative. Such resources offer a variety of means to enhance your teaching and the classroom learning environment.

Book Companion Web Site
http://psychology.wadsworth.com
Accessible from our *Psychology Resource Center,* you and your students now have cutting-edge teaching and learning tools at your fingertips—helping students master the concepts covered in this text easily and efficiently! Because no user names or passwords are required (except for password-protected instructor resources such as teaching tips and classroom activities), it's easy to access anytime, from any computer with an Internet connection. Here's what you'll find to engage and support your students in interactive learning:

Self-Study Assessments for each chapter
by Kristine Jacquin of Mississippi State University
• a *Pre-Test* that students can complete after they read the chapter to determine what they know
• *Study Plans*—automatically generated based on responses to the *Pre-Test*—that prioritize studies and direct students to Web exercises and specific pages in the book for review
• a *Post-Test* that lets them confirm what they've learned after further study

vMentor™ live Online Tutoring
Students interact one-on-one with a subject area expert who has a copy of the text

Chapter Outlines
Clearly map out the topics covered by Barlow and Durand

Learning Objectives
Provide straightforward guidance on what students need to learn

***MediaWorks* Demonstrations and Simulations (with Critical Thinking Questions)**
Walk students through key psychological concepts

Flash Cards and Crossword Puzzles
Useful for review sessions

Quizzing
Prepares students for the kinds of questions they may encounter on course quizzes, mid-terms, and finals

A Glossary

InfoTrac® College Edition
Search terms and exercises, as well as *InfoWrite,* featuring research and writing guides (with tips on APA style)

A Careers in Psychology area
Lets students explore opportunities for those with a degree in psychology

Links
To the best psychology resources on the Internet

Multimedia Manager Instructor's Resource CD-ROM
0-534-63371-4
This one-stop lecture tool makes it easy to assemble, edit, publish, and present custom lectures using Microsoft® PowerPoint®. Slides include figures and tables from the text as well as linked video clips. To add another interactive dimension to your presentation, videos from our Psychology Digital Video Library can be easily integrated into the PowerPoint slides. The CD-ROM also includes the *Instructor's Manual* and *Test Bank* as Microsoft® Word documents.

Transparency Acetates
0-534-63372-2
Approximately 100 full color images from the text.

Instructor's Manual
by John P. Forsyth, Megan M. Kelly, Tiffany Fuse, and Velma Barrios, University at Albany, SUNY

A Resource Integration Guide for each chapter of the text, as well as learning objectives, chapter outlines with overall summaries, key terms, and integrated InfoTrac® College Edition exercises, approximately 5 Classroom activities/demonstrations/lecture topics, warning signs for identifying disorders, exercises that correspond to the CNN video, Inside/Out Abnormal videos Volumes 1, 2 and 3, Deficits of Mind and Brain videos, supplementary reading material, video and internet resources, and transparency masters (including DSM-IV criteria) for each chapter of the text. The Instructor's Manual also includes information for instructors making the transition from other popular abnormal psychology textbooks to Barlow and Durand's abnormal psychology textbook.

Test Bank
by Marilyn Blumenthal and Michael Goodstone, both of State University of New York at Farmingdale
0-534-63368-4
Written by assessment specialists Marilyn Blumenthal and Michael Goodstone, the *Test Bank* includes 100 multiple-choice and 10 short answer/essay questions for each chapter of the text. Each item includes a main text page reference, is categorized by objective and question type (applied, conceptual, or factual), and marked with a designated level of difficulty. Ten questions per chapter are from the *Study Guide,* and 10 questions per chapter are available to students on the text's Book Companion Web Site. Also available in *ExamView*® format.

ExamView®
0-534-63370-6
Create, deliver, and customize tests and study guides (both print and online) in minutes with this easy-to-use assessment and tutorial system. *ExamView* offers both a Quick Test Wizard and an Online Test Wizard that guide you step-by-step through the process of creating tests, while the unique "WYSIWYG" capability allows you to see the test you are creating on the screen exactly as it will print or display online. You can build tests of up to 250 questions using up to 12 question types. Using *ExamView's* complete word processing capabilities, you can enter an unlimited number of new questions or edit existing questions.

Study Guide
by David Santagrossi, Purdue University
0-534-63366-8
Written by award-winning professor David Santagrossi, this guide includes fill-in-the-blank chapter summaries, key words to define, and a variety of questions—multiple-choice, matching, true/false, and essay—along with answers. It also includes student activities and Internet resources for each chapter of the text.

InfoTrac® College Edition
http://www.infotrac-college.com
When you adopt Barlow and Durand's text, you and your students receive four months of unlimited access to *InfoTrac College Edition.* This online database includes more than 20 years' worth of full-text articles (not abstracts) from nearly 5,000 scholarly and popular publications. Updated daily, *InfoTrac College Edition* includes such journals as *Journal of Cognitive Neuroscience, American Journal of Psychology,* and *Journal of Social Psychology* as well as such popular sources as *Time, Newsweek,* and *USA Today.* The depth and breadth of material—available 24 hours a day from any computer with Internet access—makes conducting research so easy that your students will want to use it to enhance their work in every course. Students also receive access to critical thinking and paper-writing guidelines through *InfoWrite.*

Abnormal Psychology Live 2.5 CD-ROM
This moving CD-ROM enhances students' understanding of abnormal psychology by featuring real clients talking candidly about what it is like to live with a psychological disorder. Archival footage of patient interviews is presented along with audio and visual complements to the text's integrative approach. The CD is packaged free with each *copy* of the text. Each video clip is accompanied by questions, and students can type in their answers on screen as well as print them out.

CNN® Today Video: Abnormal Psychology
Volume I: 0-534-50746-8
Volume II: 0-534-50758-1
Organized by topics covered in a typical course, these videos are divided into short segments, perfect for launching lectures and introducing key concepts. The relevant, high interest clips include eating disorders, anxiety disorders, depression treatment, and addiction topics.

Abnormal Psychology: Inside Out Videos
Vol. I: 0-534-20359-0
Vol. II: 0-534-36480-2
Vol. III: 0-534-50759-X
Vol. IV: 0-534-63369-2 *NEW!*
These VHS videos feature riveting, clinically focused diagnostic interviews with real clients. Volume I (137-minutes) includes such disorders as major depressive disorder, sexual dysfunction, panic disorder, bipolar disorder, schizophrenia, amnestic disorder, and anorexia nervosa. Skillful DSM-IV-TX-R diagnostic interviews elicit all of the characteristics of the given disorder. The interview segment includes opening commentary by Dr. John Csernansky and closing commentary by Barlow and Durand. Volume II (30 minutes) features five clients who reflect on their experiences with dissociative identity disorder, major depression disorder, HIV/AIDS and social support, gender identity disorder, and Alzheimer's. Volume III includes body dysmorphic disorder, ADHD with a child and his parents, and footage from Barlow's anxiety disorders clinic and the research program on autism for V. Mark Durand. The new Volume IV (30 minutes) features segments on post traumatic stress syndrome, phobia treatments, health, and stress.

Deficits of Mind and Brain
by Michael Posner, University of Oregon
0-534-20356-6
This 55-minute, two-part videotape on deficits of attention was produced by Perpetua Productions for the McDonnell Summer Institute in Cognitive Neuroscience, with funding provided by the Pew Charitable Trusts. Part One covers the neuropsychology of cognitive impairments that result from strokes and provides an outstanding overview of brain imaging technology, including CT and MRI. An ideal way to introduce the discussion of schizophrenia in the classroom, Part Two offers a neuropsychological view of schizophrenia, showing a number of patients with disorders and illustrating the specific cognitive problems that they experience in relation to the parts of their brains that are affected.

Casebook in Abnormal Psychology, Revised Second Edition [cover]
by Timothy Brown and David H. Barlow
0-534-36316-4
Using cases taken from the authors' case files or from case files of other working clinicians, this casebook portrays the rich and arresting nature of disorders as they are displayed in real people. Cases illustrate every major DSM-IV category and are followed by a therapy outcome section. The authors draw on an extremely current and thorough database, look at the multiple causes of disorders, and incorporate developmental and cultural issues in each case. Two complex cases are included without a diagnosis to give students an opportunity to come up with diagnoses on their own.

Looking Into Abnormal Psychology: Contemporary Readings
by Scott Lillenfeld
0-534-35416-5
This 342-page reader exposes students studying abnormal psychology to a broad sampling of the major questions and debates confronting today's psychopathology researchers. It contains 40

recent articles, compiled from popular and academic sources, that explore ongoing issues and controversies regarding mental illness and its treatment. Among the topics addressed are gender differences in depression, the biological bases of schizophrenia, the diagnosis of multiple personality disorder, the controversy regarding "recovered memories" of child abuse, and the use of Prozac and similar medications to treat mood disturbances.

The Psychology Major's Handbook
by Tara L. Kuther
0-15-508511-5
This useful handbook offers undergraduate students the information they need to make informed decisions about whether to pursue psychology as a major and career, and to succeed in psychology. The author encourages the student to become an active learner and take control of his or her education and future. The first chapter introduces the scope of psychology, the subspecialties within the field, and information on the wide range of settings in which psychologists work. Subsequent chapters help students assess their skills, abilities, and interests, as well as develop habits and strategies that promote success in psychology classes. Career opportunities at the undergraduate and graduate levels are presented so students can decide whether psychology is an appropriate major for them. Other chapters discuss the world after college, including detailed suggestions on how to find a job with a B.A., and how to apply to graduate school. The book is available at a discounted package price with the text. Contact your representative for more information.

Resource Integration Guides

Chapter 1: Abnormal Behavior in Historical Context

Class Preparation / Lecture Tools	Testing Tools / Course Management	Student Mastery / Homework and Tutorials	Beyond the Book
Instructor's Manual Includes a detailed chapter outline, learning objectives, classroom activities, demonstrations and lecture topics, supplementary reading, video and Internet resources, "Warning Signs" and "DSM-IV-TR criteria" masters, and more for Chapter 1 **Multimedia Manager Instructor's Resource CD-ROM** Allows you to create a media lecture for Chapter 1 using this Microsoft® PowerPoint® tool **Book Companion Web Site** http://psychology.wadsworth.com/barlow4e/ Online quizzes, a *Self-Study Assessment with Study Plan,* Web links, and more for Chapter 1 **CNN® Today Video: Abnormal Psychology** Vol. 1: *Introduction: The Past and Present of Mental Health* (2:24) **Transparency Acetates** Full-color images perfect for enhancing lectures	**Test Bank** Includes approximately 100 multiple-choice and 10 essay questions for Chapter 1 ExamView® **ExamView®** Computerized version of the **Test Bank** items for Chapter 1 WebTutor Advantage **WebTutor™ Advantage** Online course management tool for WebCT or Blackboard preloaded with text-specific content for Chapter 1	**Study Guide** Chapter 1 includes learning objectives, a chapter summary fill-in exercise, keywords, sample tests with rejoinders, critical-thinking activities, and more. WebTutor Advantage **WebTutor™ Advantage** Online course management tool for WebCT or Blackboard preloaded with text-specific content and media resources for Chapter 1 **Book Companion Web Site** http://psychology.wadsworth.com/barlow4e/ Online quizzes, a *Self-Study Assessment with Study Plan,* Web links, and more for Chapter 1 **Abnormal Psychology Live! Version 2.5** • *Roots of Behavior Therapy*	**Book Companion Web Site** http://psychology.wadsworth.com/barlow4e/ Online quizzes, a *Self-Study Assessment with Study Plan,* Web links, and more for Chapter 1 **InfoTrac® College Edition** http://www.infotrac-college.com *Keywords*: mental illness (attitudes), psychology (pathological history), mass hysteria, psychopathology, defense mechanisms, operant conditioning, mental health **Recommended Web Sites** Check out the Book Companion Web Site for a link to the National Institute of Mental Health

Chapter 2: An Integrative Approach to Psychopathology

Class Preparation / Lecture Tools	Testing Tools / Course Management	Student Mastery / Homework and Tutorials	Beyond the Book
Instructor's Manual Includes a detailed chapter outline, learning objectives, classroom activities, demonstrations and lecture topics, supplementary reading, video and Internet resources, "Warning Signs" and "DSM-IV-TR criteria" masters, and more for Chapter 2 **Multimedia Manager Instructor's Resource CD-ROM** Allows you to create a media lecture for Chapter 2 using this Microsoft® PowerPoint® tool **Book Companion Web Site** http://psychology.wadsworth.com/barlow4e/ Online quizzes, a *Self-Study Assessment with Study Plan*, Web links, and more for Chapter 2 **CNN® Today Video: Abnormal Psychology** Vol. 1: *An Integrative Approach to Psychopathology* (2.07) **Transparency Acetates** Full-color images perfect for enhancing lectures	**Test Bank** Includes approximately 100 multiple-choice and 10 essay questions for Chapter 2 ExamView® **ExamView®** Computerized version of the **Test Bank** items for Chapter 2 WebTutor Advantage **WebTutor™ Advantage** Online course management tool for WebCT or Blackboard preloaded with text-specific content for Chapter 2	**Study Guide** Chapter 2 includes learning objectives, a chapter summary fill-in exercise, keywords, sample tests with rejoinders, critical-thinking activities, and more. WebTutor Advantage **WebTutor™ Advantage** Online course management tool for WebCT or Blackboard preloaded with text-specific content and media resources for Chapter 2 **Book Companion Web Site** http://psychology.wadsworth.com/barlow4e/ Online quizzes, a *Self-Study Assessment with Study Plan*, Web links, and more for Chapter 2 **Abnormal Psychology Live! Version 2.5** • *Integrative Approach*	**Book Companion Web Site** http://psychology.wadsworth.com/barlow4e/ Online quizzes, a *Self-Study Assessment with Study Plan*, Web links, and more for Chapter 2 **InfoTrac® College Edition** http://www.infotrac-college.com *Keywords*: nature and nurture (periodicals), amygdala (periodicals), neuroscience, behavior genetics, cognitive science, psychosocial development, developmental psychopathology, observational learning **Recommended Web Sites** Check out the Book Companion Web Site for links to these sites: •The Whole Brain Atlas •Albert Bandura

Chapter 3: Clinical Assessment and Diagnosis

Class Preparation / Lecture Tools	Testing Tools / Course Management	Student Mastery / Homework and Tutorials	Beyond the Book
Instructor's Manual Includes a detailed chapter outline, learning objectives, classroom activities, demonstrations and lecture topics, supplementary reading, video and Internet resources, "Warning Signs" and "DSM-IV-TR criteria" masters, and more for Chapter 3 **Multimedia Manager Instructor's Resource CD-ROM** Allows you to create a media lecture for Chapter 3 using this Microsoft® PowerPoint® tool **Book Companion Web Site** http://psychology.wadsworth.com/barlow4e/ Online quizzes, a *Self-Study Assessment with Study Plan*, Web links, and more for Chapter 3 **CNN® Today Video: Abnormal Psychology** Vol. 1: *Clinical Assessment and Diagnosis* (1:82) **Transparency Acetates** Full-color images perfect for enhancing lectures	**Test Bank** Includes approximately 100 multiple-choice and 10 essay questions for Chapter 3 ExamView® **ExamView®** Computerized version of the **Test Bank** items Chapter 3 WebTUTOR Advantage **WebTutor™ Advantage** Online course management tool for WebCT or Blackboard preloaded with text-specific content for Chapter 3	**Study Guide** Chapter 3 includes learning objectives, a chapter summary fill-in exercise, keywords, sample tests with rejoinders, critical-thinking activities, and more. WebTUTOR Advantage **WebTutor™ Advantage** Online course management tool for WebCT or Blackboard preloaded with text-specific content and media resources for Chapter 3 **Book Companion Web Site** http://psychology.wadsworth.com/barlow4e/ Online quizzes, a *Self-Study Assessment with Study Plan*, Web links, and more for Chapter 3 **Abnormal Psychology Live! Version 2.5** •*Arriving at a Diagnosis* •*Psychological Assessment*	**Book Companion Web Site** http://psychology.wadsworth.com/barlow4e/ Online quizzes, a *Self-Study Assessment with Study Plan*, Web links, and more for Chapter 3 **InfoTrac® College Edition** http://www.infotrac-college.com *Keywords*: mental illness (public opinion), placebo effect, psychological assessment, Diagnostic and Statistical Manual, neuropsychological testing

Chapter 4: Research Methods			
Class Preparation / Lecture Tools	**Testing Tools / Course Management**	**Student Mastery / Homework and Tutorials**	**Beyond the Book**
Instructor's Manual Includes a detailed chapter outline, learning objectives, classroom activities, demonstrations and lecture topics, supplementary reading, video and Internet resources, "Warning Signs" and "DSM-IV-TR criteria" masters, and more for Chapter 4 **Multimedia Manager Instructor's Resource CD-ROM** Allows you to create a media lecture for Chapter 4 using this Microsoft® PowerPoint® tool **Book Companion Web Site** http://psychology.wadsworth.com/barlow4e/ Online quizzes, a *Self-Study Assessment with Study Plan,* Web links, and more for Chapter 4 **Abnormal Psychology Inside Out** Vol. III: *Research Methods* (13:10) **Transparency Acetates** Full-color images perfect for enhancing lectures	**Test Bank** Includes approximately 100 multiplechoice and 10 essay questions for Chapter 4 ExamView® **ExamView®** Computerized version of the **Test Bank** items for Chapter 4 WebTutor Advantage **WebTutor™ Advantage** Online course management tool for WebCT or Blackboard preloaded with text-specific content for Chapter 4	**Study Guide** Chapter 4 includes learning objectives, a chapter summary fill-in exercise, keywords, sample tests with rejoinders, criticalthinking activities, and more. WebTutor Advantage **WebTutor™ Advantage** Online course management tool for WebCT or Blackboard preloaded with text-specific content and media resources for Chapter 4 **Book Companion Web Site** http://psychology.wadsworth.com/barlow4e/ Online quizzes, a *Self-Study Assessment with Study Plan,* Web links, and more for Chapter 4 **Abnormal Psychology Live! Version 2.5** •*Research Methods*	**Book Companion Web Site** http://psychology.wadsworth.com/barlow4e/ Online quizzes, a *Self-Study Assessment with Study Plan,* Web links, and more for Chapter 4 **InfoTrac® College Edition** http://www.infotrac-college.com *Keywords:* placebo effect, research methods, experimental design, epidemiology, twin studies, cross-sectional design **Recommended Web Sites** Check out the Book Companion Web Site for link to the sites •APA Ethics Office •Research Design Explained

Chapter 5: Anxiety Disorders			
Class Preparation / Lecture Tools	**Testing Tools / Course Management**	**Student Mastery / Homework and Tutorials**	**Beyond the Book**
Instructor's Manual Includes a detailed chapter outline, learning objectives, classroom activities, demonstrations and lecture topics, supplementary reading, video and Internet resources, "Warning Signs" and "DSM-IV-TR criteria" masters, and more for Chapter 5 **Multimedia Manager Instructor's Resource CD-ROM** Allows you to create a media lecture for Chapter 5 using this Microsoft® PowerPoint® tool **Book Companion Web Site** http://psychology.wadsworth.com/barlow4e/ Online quizzes, a *Self-Study Assessment with Study Plan,* Web links, and more for Chapter 5 **CNN® Today Video: Abnormal Psychology** Vol. 1: *Anxiety Disorders: Panic Attacks* (2:75) Vol. 2: *Anxiety Post 9/11* (2:32) **Abnormal Psychology Inside Out** Vol. IV: *Brief Behavioral Treatment of Specific Phobia (Parts 1–3) (12:36), Virtual Reality: A New Approach to Treatment for Anxiety Disorders (5:39)* **Transparency Acetates** Full-color images perfect for enhancing lectures	**Test Bank** Includes approximately 100 multiple-choice and 10 essay questions for Chapter 5 ExamView® **ExamView®** Computerized version of the **Test Bank** items for Chapter 5 WebTUTOR Advantage **WebTutor™ Advantage** Online course management tool for WebCT or Blackboard preloaded with text-specific content for Chapter 5	**Study Guide** Chapter 5 includes learning objectives, a chapter summary fill-in exercise, keywords, sample tests with rejoinders, critical-thinking activities, and more. WebTUTOR Advantage **WebTutor™ Advantage** Online course management tool for WebCT or Blackboard preloaded with text-specific content and media resources for Chapter 5 **Book Companion Web Site** http://psychology.wadsworth.com/barlow4e/ Online quizzes, a *Self-Study Assessment with Study Plan,* Web links, and more for Chapter 5 **Abnormal Psychology Live! Version 2.5** • *Panic Disorder: Steve* • *Obsessive Compulsive Disorder: Chuck* • *Rapid Behavioral Treatment of Specific Phobia (Parts 1–3)* • *Virtual Reality: A New Approach Treatment for Anxiety Disorders*	**Book Companion Web Site** http://psychology.wadsworth.com/barlow4e/ Online quizzes, a *Self-Study Assessment with Study Plan,* Web links, and more for Chapter 5 **InfoTrac® College Edition** http://www.infotrac-college.com *Keywords*: anxiety, panic disorder, phobia, generalized anxiety disorder, agoraphobia, separation anxiety disorder, posttraumatic stress disorder, obsessive-compulsive disorder **Casebook in Abnormal Psychology,** Chapters 1–5 **Looking into Abnormal Psychology** • Current Perspectives on Panic and Panic Disorder **Recommended Web Sites** Check out the Book Companion Web Site for links to these sites: • The Phobia List • Obsessive-Compulsive Foundation

Chapter 6: Somatoform and Dissociative Disorders

Class Preparation / Lecture Tools	Testing Tools / Course Management	Student Mastery / Homework and Tutorials	Beyond the Book
Instructor's Manual Includes a detailed chapter outline, learning objectives, classroom activities, demonstrations and lecture topics, supplementary reading, video and Internet resources, "Warning Signs" and "DSM-IV-TR criteria" masters, and more for Chapter 6 **Multimedia Manager Instructor's Resource CD-ROM** Allows you to create a media lecture for Chapter 6 using this Microsoft® PowerPoint® tool **Book Companion Web Site** http://psychology.wadsworth.com/barlow4e/ Online quizzes, a *Self-Study Assessment with Study Plan*, Web links, and more for Chapter 6 **Abnormal Psychology Inside Out** Vol. III: *Body Dysmorphic Disorder* (7:40) **Transparency Acetates** Full-color images perfect for enhancing lectures	**Test Bank** Includes approximately 100 multiple-choice and 10 essay questions for Chapter 6 ExamView® **ExamView®** Computerized version of the **Test Bank** items for Chapter 6 WebTUTOR Advantage **WebTutor™ Advantage** Online course management tool for WebCT or Blackboard preloaded with text-specific content for Chapter 6	**Study Guide** Chapter 6 includes learning objectives, a chapter summary fill-in exercise, keywords, sample tests with rejoinders, critical-thinking activities, and more. WebTUTOR Advantage **WebTutor™ Advantage** Online course management tool for WebCT or Blackboard preloaded with text-specific content and media resources for Chapter 6 **Book Companion Web Site** http://psychology.wadsworth.com/barlow4e/ Online quizzes, a *Self-Study Assessment with Study Plan*, Web links, and more for Chapter 6 **Abnormal Psychology Live! Version 2.5** • *Dissociative Identity Disorder: Rachel* • *Body Dysmorphic Disorder: Doug*	**Book Companion Web Site** http://psychology.wadsworth.com/barlow4e/ Online quizzes, a *Self-Study Assessment with Study Plan*, Web links, and more for Chapter 6 **InfoTrac® College Edition** http://www.infotrac-college.com *Keywords*: somatoform disorders, dissociation (psychology), body dysmorphic disorder, dissociative identity disorder, dissociative, factitious disorder, somatization **Casebook in Abnormal Psychology** Chapter 7 **Looking into Abnormal Psychology** • The Mind of a Hypochondriac

Chapter 7: Mood Disorders and Suicide

Class Preparation / Lecture Tools	Testing Tools / Course Management	Student Mastery / Homework and Tutorials	Beyond the Book
Instructor's Manual Includes a detailed chapter outline, learning objectives, classroom activities, demonstrations and lecture topics, supplementary reading, video and Internet resources, "Warning Signs" and "DSM-IV-TR criteria" masters, and more for Chapter 7 **Multimedia Manager Instructor's Resource CD-ROM** Allows you to create a media lecture for Chapter 7 using this Microsoft® PowerPoint® tool **Book Companion Web Site** http://psychology.wadsworth.com/barlow4e/ Online quizzes, a *Self-Study Assessment with Study Plan*, Web links, and more for Chapter 7 **CNN® Today Video: Abnormal Psychology** Vol. 1: *Depression Treatment* (2:04) Vol. 2: *Depression and School Violence* (2:28) **Transparency Acetates** Full-color images perfect for enhancing lectures	**Test Bank** Includes approximately 100 multiple-choice and 10 essay questions for Chapter 7 ExamView® **ExamView®** Computerized version of the **Test Bank** items for Chapter 7 WebTUTOR Advantage **WebTutor™ Advantage** Online course management tool for WebCT or Blackboard preloaded with text-specific content for Chapter 7	**Study Guide** Chapter 7 includes learning objectives, a chapter summary fill-in exercise, keywords, sample tests with rejoinders, critical-thinking activities, and more. WebTUTOR Advantage **WebTutor™ Advantage** Online course management tool for WebCT or Blackboard preloaded with text-specific content and media resources for Chapter 7 **Book Companion Web Site** http://psychology.wadsworth.com/barlow4e/ Online quizzes, a *Self-Study Assessment with Study Plan*, Web links, and more for Chapter 7 **Abnormal Psychology Live! Version 2.5** • *Major Depressive Disorder: Barbara* • *Major Depressive Disorder: Evelyn* • *Bipolar Disorder: Mary*	**Book Companion Web Site** http://psychology.wadsworth.com/barlow4e/ Online quizzes, a *Self-Study Assessment with Study Plan*, Web links, and more for Chapter 7 **InfoTrac® College Edition** http://www.infotrac-college.com *Keywords*: major depression, bipolar disorder, seasonal affective disorder, mood disorder, mania, suicide, dysphoria, delusions, electroconvulsive therapy, cognitive therapy **Casebook in Abnormal Psychology** Chapters 8 and 9 **Looking into Abnormal Psychology** • Women and Depression • Manic-Depressive Illness and Creativity **Recommended Web Sites** Check out the Book Companion Web Site for links to these sites: • Depression Central • National Institute of Mental Health

Chapter 8: Eating and Sleep Disorders

Class Preparation / Lecture Tools	Testing Tools / Course Management	Student Mastery / Homework and Tutorials	Beyond the Book
Instructor's Manual Includes a detailed chapter outline, learning objectives, classroom activities, demonstrations and lecture topics, supplementary reading, video and Internet resources, "Warning Signs" and "DSM-IV-TR criteria" masters, and more for Chapter 8 **Multimedia Manager Instructor's Resource CD-ROM** Allows you to create a media lecture for Chapter 8 using this Microsoft® PowerPoint® tool **Book Companion Web Site** http://psychology.wadsworth.com/barlow4e/ Online quizzes, a *Self-Study Assessment with Study Plan,* Web links, and more for Chapter 8 **CNN® Today Video: Abnormal Psychology** Vol. 1: *Hollywood Thin* (2:40) **Transparency Acetates** Full-color images perfect for enhancing lectures	**Test Bank** Includes approximately 100 multiple-choice and 10 essay questions for Chapter 8 ExamView® **ExamView®** Computerized version of the **Test Bank** items for Chapter 8 WebTUTOR Advantage **WebTutor™ Advantage** Online course management tool for WebCT or Blackboard preloaded with text-specific content for Chapter 8	**Study Guide** Chapter 8 includes learning objectives, a chapter summary fill-in exercise, keywords, sample tests with rejoinders, critical-thinking activities, and more. WebTUTOR Advantage **WebTutor™ Advantage** Online course management tool for WebCT or Blackboard preloaded with text-specific content and media resources for Chapter 8 **Book Companion Web Site** http://psychology.wadsworth.com/barlow4e/ Online quizzes, a *Self-Study Assessment with Study Plan,* Web links, and more for Chapter 8 **Abnormal Psychology Live! Version 2.5** • *Anorexia Nervosa: Susan* • *Anorexia Nervosa/ Bulimia: Twins* • *Sleep Cycle*	**Book Companion Web Site** http://psychology.wadsworth.com/barlow4e/ Online quizzes, a *Self-Study Assessment with Study Plan,* Web links, and more for Chapter 8 **InfoTrac® College Edition** http://www.infotrac-college.com *Keywords*: anorexia nervosa, body image, bulimia, compulsive eating, eating disorders, narcolepsy, sleep apnea syndromes, sleep-wake cycle, rapid eye movement, insomnia, obesity, obesity in children, failure to thrive **Casebook in Abnormal Psychology** Chapter 10 **Looking into Abnormal Psychology** • The Pressure to Lose **Recommended Web Sites** Check out the Book Companion Web Site for links to these sites: • Medline Plus Sleep Disorders • Tips for Healthy Sleep

Chapter 9: Physical Disorders and Health Psychology			
Class Preparation / Lecture Tools	**Testing Tools / Course Management**	**Student Mastery / Homework and Tutorials**	**Beyond the Book**
Instructor's Manual Includes a detailed chapter outline, learning objectives, classroom activities, demonstrations and lecture topics, supplementary reading, video and Internet resources, "Warning Signs" and "DSM-IV-TR criteria" masters, and more for Chapter 9 **Multimedia Manager Instructor's Resource CD-ROM** Allows you to create a media lecture for Chapter 9 using this Microsoft® PowerPoint® tool **Book Companion Web Site** http://psychology.wadsworth.com/barlow4e/ Online quizzes, a *Self-Study Assessment with Study Plan*, Web links, and more for Chapter 9 **CNN® Today Video: Abnormal Psychology** Vol. 1: *Stressful Heart* (2:04) **Abnormal Psychology Inside Out** Vol. IV: *Studying the Effects of Emotions on Physical Health (5:10), Breast Cancer Support and Education (3:34), Obesity and Weight Control (5:57)* **Transparency Acetates** Full-color images perfect for enhancing lectures	**Test Bank** Includes approximately 100 multiple-choice and 10 essay questions for Chapter 9 ExamView® **ExamView®** Computerized version of the **Test Bank** items for Chapter 9 WebTUTOR Advantage **WebTutor™ Advantage** Online course management tool for WebCT or Blackboard preloaded with text-specific content for Chapter 9	**Study Guide** Chapter 9 includes learning objectives, a chapter summary fill-in exercise, keywords, sample tests with rejoinders, critical-thinking activities, and more. WebTUTOR Advantage **WebTutor™ Advantage** Online course management tool for WebCT or Blackboard preloaded with text-specific content and media resources for Chapter 9 **Book Companion Web Site** http://psychology.wadsworth.com/barlow4e/ Online quizzes, a *Self-Study Assessment with Study Plan*, Web links, and more for Chapter 9 **Abnormal Psychology Live! Version 2.5** • *Social Support/HIV: Orel* • *Studying the Effects of Emotions on Physical Health* • *Breast Cancer Support and Education* • *Research on Exercise and Weight Control*	**Book Companion Web Site)** http://psychology.wadsworth.com/barlow4e/ Online quizzes, a *Self-Study Assessment with Study Plan*, Web links, and more for Chapter 9 **InfoTrac® College Edition** http://www.infotrac-college.com *Keywords*: phantom limb pain, chronic fatigue syndrome (diagnosis), biofeedback training, stress (physiology), self-efficacy (psychology), chronic fatigue syndrome, intractable pain, acute pain, coronary heart disease, hypertension, cardiovascular disease nursing, cancer, stroke (disease), rheumatoid arthritis, autoimmune disease, immune system **Looking into Abnormal Psychology** • Hotheads and Heart Attacks **Recommended Web Sites** Check out the Book Companion Web Site for links to these sites: • Society of Behavioral Medicine • Diseases and Disorders • The American Heart Association

Chapter 10: Sexual and Gender Identity Disorders

Class Preparation / Lecture Tools	Testing Tools / Course Management	Student Mastery / Homework and Tutorials	Beyond the Book
Instructor's Manual Includes a detailed chapter outline, learning objectives, classroom activities, demonstrations and lecture topics, supplementary reading, video and Internet resources, "Warning Signs" and "DSM-IV-TR criteria" masters, and more for Chapter 10 **Multimedia Manager Instructor's Resource CD-ROM** Allows you to create a media lecture for Chapter 10 using this Microsoft® PowerPoint® tool **Book Companion Web Site** http://psychology.wadsworth.com/barlow4e/ Online quizzes, a *Self-Study Assessment with Study Plan*, Web links, and more for Chapter 10 **CNN® Today Video: Abnormal Psychology** Vol. 1: *Viagra Failures* (1:83) **Transparency Acetates** Full-color images perfect for enhancing lectures	**Test Bank** Includes approximately 100 multiple-choice and 10 essay questions for Chapter 10 ExamView® **ExamView®** Computerized version of the **Test Bank** items Chapter 10 WebTutor Advantage **WebTutor™ Advantage** Online course management tool for WebCT or Blackboard preloaded with text-specific content for Chapter 10	**Study Guide** Chapter 10 includes learning objectives, a chapter summary fill-in exercise, keywords, sample tests with rejoinders, critical-thinking activities, and more. WebTutor Advantage **WebTutor™ Advantage** Online course management tool for WebCT or Blackboard preloaded with text-specific content and media resources for Chapter 10 **Book Companion Web Site** http://psychology.wadsworth.com/barlow4e/ Online quizzes, a *Self-Study Assessment with Study Plan*, Web links, and more for Chapter 10 **Abnormal Psychology Live! Version 2.5** • *Erectile Dysfunction: Clark* • *Changing Over: Jessica*	**Book Companion Web Site** http://psychology.wadsworth.com/barlow4e/ Online quizzes, a *Self-Study Assessment with Study Plan*, Web links, and more for Chapter 10 **InfoTrac® College Edition** http://www.infotrac-college.com *Keywords*: sexual disorders, erectile dysfunction, psychosexual therapy, sensate focus, premature ejaculation, paraphilia, fetishism, exhibitionism, pedophilia, child sexual abuse, incest, sex psychology, sadomasochism **Casebook in Abnormal Psychology** Chapters 11 and 12 **Looking into Abnormal Psychology** • Have Periods, Will Seek Therapy **Recommended Web Sites** Check out the Book Companion Web Site for links to these sites: • His and Her Health • Sexual Health

Chapter 11: Substance-Related and Impulse Control Disorders

Class Preparation / Lecture Tools	Testing Tools / Course Management	Student Mastery / Homework and Tutorials	Beyond the Book
Instructor's Manual Includes a detailed chapter outline, learning objectives, classroom activities, demonstrations and lecture topics, supplementary reading, video and Internet resources, "Warning Signs" and "DSM-IV-TR criteria" masters, and more for Chapter 11 **Multimedia Manager Instructor's Resource CD-ROM** Allows you to create a media lecture for Chapter 11 using this Microsoft® PowerPoint® tool **Book Companion Web Site** http://psychology.wadsworth.com/barlow4e/ Online quizzes, a *Self-Study Assessment with Study Plan,* Web links, and more for Chapter 11 **CNN® Today Video: Abnormal Psychology** Vol. 1: *Marijuana Brains* (2:40), *Fighting Addictions* (2:13) **Abnormal Psychology Inside Out** Vol. 4: *Nicotine Dependence: Testing a Theory in Animals and Humans (4:55)* **Transparency Acetates** Full-color images perfect for enhancing lectures	**Test Bank** Includes approximately 100 multiple-choice and 10 essay questions for Chapter 11 ExamView® **ExamView®** Computerized version of the **Test Bank** items Chapter 11 WebTutor Advantage **WebTutor™ Advantage** Online course management tool for WebCT or Blackboard preloaded with text-specific content for Chapter 11	**Study Guide** Chapter 11 includes learning objectives, a chapter summary fill-in exercise, keywords, sample tests with rejoinders, critical-thinking activities, and more. WebTutor Advantage **WebTutor™ Advantage** Online course management tool for WebCT or Blackboard preloaded with text-specific content and media resources for Chapter 11 **Book Companion Web Site** http://psychology.wadsworth.com/barlow4e/ Online quizzes, a *Self-Study Assessment with Study Plan,* Web links, and more for Chapter 11 **Abnormal Psychology Live! Version 2.5** • *Substance Use Disorder: Tim* • *Nicotine Dependence: Testing a Theory in Animals and Humans (parts 1–2)*	**Book Companion Web Site** http://psychology.wadsworth.com/barlow4e/ Online quizzes, a *Self-Study Assessment with Study Plan,* Web links, and more for Chapter 11 **InfoTrac® College Edition** http://www.infotrac-college.com *Keywords:* drug abuse, drug addicts, drug withdrawal symptoms, substance abuse, substance dependence, stimulants, narcotics, alcohol use disorders, fetal alcohol syndrome **Casebook in Abnormal Psychology** Chapter 13 **Recommended Web Sites** Check out the Book Companion Web Site for links to these sites: • National Institute on Drug Abuse • NIDA Teaching Aids

Chapter 12: Personality Disorders

Class Preparation / Lecture Tools	Testing Tools / Course Management	Student Mastery / Homework and Tutorials	Beyond the Book
Instructor's Manual Includes a detailed chapter outline, learning objectives, classroom activities, demonstrations and lecture topics, supplementary reading, video and Internet resources, "Warning Signs" and "DSM-IV-TR criteria" masters, and more for Chapter 12 **Multimedia Manager Instructor's Resource CD-ROM** Allows you to create a media lecture for Chapter 12 using this Microsoft® PowerPoint® tool **Book Companion Web Site** http://psychology.wadsworth.com/barlow4e/ Online quizzes, a *Self-Study Assessment with Study Plan*, Web links, and more for Chapter 12 **Transparency Acetates** Full-color images perfect for enhancing lectures	**Test Bank** Includes approximately 100 multiple-choice and 10 essay questions for Chapter 12 ExamView® **ExamView®** Computerized version of the **Test Bank** items for Chapter 12 WebTutor Advantage **WebTutor™ Advantage** Online course management tool for WebCT or Blackboard preloaded with text-specific content for Chapter 12	**Study Guide** Chapter 12 includes learning objectives, a chapter summary fill-in exercise, keywords, sample tests with rejoinders, critical-thinking activities, and more. WebTutor Advantage **WebTutor™ Advantage** Online course management tool for WebCT or Blackboard preloaded with text-specific content and media resources for Chapter 12 **Book Companion Web Site** http://psychology.wadsworth.com/barlow4e/ Online quizzes, a *Self-Study Assessment with Study Plan*, Web links, and more for Chapter 12 **Abnormal Psychology Live! Version 2.5** • *Antisocial Personality Disorder* • *Borderline Personality Disorder: Overview* • *Borderline Personality Disorder: Client Interview*	**Book Companion Web Site** http://psychology.wadsworth.com/barlow4e/ Online quizzes, a *Self-Study Assessment with Study Plan*, Web links, and more for Chapter 12 **Casebook in Abnormal Psychology** Chapter 14 **Looking into Abnormal Psychology** • Piecing Together Personality **Recommended Web Sites** Check out the Book Companion Web Site for links to these sites: • Internet Mental Health • Health Center

Chapter 13: Schizophrenia and Other Psychotic Disorders

Class Preparation / Lecture Tools	Testing Tools / Course Management	Student Mastery / Homework and Tutorials	Beyond the Book
Instructor's Manual Includes a detailed chapter outline, learning objectives, classroom activities, demonstrations and lecture topics, supplementary reading, video and Internet resources, "Warning Signs" and "DSM-IV-TR criteria" masters, and more for Chapter 13 **Multimedia Manager Instructor's Resource CD-ROM** Allows you to create a media lecture for Chapter 13 using this Microsoft® PowerPoint® tool **Book Companion Web Site** http://psychology.wadsworth.com/barlow4e/ Online quizzes, a *Self-Study Assessment with Study Plan*, Web links, and more for Chapter 13 **CNN® Today Video: Abnormal Psychology** Vol. 1: *Schizophrenia Drug* (2:72) Vol. 2: *Promising Future for a Person with Schizophrenia* (4:33) **Transparency Acetates** Full-color images perfect for enhancing lectures	**Test Bank** Includes approximately 100 multiple-choice and 10 essay questions for Chapter 13 ExamView® **ExamView®** Computerized version of the **Test Bank** items for Chapter 13 WebTUTOR Advantage **WebTutor™ Advantage** Online course management tool for WebCT or Blackboard preloaded with text-specific content for Chapter 13	**Study Guide** Chapter 13 includes learning objectives, a chapter summary fill-in exercise, keywords, sample tests with rejoinders, critical-thinking activities, and more. WebTUTOR Advantage **WebTutor™ Advantage** Online course management tool for WebCT or Blackboard preloaded with text-specific content and media resources for Chapter 13 **Book Companion Web Site** http://psychology.wadsworth.com/barlow4e/ Online quizzes, a *Self-Study Assessment with Study Plan*, Web links, and more for Chapter 13 **Abnormal Psychology Live! Version 2.5** • *Schizophrenia: Etta* • *Positive and Negative Symptoms* • *Common Symptoms*	**Book Companion Web Site** http://psychology.wadsworth.com/barlow4e/ Online quizzes, a *Self-Study Assessment with Study Plan*, Web links, and more for Chapter 13 **InfoTrac® College Edition** http://www.infotrac-college.com *Keywords*: schizophrenia, paranoia, psychoses, dementia praecox, hallucinations, delusions **Casebook in Abnormal Psychology** Chapter 15 **Looking into Abnormal Psychology** Part II **Recommended Web Sites** Check out the Book Companion Web Site for links to these sites: • Internet Mental Health/Schizophrenia • Schizophrenia Information Center

Chapter 14: Developmental Disorders

Class Preparation / Lecture Tools	Testing Tools / Course Management	Student Mastery / Homework and Tutorials	Beyond the Book
Instructor's Manual Includes a detailed chapter outline, learning objectives, classroom activities, demonstrations and lecture topics, supplementary reading, video and Internet resources, "Warning Signs" and "DSM-IV-TR criteria" masters, and more for Chapter 14 **Multimedia Manager Instructor's Resource CD-ROM** Allows you to create a media lecture for Chapter 14 using this Microsoft® PowerPoint® tool **Book Companion Web Site** http://psychology.wadsworth.com/barlow4e/ Online quizzes, a *Self-Study Assessment with Study Plan,* Web links, and more for Chapter 14 **CNN® Today Video: Abnormal Psychology** Vol. 1: *Learning Disabilities* (3:97) **Abnormal Psychology Inside Out** Vol. III: *Attention Deficit Hyperactivity Disorder (14:57), Autism: The Nature of the Disorder (4:38), Autism: Christina (4:45)* Vol. IV: *Rebecca: A First-Grader with Autism (2:43), Lauren: A Kindergartner with Down Syndrome (3:48), Edward: ADHD (1:28)* **Transparency Acetates** Full-color images perfect for enhancing lectures	**Test Bank** Includes approximately 100 multiple-choice and 10 essay questions for Chapter 14 ExamView® **ExamView®** Computerized version of the **Test Bank** items for Chapter 14 WebTutor Advantage **WebTutor™ Advantage** Online course management tool for WebCT or Blackboard preloaded with text-specific content for Chapter 14	**Study Guide** Chapter 14 includes learning objectives, a chapter summary fill-in exercise, keywords, sample tests with rejoinders, critical-thinking activities, and more. WebTutor Advantage **WebTutor™ Advantage** Online course management tool for WebCT or Blackboard preloaded with text-specific content and media resources for Chapter 14 **Book Companion Web Site** http://psychology.wadsworth.com/barlow4e/ Online quizzes, a *Self-Study Assessment with Study Plan,* Web links, and more for Chapter 14 **Abnormal Psychology Live! Version 2.5** • *ADHD: Sean* • *Life Skills Training* • *Bullying Prevention* • *Autism: Christina* • *Autism: The Nature of the Disorder* • *Rebecca: A First-Grader with Autism* • *Lauren: A Kindergartner with Down Syndrome* • *Edward: ADHD*	**Book Companion Web Site** http://psychology.wadsworth.com/barlow4e/ Online quizzes, a *Self-Study Assessment with Study Plan,* Web links, and more for Chapter 14 **InfoTrac® College Edition** http://www.infotrac-college.com *Keywords*: attention deficit/hyperactivity disorder, language acquisition, language disorders in children, pervasive developmental disorder, mental retardation, Down syndrome, behavior disorders in children, autism, autistic children, Asperger's syndrome, prenatal screening, learning disabilities **Casebook in Abnormal Psychology** Chapter 16 **Looking into Abnormal Psychology** Part II **Recommended Web Sites** Check out the Book Companion Web Site for links to these sites: • Down Syndrome • Division of Early Childhood

Chapter 15: Cognitive Disorders

Class Preparation / Lecture Tools	Testing Tools / Course Management	Student Mastery / Homework and Tutorials	Beyond the Book
Instructor's Manual Includes a detailed chapter outline, learning objectives, classroom activities, demonstrations and lecture topics, supplementary reading, video and Internet resources, "Warning Signs" and "DSM-IV-TR criteria" masters, and more for Chapter 15 **Multimedia Manager Instructor's Resource CD-ROM** Allows you to create a media lecture for Chapter 15 using this Microsoft® PowerPoint® tool **Book Companion Web Site** http://psychology.wadsworth.com/barlow4e/ Online quizzes, a *Self-Study Assessment with Study Plan,* Web links, and more for Chapter 15 **CNN® Today Video: Abnormal Psychology** Vol. 2: *Alzheimer's Vaccine* (2:10), *Alzheimer's Debate* (2:09) **Abnormal Psychology Inside Out** Vol. IV: *Computer Simulations and Senile Dementia (3:44)* **Transparency Acetates** Full-color images perfect for enhancing lectures	**Test Bank** Includes approximately 100 multiple-choice and 10 essay questions for Chapter 15 ExamView® **ExamView®** Computerized version of the **Test Bank** items for Chapter 15 WebTUTOR® Advantage **WebTutor™ Advantage** Online course management tool for WebCT or Blackboard preloaded with text-specific content for Chapter 15	**Study Guide** Chapter 15 includes learning objectives, a chapter summary fill-in exercise, keywords, sample tests with rejoinders, critical-thinking activities, and more. WebTUTOR® Advantage **WebTutor™ Advantage** Online course management tool for WebCT or Blackboard preloaded with text-specific content and media resources for Chapter 15 **Book Companion Web Site** http://psychology.wadsworth.com/barlow4e/ Online quizzes, a *Self-Study Assessment with Study Plan,* Web links, and more for Chapter 15 **Abnormal Psychology Live! Version 2.5** • *Alzheimer's Disease: Tom* • *Amnestic Disorder: Mike* • *Computer Simulations and Senile Dementia (parts 1–2)*	**Book Companion Web Site** http://psychology.wadsworth.com/barlow4e/ Online quizzes, a *Self-Study Assessment with Study Plan,* Web links, and more for Chapter 15 **InfoTrac® College Edition** http://www.infotrac-college.com *Keywords:* delirium, dementia, Alzheimer's disease, head trauma, Parkinson's disease, Huntington's cholera, Creutzfeldt-Jakob disease **Recommended Web Sites** Check out the Book Companion Web Site for links to these sites: • Alzheimer's Association • Internet Mental Health

Chapter 16: Mental Health Services: Legal, Ethical, and Professional Issues

Class Preparation / Lecture Tools	Testing Tools / Course Management	Student Mastery / Homework and Tutorials	Beyond the Book
Instructor's Manual Includes a detailed chapter outline, learning objectives, classroom activities, demonstrations and lecture topics, supplementary reading, video and Internet resources, "Warning Signs" and "DSM-IV-TR criteria" masters, and more for Chapter 16 **Multimedia Manager Instructor's Resource CD-ROM** Allows you to create a media lecture for Chapter 16 using this Microsoft® PowerPoint® tool **Book Companion Web Site** http://psychology.wadsworth.com/barlow4e/ Online quizzes, a *Self-Study Assessment with Study Plan,* Web links, and more for Chapter 16 **CNN® Today Video: Abnormal Psychology** Vol. 1: *Mental Health Services: Britain Bedlam* (2:98) Vol. 2: *Insanity Defense* (2:41) **Transparency Acetates** Full-color images perfect for enhancing lectures	**Test Bank** Includes approximately 100 multiple-choice and 10 essay questions for Chapter 16 ExamView® **ExamView®** Computerized version of the **Test Bank** items for Chapter 16 WebTUTOR Advantage **WebTutor™ Advantage** Online course management tool for WebCT or Blackboard preloaded with text-specific content for Chapter 16	**Study Guide** Chapter 16 includes learning objectives, a chapter summary fill-in exercise, keywords, sample tests with rejoinders, critical-thinking activities, and more. WebTUTOR Advantage **WebTutor™ Advantage** Online course management tool for WebCT or Blackboard preloaded with text-specific content and media resources for Chapter 16 **Book Companion Web Site** http://psychology.wadsworth.com/barlow4e/ Online quizzes, a *Self-Study Assessment with Study Plan,* Web links, and more for Chapter 16 **Abnormal Psychology Live! Version 2.5** • *False Memories*	**Book Companion Web Site** http://psychology.wadsworth.com/barlow4e/ Online quizzes, a *Self-Study Assessment with Study Plan,* Web links, and more for Chapter 16 **InfoTrac® College Edition** http://www.infotrac-college.com *Keywords:* assessment of decision-making capacity, criminal commitment **Looking into Abnormal Psychology** • Seeking the Criminal Element **Recommended Web Sites** Check out the Book Companion Web Site for links to these sites: • APA Ethics Office • Psychiatry and the Law

CHAPTER ONE

ABNORMAL BEHAVIOR IN HISTORICAL CONTEXT

LEARNING OBJECTIVES

1. Define abnormal behavior (psychological disorder) and describe psychological dysfunction, distress, and atypical or unexpected cultural response.
2. Describe a contemporary scientific approach to abnormal behavior, including the background and training of mental-health care professionals, the scientist-practitioner model, and the domains of clinical description.
3. Place abnormal behavior in historical context by comparing and contrasting the historical views of abnormal behavior, including supernatural, biological and psychological (including psychoanalysis, humanistic, and behavioral) explanations.
4. Explain the importance of science and the scientific method as applied to abnormal behavior.
5. Describe the multidimensional-integrative approach to diagnosing and evaluating abnormal behavior and explain why it is important.

LECTURE OUTLINE

I. Understanding Psychopathology
   A. The Case of Judy: The Girl who Fainted at the Sight of Blood
      1. Use the case of Judy or a similar case to illustrate the definition of a psychological disorder below.

   B. A **psychological disorder,** or abnormal behavior, is defined as some *psychological dysfunction* associated with *distress or impairment in functioning that is not a typical or culturally expected response.*
      1. **Psychological dysfunction** is a breakdown in cognitive, emotional, or behavioral functioning. Provide examples of each.
      2. **Distress** occurs when a person is extremely upset.
      3. An **atypical or not culturally expected** response refers to those behaviors or attitudes which do not occur in a society very frequently.
      4. Illustrate how each of the features of the definition (1-3) is inadequate when considered in isolation.

   C. An Accepted Definition of a Psychological Disorder
      1. As defined in the DSM-IV-TR, **an accepted definition** of abnormal behavior is *behavioral, emotional or cognitive dysfunctions that are unexpected in their cultural context and associated with personal distress or substantial impairment in functioning.*

2. The planning process for the 5th edition of the DSM (DSM-V) has begun, and three research questions form the basis for the inclusion of psychological disorders.
    a. An evaluation of the degree to which specified behaviors conform (or not) to our previously understood definitions of disorders will be conducted.
    b. A survey process of mental health practitioners will be utilized to search for commonalities in abnormal behavior across cultures.
    c. Using the same survey process, mental health practitioners will provide information about what separates individuals who truly meet criteria for the disorder from others who show milder forms of the same problem.

II. The Science of Psychopathology

A. Mental Health Care Professionals (Background, Training, & Approach)
1. Clinical and counseling psychologists
2. Psychiatrists
3. Psychiatric social workers
4. Social workers
5. Psychiatric nurses
6. Marriage and family therapists

B. The Scientist-Practitioner Framework
1. The **scientist-practitioner** is a mental health professional who takes a scientific approach to their clinical work.
2. The function of a scientist-practitioner
    a. Consumer of science
    b. Evaluator of science
    c. Creator of science

C. Clinical Description of Abnormal Behavior
1. A **presenting problem** typically refers to one first noted as the reason for coming to a clinical setting.
2. One important function of clinical description is to specify what makes a disorder different from normal behavior and other disorders.
3. **Prevalence** refers to the number of people in the population as a whole who have the disorder.
4. **Incidence** refers to the number of new cases of a disorder occurring during a specific period of time (e.g., a year)
5. **Course** refers to the pattern of the disorder in time can be described as chronic, episodic, or time-limited. Related to **prognosis**.
6. **Acute onset** refers to disorders that begin suddenly, whereas **insidious onset** refers to disorders that develop gradually over time.
7. Important associated features (e.g., age, developmental stage, ethnicity, race).

D. Causation, Treatment, and Outcome in Psychopathology

1. **Etiology** refers to factors or dimensions that cause psychological disorders. Such factors include biological, psychological, and social dimensions (covered in detail in Chapter 2 of the textbook).
2. **Treatment** can include psychological, psychopharmacological, or some combination of the two. **Successful outcome** can assist in making inferences about the variables leading to and maintaining a disorder, but not in the determination of the actual causes of a disorder (e.g., aspirin alleviates headache, but headache is not caused by deficits of aspirin in the brain).

III. Historical Conceptions of Abnormal Behavior

A. Overview of Supernatural, Biological, and Psychological Traditions

B. The Supernatural Tradition

1. Deviant behavior as battle between "good" vs. "evil"
    a. A popular opinion during the Middle Ages purported that psychopathology was due to the presence of evil demons. As a result, treatment included **exorcism**, or tortuous, drastic action to dispossess a spirit from a human body.
    b. 15th Century was characterized by the view that the causes of madness and other evils was due to sorcery, witches, and evil. Though some increasingly viewed abnormality as purely natural, physical phenomenon (i.e., as an illness).
2. An interesting phenomenon of the Middle Ages was **mass hysteria** (also known as **Saint Vitus' Dance** or **Tarantism**), which is characterized by outbreaks of strange behavior on a grand scale.
3. **Paracelsus**, a Swiss physician who lived during the 16th century, introduced the idea that the movement of the moon and stars affected people's psychological functioning; this theory inspired the use of the word *lunatic* (Latin word for moon, *luna*) to describe those who exhibited behavioral disorders. Many of his views still persist today.

C. The Biological Tradition

1. The Greek physician **Hippocrates** (460-377 B.C.), the father of modern medicine, presumed that psychological disorders could be conceptualized as a brain or hereditary disease, while recognizing the importance of psychological and interpersonal factors in psychopathology. Hippocrates also coined the term **hysteria** and believed the cause to be due to a wandering uterus, and the cure marriage and pregnancy. A Roman physician **Galen** (129-198 A.D.) expanded upon the work of Hippocrates, and the Hippocratic-Galenic approach to psychopathology extended to the 19th century.
    a. A legacy of this approach was the **humoral theory** of mental disorder (i.e., blood, black bile, yellow bile, phlegm)– a view that foreshadowed modern views linking psychological disorders with chemical imbalances in the brain.
2. Symptoms associated with advanced **syphilis**, a sexually transmitted disease caused by a bacterial microorganism, are similar to symptoms associated with

schizophrenia and other psychotic disorders. During the 19th century, syphilis was discovered to be a cause of *general paresis* (a disorder characterized by both behavioral and cognitive symptoms). Eventually scientists (Pasteur) discovered that syphilis could be cured by penicillin, which in turn led many mental health professionals to believe that similar cures could be discovered for all psychological disorders.

3. **John P. Grey**, and American Psychiatrist, believed that insanity was always due to physical causes and that mentally ill patients should be treated like the physically ill. Reformers, such as **Dorothea Dix,** stated that the treatment of those with mental illness should parallel the treatment of those with physical illness. As a result, mental hospital conditions improved significantly and many advocated the practice of "deinstitutionalization."
4. Biological treatments for mental disorders in the 1930's (such as insulin, ECT, and brain surgery) were periodically administered to persons with psychoses to calm them (leading to insulin shock therapy and lobotomy). In addition, **Joseph von Meduna** thought that schizophrenia was rare in persons with epilepsy; hence, the deliberate induction of brain seizures was soon considered useful.
5. The first effective drugs for treating severe psychotic disorders emerged in the 1950's. The discovery of *rauwolfia serpentina* (**reserpine**), **neuroleptics**, and major tranquilizers proved useful for treating hallucinations, delusions, agitation, and aggression.
6. The consequences of the early biogenic approach to psychopathology included an ironic tendency not to pursue new drug treatments. Instead, more effort was devoted to diagnosis, legal issues, and the study of brain pathology itself.
7. **Emil Kraepelin** became a dominant figure in the field of diagnosis and classification; a central theme of his approach was that separate, discriminantly valid syndromes could be culled, with each comprising different symptoms, course, and onset.
8. By the end of the 1800's, a scientific approach to psychological disorders and their classification was couched as a search for biological causes and medicalized and humane treatments.

D. The Psychological Tradition

1. Psychosocial models of mental disorder did not predominate until the 18th century with the advent of **moral therapy** (originated by a well known French psychiatrist **Philippe Pinel** and his former patient **Jean-Baptiste Pussin**) – the practice of allowing patients to be treated in settings as normal as possible to encourage and reinforce social interaction.
2. **William Tuke** followed Pinel's lead in England, and **Benjamin Rush** (founder of American Psychiatry) introduced moral therapy in his early work at Pennsylvania Hospital. The rise of moral therapy in England and the United States is what made institutions habitable and even therapeutic.
3. The decline of moral therapy and humane treatment was precipitated by factors such as the belief that psychopathology was caused by incurable brain pathology; also, providing individual attention to increasing numbers of

patients with mental illness (an important practice of moral therapists) was becoming impossible with limited hospital staffing.

4. Although the psychodynamic model partially grew out of the work of **Anton Mesmer** (father of hypnosis) and **Jean Charcot**, it is largely the result of the work of **Sigmund Freud** and **Josef Breuer**.
5. Psychoanalytic Theory
    a. Freud developed a comprehensive theory on the development and structure of personality, including hypothesis about how both can lead to psychopathology. Freud believed that mind was composed of the **id, ego**, and **superego**. The id operates on the **pleasure principle**, or the maximization of pleasure and minimization of competing tension. The id was thought to be the source of sexual and aggressive thoughts and behaviors. The ego was thought to develop a few months after birth to realistically address one's environment; it operates on the **reality principle** via the secondary process, with an emphasis on logical and reasonable thought. The superego (conscience) develops last and represents the moral standards instilled by parents or other important influences. The primary purpose of the superego is to suppress id drives.
    b. When the id or superego gather enough strength to challenge the conscious ego, anxiety results. To ward off anxiety, the ego may employ **defense mechanisms**, or unconscious protective processes to keep intrapsychic conflicts in check. Though Freud initially introduced the idea of defense mechanisms, it was his daughter Anna Freud that developed them.
    c. Examples of defense mechanisms include **displacement** (i.e., redirecting anger on a less threatening object or person); **denial** (i.e., refusal to acknowledge some aspect of objective reality or subject experience that is apparent to others); **projection** (i.e., falsely attributing one's unacceptable feelings, impulses, or thoughts on another individual or object); **rationalization** (i.e., concealing true motivations for actions, thoughts, or feelings through elaborate reassuring or self-serving but incorrect explanations); **reaction formation** (i.e., substituting behavior, thoughts, or feelings that are direct opposites of unacceptable ones); **repression** (i.e., blocking disturbing wishes, thoughts, or experiences from conscious awareness); and **sublimation** (i.e., directing potentially maladaptive feelings or impulses into socially accepted behavior).
    d. Freud also theorized that people progress through **psychosexual developmental stages**. The oral, anal, phallic, latency, and genital stages represent distinct patterns of gratifying libidinal needs. The most controversial developmental stage is the phallic stage.
6. Later Developments in Psychoanalytic Thought: Neo-Freudians
    a. The Neo-Freudians adapted the classic psychoanalytic approach and modified and developed it in a number of different directions. For example, **Anna Freud** developed **self-psychology** to emphasize the

influence of the ego in defining behavior, while **Melanie Klein** and **Otto Kernberg** developed **object relations**, (the study of how children incorporate (introject) the images, memories, and values of significant others (objects).

   b. Other theorists rejected the classic psychoanalytic approach and developed their own principles. For example, **Carl Jung**, rejected many of the sexual aspects of Freud's theory, and introduced the concept of **collective unconscious**, or a source of accumulated wisdom stored in human memory and passed from one generation to the next. In addition, **Alfred Adler** focused on feelings of inferiority, superiority, and a drive toward self-actualization. Finally, **Karen Horney**, **Erich Fromm**, and **Erik Erickson** concentrated on life-span development and societal influences on behavior.
   c. Psychoanalytic theory is intertwined into psychodynamic therapy. The goal of this approach is to help a person understand the true nature of his/her intrapsychic conflicts and psychological problems. Several techniques, such as **free association** and **dream analysis**, are used by the psychoanalyst to help reveal such conflicts to the client. The relationship between therapist and client in psychoanalysis is very important, for it is here where **transference** (i.e., when the patient begins to relate to the therapist as they did with important people in their lives) and **countertransference** (i.e., where the therapist projects their own personal issues and feelings, usually positive, onto the patient) play out. Therapy is often long term, taking 4-5 weekly sessions over a period of 2 to 5 years.

7. Humanistic Theory
   a. Primary humanistic theorists include **Carl Rogers**, **Abraham Maslow**, and **Fritz Perls**. A major theme running through this work is the view that people are basically good.
   b. A central concept of this approach is **self-actualization**, or the assumption that all people strive to reach their highest potential. With freedom and support, one's drive toward self-actualization can be highly successful. If this drive is thwarted, however, psychological problems may develop. Unlike psychoanalysis, the therapist takes a passive role, makes very few interpretations, and attempts to convey to the client a sense of **unconditional positive regard**.
8. The Behavioral Model
   a. The behavioral, cognitive-behavioral, or social learning model was derived from a scientific approach to the study of psychopathology
   b. **Ivan Pavlov** discovered a simple form of learning, known as **classical conditioning**, where a neutral stimulus is paired with a response until it elicits that (conditioned) response (e.g., phobias, nausea associated with chemotherapy, food aversions).
   c. **John Watson** stated that the field of psychology should be based on scientific analyses of observable and measurable behavior. Such analyses could be used in the prediction and control of behavior.

Watson is credited with creating the school of Behaviorism, whereas one of his students, **Mary Cover Jones**, can be credited for providing one of the first demonstrations of successful treatment (via extinction) of fear of furry objects in a 2 year old boy named Peter.

d. In the mid-20th century, **Joseph Wolpe** developed therapeutic procedures based on the work of these early behaviorists, particularly the work of Pavlov and Hull. In **systematic desensitization**, for example, a person may extinguish fear by practicing relaxation and pairing it with the phobic stimulus. Such a process could be done through imagining the stimulus (in vivo).

e. **B. F. Skinner** was strongly influenced by Watson's conviction that a science of psychology must take as its subject matter behavior, but unlike Watson also believed that the task of psychology was to account for all behavior, even behavior that can not be observed directly (e.g., thoughts, feelings). Skinner developed the field of behavior analysis and concepts related to **operant conditioning** (i.e., learning which occurs when responses are modified as a function of the **consequence** of the response). Skinner maintained that this principle was applicable to daily learning in particular but also to society and culture in general. Though Skinner was not a behavior therapist, many of his technologies and concepts form the core of several contemporary behavior therapies.

IV. The Present: The Scientific Method and an Integrative Approach

A. The view that psychopathology is determined by different processes does have an historical basis, and recent evidence suggests a strong reciprocal influence among biological, psychological, and social factors. No account alone is complete. Therefore, this textbook is devoted to an integrative multidimensional approach in describing various topics.

OVERALL SUMMARY

This chapter presents an overview of past and future conceptions of abnormal behavior. Specifically, the chapter introduces the concept of abnormal behavior and its definitional components, outlines some primary professions in the field and terms for understanding psychological disorders, describes biological, psychological, and supernatural models of abnormal behavior in a historical context, and summarizes a multidimensional integrative scientific approach for understanding psychopathology.

KEY TERMS

Behaviorism (p. 16)
Behavioral model (p. 22)
Behavior therapy (p. 24)
Catharsis (p. 17)
Classical conditioning (p. 22)

Clinical description (p. 6)
Collective unconscious (p. 20)
Course (p. 6)
Defense mechanisms (p. 18)
Dream analysis (p. 20)
Ego (p. 18)
Ego psychology (p. 20)
Etiology (p. 7)
Extinction (p. 23)
Free association (p. 20)
Id (p. 18)
Incidence (p. 6)
Intrapsychic conflicts (p. 18)
Introspection (p. 23)
Mental hygiene movement (p. 15)
Moral therapy (p. 14)
Neuroses (p. 19)
Object relations (p. 20)
Person-centered therapy (p. 22)
Phobia (p. 2)
Presenting problem (p. 6)
Prevalence (p. 6)
Prognosis (p. 7)
Psychoanalysis (p. 16)
Psychoanalyst (p. 21)
Psychoanalytic model (p. 18)
Psychodynamic psychotherapy (p. 21)
Psychological disorder (p. 2)
Psychopathology (p. 5)
Psychosexual stages of development (p. 19)
Psychosocial (p. 14)
Reinforcement (p. 24)
Scientist-practitioner (p. 5)
Self-actualizing (p. 21)
Shaping (p. 25)
Superego (p. 18)
Systematic desensitization (p. 24)
Transference (p. 21)
Unconditional positive regard (p. 22)
Unconscious (p. 17)

INFOTRAC KEY TERM EXERCISES

Each exercise is linked to key terms from the Wadsworth InfoTrac on-line searchable database. Key terms must be entered exactly as written.

Exercise 1: **Medieval Mass Hysteria: Fact or Fiction?**
Article: A63693007
Citation: (Rethinking the Dancing Mania). Robert E. Batholomew
Skeptical Inquirer, July 2000 v24 i4 p42

Though medieval dance frenzies (i.e., St. Vitus's dance or Tartanism) have long been regarded as a classic example of stress-induced mental disorder affecting mostly women, there is much evidence to the contrary. Review the InfoTrac article on this topic and answer the following questions: (a) where most dancers crazy?, (b) was there a spontaneous, uncontrollable urge to dance?, and (c) where most dancers hysterical females? Lastly, what does the author suggest as the likely cause of dance manias? Be sure to justify your response to each question with appropriate arguments/evidence from the article. Limit your answer to 3-5 typed double-spaced pages.

Exercise 2: The Stigma of Mental Illness
Key Terms: *Mental Illness, Attitudes*

Many persons who fit the definition of psychological disorder in the textbook feel stigmatized by society. Yet, the same sort of stigmatization does not normally occur with most physical diseases. Review the InfoTrac articles on this topic and prepare a 3-5 typed double-spaced page essay where you address the following points: (a) What does it mean to be stigmatized?; (b) What forms does stigmatization take regarding mental illness?, (c) why does stigmatization exist with regard to mental illness?, (d) and what steps would you prose to reduce the sense of shame and stigmatization often experienced by those suffering from psychological disorders? In formulating your answer, you may want to consider how most physical diseases differ from psychological disorders in terms of how society responds to persons suffering from them, and how you might feel with a diagnosis of a psychological disorder (e.g., a phobia) vs. a diagnosis of, say "a severe case of the flu."

Exercise 3 (Future Trend): Alternative Therapies and Psychology's Battle for Legitimacy

In recent years there has been a proliferation of alternative treatments for various psychological problems. This list includes various herbal and homeopathic remedies (e.g., St. John's Wort), rebirthing therapy, and more recently Thought Field Therapy. Proponents of such treatments claim that they are far superior to standard treatments both in terms of effectiveness and efficiency. Opponents, however, are quick to point out that such claims are well ahead of the data. Moreover, there is the issue of whether the largely unregulated availability of such treatments is good for psychology in general. Here you may have students select one of several "new wave" alternative treatments for psychological disorders and evaluate the evidence pro and con supporting them. This activity could be arranged as an in-class debate, or in the form of a brief paper. The goal, however, is to help students become critical consumers about knowledge claims. Below are several InfoTrac articles that may serve as good starting points.

Gaudiano, B. A., & Herbert, J. D. (2000). Can we really tap our problems away?: A critical analysis of Thought Field Therapy. Skeptical Inquirer, v24 i4, p29.

Sampson, W. (1997). Inconsistencies and errors in alternative medicine research. Skeptical Inquirer, v21 n5, p35(4).

CLASSROOM ACTIVITIES, DEMONSTRATIONS, AND LECTURE TOPICS

1. **Activity: Distinguishing Normal From Abnormal Behavior**. An exercise that helps students recognize the difficulty of distinguishing normal from abnormal behavior is to begin by presenting a small amount of information about a case. If your class is large, break your students into groups of 4-5. Instruct each group to list the top four questions they would want to know about the case to evaluate the behavior. For example, present the following information:

   Case #1: Tom is uncomfortable riding escalators. As a result, Tom avoids using any escalator.
   (After your students have explored the case, encourage them to ask the following types of questions):
   a. How old is Tom? Is it more "normal" for Tom to fear escalators if he is a child versus an adult? Discuss developmental issues.
   b. What culture does Tom come from? Has he ever had exposure to an escalator? Cultural contexts must always be considered when evaluating abnormal behavior.
   c. How does Tom manage his fear? What symptoms does he have?
   d. To what extent does Tom avoid using escalators? Does his fear significantly interfere with his life? Also ask if your students would consider the behavior more abnormal if he had a fear of flying in airplanes versus escalators. In other words, at one point would the behavior be considered an abnormal fear versus a normal fear?

   Case #2: Rachel has been caught urinating in the corner of her bedroom. Is her behavior abnormal?
   (Encourage students to ask):
   a. How old is Rachel? The clinical picture is very different if Rachel is one year old than if she is 13 years old. Discuss the importance of understanding developmental psychology.
   b. How many times has she engaged in the behavior? A pattern of behavior may be viewed differently than if it is a rare occurrence.
   c. Does Rachel have a medical condition? Is she on any medications? Rachel may have a medical or organic condition that accounts for her behavior. Ask your students if identifying an organic condition would change their perception of Rachel. Discuss the implication of assigning less social stigma to medical versus psychiatric patients.
   d. Has Rachel experienced a recent trauma, or is she exposed to unusual stressors?
   e. How does Rachel feel about her behavior? How does she explain it?

   Examples such as these stimulate students to explore cases more fully before making snap judgments about people's behavior, and illustrate the complexity in teasing out normal from abnormal behavior.

2. **Activity: What is Normal vs. Abnormal?** A similar exercise is to break students into groups and have them work with HANDOUT 1.1. Students should complete the handout on their own, and then discuss their opinions.

3. **Activity: Examples of Conditioning in Everyday Life**. To illustrate learning theory, ask your students to apply what they have learned about conditioning and behavior therapy to their own lives. Students may choose a behavior they would like to change or eliminate, or may identify a new behavior they would like to acquire. Ask them to keep a journal of the conditioning technique they are using and the exact procedure they are employing. For example, a student may want to stop biting her nails. She could keep a journal to describe if she is using a classical or operant procedure and monitor the progress (or success!) of the conditioning.

4. **Activity: The Blind Men and the Human Elephant**. To illustrate the importance of taking an integrative, multidimensional approach and the dangers of scientific tunnel vision, read John G. Saxe's (1963) poem "The Blind Men and the Elephant." The poem is available from several sites on the web (using the complete search phrase "Saxe's Blind Men and the Elephant"), but here are two: *http://www.wordfocus.com/ word-act-blindmen.html* or *http://www.kheper.auz.com/realities/blind_men_and_elephant/ Saxe.html*. Then have students discuss what behaving as one of the blind men would look like from a supernatural, biological, or psychological perspective (include psychoanalytic, behavioral, humanistic views). Use human behavior in place of the elephant illustrated in the poem. Try wearing a Turban, a robe, or using other props while reading the poem as a means to elicit humor and to make the message stick.

5. **Activity: Myths, Magic, & Placebos: What Do They Have to Do With Having Rocks in Your Head?** When you discuss material dealing with treatment of the mentally ill during the Middle Ages, see whether students know where the phrase "rocks in your head" originated. This phrase originated during the Middle Ages, where city street vendors would commonly perform pseudosurgery on street corners. Troubled persons with symptoms associated with mental illness would often frequent the vendors for relief. The vendors, in turn, would make a minor incision on the skull, while an accomplice would sneak the surgeon a few small stones. The surgeon would then pretend to have taken the stones from the patient's head. The stones were claimed to be the cause of the person's problems and that the person was now cured. A similar variant on this theme is quite popular with modern magicians and some faith healers who purport to painlessly remove diseased organs from the bodies their subjects. The procedure involves an elaborate ritual, accompanied by chicken or beef blood and associated meat parts. The magic rests in the illusion of the magician's arm twisting and turning into the blood-covered exposed belly of the subject and the slow removal of what appears to look like a body part. Ask students to think about other examples of modern-day cures that they have heard in the media or that they may have experienced themselves. This is a good place to tie in the concept of the Placebo Effect, and perhaps open up a discussion about the role of beliefs and expectancies in producing and alleviating medical and psychological forms of distress and suffering.

HANDOUT 1.1:
WHAT IS ABNORMAL?

Consider the following situations. Most people would consider at least some of the actions of the people involved to be abnormal. What do you think? Think about each one as you read through the list. Then, talk with your group about your judgments. When you are through talking about each, elect a group spokesperson who will take notes on the reasons that the group members come up with as to why you did or did not consider each situation to be abnormal. You will have to "dig" mentally to put some of these reasons into words.

1. Your uncle consumes a quart of whiskey per day; he has trouble remembering the names of those around him.

2. Your grandmother believes that part of her body is missing and cries out about this missing part all day long. You show her the part that is missing but she refuses to acknowledge this contradictory information.

3. Your neighbor has vague physical complaints and sees 2-3 doctors weekly.

4. Your neighbor sweeps, washes, and scrubs his driveway daily.

5. Your cousin is pregnant, and she is dieting (800 calories per day) so that she will not get "too fat" with the pregnancy. She has had this type of behavioral response since she was 13 years old.

6. A woman's husband dies within the past year. The widow appears to talk to herself in the yard, doesn't wash herself or dress in clean clothes, and has evidently lost a lot of weight.

7. A 10 year old wants to have his entire body tattooed.

8. A 23 year old female smokes 4-5 marijuana joints a day, is a straight A student in college, has a successful job, and a solid long-term relationship.

9. A person experiences several unexpected panic attacks each week, but it otherwise happily married, functions well at work, and leads an active recreational lifestyle.

10. A 35 year old happily married man who enjoys wearing women's clothes and underwear on the weekends when he and his wife go out on the town.

SUPPLEMENTARY READING MATERIAL FOR CHAPTER ONE

(= These sources can be found on "*Infotrac, the online library*" provided by Wadsworth and Brooks/Cole Publishing.)

Bjork, D. W. (1993). B.F. Skinner: A life. New York: Basic.

Bolles, R. C. (1993). The story of psychology: A thematic history. Pacific Grove, CA: Brooks/Cole.

Grob, G. (1994). The mad among us: A history of the care of America's mentally ill. New York: MacMillan.

Hatfield, A. B., & Lefley, H. P. (1993). Surviving mental illness. New York: Guilford.

Hunt, M. M. (1993). The story of psychology. New York: Doubleday.

Shorter, E. (1997). A history of psychiatry: From the era of asylum to the age of prozac. New York: Wiley. Only reviews of this book are available on InfoTrac.

Watson, R. I. (1991). The great psychologists: A history of psychological thought. (5th ed.). Reading, MA: Addison Wesley Longman. Traces the history of psychology by examining the work of its' pioneers.

Weitz, R. D. (1992). A half century of psychological practice. Professional Psychology: Research and Practice, 23, 448-452.

Windholz, G. (1995). Pavlov on the Conditioned Reflex Method and its limitations. American Journal of Psychology, 108 (4), 575-588.

Windholz, G. (1998). Pavlov's conceptualization of voluntary movements within the framework of the theory of higher nervous activity. American Journal of Psychology, 111(3), 435-439.

SUPPLEMENTARY VIDEO RESOURCES FOR CHAPTER ONE

Abnormal behavior: A mental hospital. (CRM/McGraw-Hill Films, 110 15th Street, Del Mar, CA 92014). Portrays life in a modern mental hospital, including views of schizophrenics and of a patient receiving ECT. (28 min)

Adlerian therapy. (Insight Media: 2162 Broadway, New York, NY 10024/ (800)-233-9910). Dr. Jon Carlson examines and demonstrates Adlerian therapy (also known as individual psychology). (100 min)

B. F. Skinner and behavior change: Research, practice, and promise. (Research Press: Department 95, P.O. Box 9177, Champaign, IL 61826/ (800)-519-2707). This video features a discussion with B. F. Skinner and addresses some controversial issues related to behavioral psychology. (45 min)

Carl Rogers. (Insight Media: 2162 Broadway, New York, NY 10024/ (800)-233-9910). Carl Rogers discusses the humanistic model of personality as well as his views on encounter groups, education and other issues facing psychologists. (2 programs, each 50 min)

CNN today: Abnormal psychology 2000, vol. 1. (*Available through your International Thomson Learning representative).* The segment titled "Introduction: The Past Mental Health History" provides a brief presentation of the first mental health hospitals, the inhumane conditions they were present in such hospitals, and the horrible restraining devices used at the time. (2 min 24 sec)

Freud: The hidden nature of man. (Insight Media: 2162 Broadway, New York, NY 10024/ (800)-233-9910). Through interviews with Sigmund Freud himself, this video explores the concepts of psychoanalysis. (29 min)

Is mental illness a myth? (NMAC-T 2031). Debates whether mental illness is a physical disease or a collection of socially learned behaviors. Panelists include Thomas Szasz, Nathan Kline, and F. C. Redlich. (29 min)

Keltie's beard: A woman's story (1983, FL). About a woman with heavy facial hair that she chooses not to cut. Useful in discussing the criteria for abnormal behavior (film and video, 9 min).

Man facing southeast. (Hollywood, Drama). Fascinating Argentine film about a man with no identity who shows up at a psychiatric hospital claiming to be from another planet. It seems that this is not just another patient, and neither the hospital staff nor the film's audience every figure out exactly what is happening.

Out of sight. (From the PBS *Madness* series; PBS Video Catalog, 1-800-344-3337). Discusses the development of institutions for the mentally ill and traces custodial care practices of the mentally disturbed. (VHS, color, 60 min)

Pavlov: The conditioned reflex. (Films for the Humanities and Sciences: P.O. Box 2053, Princeton, NJ 08543-2053/ (800)-257-5126). A documentary focusing on the classic work of Ivan Pavlov, this video includes rare footage of his investigations on the conditioned reflex. (25 min)

The dark side of the moon. (Fanlight Productions, 1-800-937-4113). Chronicles the lives of three men with mental disorders from living on the streets to becoming useful members of society. They now work to help other people in similar situations. (VHS, color, 25 min)

To define true madness. (From the PBS *Madness* series; PBS Video Catalog, 1-800-344-3337). Examines mental illness through history and considers the progress made to understand psychological disorders. (VHS, color, 60 min)

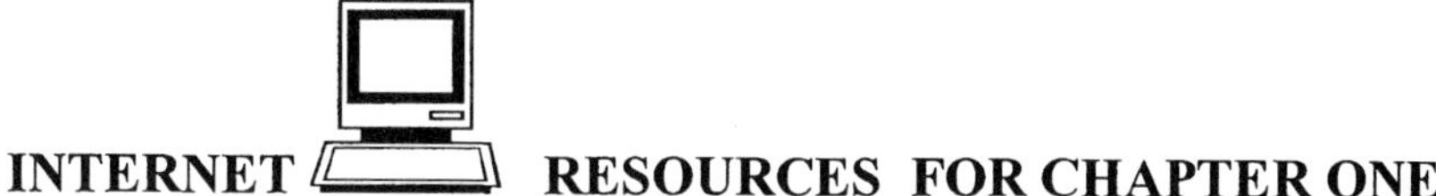

INTERNET RESOURCES FOR CHAPTER ONE

Abnormal Psychology News
http://taxa.psyc.missouri.edu/abnormal/

This is a collection of articles, primarily newspaper articles, relevant to abnormal psychology. They are highly variable in quality, but nearly all come from top news sources and journals. This site is one that you will likely want to refer to time again throughout your teaching!

Abraham Maslow
http://www.ship.edu/~cgboeree/maslow.html

A short biography of Abraham Maslow as well as an elaborate explanation of his humanistic theory can be found at this web site.

American Psychiatric Association
http://www.psych.org/

APA's web site contains psychology-related links, information on legal cases that have affected psychiatry, continuing education for therapists, and much more.

Internet Mental Health
http://www.mentalhealth.com/

A comprehensive site containing information related to the assessment, diagnosis, and treatment of mental illness.

Mental Health History
http://www.mdx.ac.uk/www/study/mhhhome.htm

An interesting site containing a timeline tracing the history of mental health care and asylums, asylum care, and community care.

National Alliance for the Mentally Ill
http://www.nami.org/
Links, membership information, and searchable indexes of mental disorders.

Personality Theories
http://www.ship.edu/~cgboeree/perscontents.html
This is an electronic textbook ("e-text") created for undergraduate and graduate courses in Personality Theory.

Sigmund Freud Museum Vienna Homepage
http://freud.t0.or.at/freud/index-e.htm
Includes a chronology of events in Freud's life and in the history of psychoanalysis plus excellent descriptions of psychoanalytic terminology.

The History of Psychology Web Site
http://elvers.stjoe.udayton.edu/history/welcome.htm
Links to many psychology-related web pages on the internet.

The National Institute of Mental Health
http://www.nimh.nih.gov
The NIMH web site offers information about diagnosis and treatment of several mental health disorders.

Today in the History of Psychology
http://www.cwu.edu/~warren/today.html
The American Psychological Association created this web site which allows the user to access information on the history of psychology by selecting a date on the calendar.

WARNING SIGNS FOR PSYCHOLOGICAL DISORDERS IN ADULTS

- Confused thinking
- Prolonged depression (sadness or irritability)
- Feelings of extreme highs and lows
- Excessive fears, worries and anxieties
- Social withdrawal
- Dramatic changes in eating or sleeping habits
- Strong feelings of anger
- Delusions or hallucinations
- Growing inability to cope with daily problems and activities
- Suicidal thoughts
- Denial of obvious problems
- Numerous unexplained physical ailments
- Substance abuse

WARNING SIGNS FOR PSYCHOLOGICAL DISORDERS IN YOUNGER CHILDREN

- Changes in school performance
- Poor grades despite strong efforts
- Excessive worry or anxiety (i.e. refusing to go to bed or school)
- Hyperactivity
- Persistent nightmares
- Persistent disobedience or aggression
- Frequent temper tantrums

WARNING SIGNS FOR PSYCHOLOGICAL DISORDERS IN OLDER CHILDREN AND PRE-ADOLESCENTS

- Substance abuse
- Inability to cope with problems and daily activities
- Change in sleeping and/or eating habits
- Excessive complaints of physical ailments
- Defiance of authority, truancy, theft, and/or vandalism
- Intense fear of weight gain
- Prolonged negative mood, accompanied by poor appetite or thoughts of death
- Frequent outbursts of anger

CHAPTER TWO

AN INTEGRATIVE APPROACH TO PSYCHOPATHOLOGY

LEARNING OBJECTIVES

1. Distinguish between multidimensional vs. unidimensional models of causality.
2. Identify the main influences comprising the multidimensional model.
3. Define and describe how genes interact with environmental factors to affect behavior.
4. Identify the different models proposed to describe how genes interact with environmental factors to affect behavior.
5. Identify the functions of different brain regions and their role in psychopathology.
6. Explain the role of neurotransmitters and their involvement in abnormal behavior.
7. Compare and contrast the behavioral and cognitive theories and how they are used to explain the origins of mental illness.
8. Describe emotional, social, and cultural influences on abnormal behavior.
9. Be sure that students understand the specific components of a multidimensional, integrative approach to psychopathology (i.e., biological, psychological, emotional, interpersonal, and developmental).

OUTLINE

I. One-Dimensional or Multidimensional Models

A. **One-dimensional models** posit single causes of psychopathology (e.g., its all conditioning, its all biology, its all social or psychological). Note that there are few one-dimensional models in the sense used in the textbook. For instance, even behavioral types rarely (if ever) ascribe to a one-cause model of conditioning; though they will tend to conceptualize most psychopathology as explained by conditioning or learning processes. You can use this to illustrate how one's conceptual system will greatly influence how one goes about explaining psychopathology, and that particularly conceptual systems (e.g., behavioral, cognitive, biological, neurobiological) are quite complex in themselves.

B. **Multi-dimensional models** are systemic and often interdisciplinary, and hold that a system of different reciprocal influences (i.e., biological, cognitive, learning, emotional, social, cultural, developmental) interact in complex ways to yield the major etiological and maintaining processes responsible for abnormal behavior. As such, any biological or environmental influence can become part of this system and cannot be considered in an isolated context. Consider the causes of Judy's phobia, or another case example of your choosing, in the context of a multi-dimensional vs. unidimensional framework.

II. Genetic Contributions to Psychopathology

A. **Gregor Mendel's** work in the 19th century initially demonstrated that our physical characteristics are largely determined by genetic endowment. Examples include hair and eye color. With respect to mental disorder, genetic influences are predominant in some cases (e.g., Huntington's disease and PKU).

B. The Nature of Genes

1. **Genes** are long molecules of **deoxyribonucleic acid** (**DNA**) that are located at various **chromosomal** sites within the cell nucleus. Problems sometimes develop when the normal contingent of 46 human chromosomes (arranged in 23 pairs) is disturbed (an example is **Down's syndrome** or trisomy 21, where a person inherits an extra chromosome on the 21st pair).
2. The DNA molecular structure of genes is referred to as a **double helix** or spiral ladder. The first 22 pairs of chromosomes program development of body and brain and the last pair, called the sex chromosomes, determines sex phenotype. A **defective gene** results if something is wrong with respect to the ordering of DNA molecules on the double helix. A **dominant gene** is one of the pair of genes that determine a particular trait and the effect can be quite noticeable. A **recessive gene**, by contrast, must be paired with another recessive gene to determine a trait.
3. Genes seldom determine our physical development in any absolute way and the same is true for psychopathology. Much of human development and behavior is **polygenic** (i.e., influences by many genes that individually exert a tiny effect). Because of this, scientists look for patterns of influence across genes using a procedure called **quantitative genetics**.

C. New Developments in the Study of Genes and Behavior

1. The best estimate for genetic contribution to enduring personality traits and cognitive abilities in humans is about 50%. With respect to psychological disorders, genetic influences seem to account for less than half the etiological explanation; however, **no individual genes** have been identified relating to any major psychological disorders.
2. More important questions now are how genetic and environmental factors interact to influence the development, maintenance, and treatment of psychological disorders.

D. The Interaction of Genetic and Environmental Effects

1. An example of gene-environment interaction was proposed by **Eric Kandel**, who stated that the process of learning may change the genetic structure of cells. This may occur when environmental processes turn on dormant genes and changes in the brain's biochemical functioning. This view lends support to the notion that we are less hardwired than previously thought.
2. The **diathesis-stress model**
    a. According to this model of gene-environment interaction, persons inherit from multiple genes tendencies to express certain traits or

behaviors (diathesis), which may then be activated under certain environmental events such as stress. Examples include blood-injury-injection phobia and alcoholism. The diathesis or **vulnerability** does *not* necessarily lead to a disorder unless some specific life event occurs.
   b. A person with a large diathesis would, according to this model, require a smaller amount of stress for a disorder to develop compared to someone with a relatively smaller diathesis to begin with.
3. **Reciprocal gene-environment model**
   a. This model states that persons are believed to have a genetically determined tendency to create the very environmental risk factors that trigger genetic vulnerabilities.
   b. Such a model may be used to explain depression, divorce, and personality characteristics such as impulsivity.
4. **Non-genomic "inheritance"** of behavior
   a. Related to research suggesting that there has been an overemphasis on the role of genetic influence on personality, temperament, and their contribution to the development of psychological disorders. Examples include research on genetically identical mice (including rats and rhesus monkeys using cross fostering strategies) reared in identical environments, but perform and behave quite differently on several experimental tasks above what genes would suggest.
   b. The moral is that it is even too simplistic to say that the genetic contributions to personality traits or psychopathology is 50%; one must consider the heritable contribution in the context of an individual's past and present environment.

III. Neuroscience and its Contributions to Psychopathology

A. The field of **neuroscience** focuses on understanding the role of the nervous system in disease and behavior. Knowing how the nervous system and particularly the brain works is central to understanding behavior, emotion, and cognitive processes.

B. The **central nervous system (CNS)**
1. Consists of the **brain** and **spinal cord** and processes all information received from our sense organs and reacts as necessary.
2. **Neurons** control every thought and action, the brain contains an average of 140 billion neurons.
   a. The typical neuron contains a central cell body with two different kinds of branches. One set of branches, **dendrites**, extend from the cell body to receive chemical messages from other nerve cells which are converted into electrical impulses. The other branch, the **axon**, transmits these impulses to other neurons. Any one nerve cell is linked with multiple others.
   b. Neurons themselves operate electrically, but communicate with other neurons chemically. The **synaptic cleft** is a small space that exists between the axon of one neuron and the dendrites of another. It is here

where neurons communicate with one another via release of neurotransmitters from dendrites of other neurons.

c. **Neurotransmitters** are the chemicals released from one nerve cell to another across the synaptic cleft. Major neurotransmitters implicated in psychopathology include **norepinephrine** (or noradrenaline), **serotonin**, **dopamine**, and **gamma aminobutyric acid** (GABA).

C. The Structure of the Brain

1. The **brain** is divided into two parts. The lower **brain stem** is the most primitive part and is responsible for most of the automatic functions necessary for survival (e.g., breathing, sleeping, moving). The more advanced brain systems are located in the **forebrain**.
    a. The **hindbrain** is the lowest part of the brainstem, and contains the **medulla**, **pons**, and **cerebellum** (motor coordination). These structures control activities such as breathing, heartbeat, and digestion.
    b. The **midbrain** coordinates movement with sensory input and contains parts of the **reticular activating system (RAS)**. The RAS contributes to arousal, tension, and waking and sleeping.
    c. At the very top of the brain stem (i.e., above the hindbrain) lies the **diencephalon**, which contains the **thalamus** and **hypothalamus**; these structures help transmit information to the forebrain and are integral to behavior and emotion.
    d. At the very base of the forebrain (just above the thalamus and hypothalamus) is the **telencephalon**, containing the **limbic system**. Limbic means "border," and this system figures prominently in much of psychopathology. It includes the following structures: **hippocampus (sea horse)**, **cingulate gyrus (girdle)**, **septum (partition)**, and **amygdala (almond)**. Emotional expression, impulse control, sex, aggression, hunger, and thirst are controlled by this part of the brain. Another area at the base of the forebrain is the **basal ganglia**, including the **caudate (tailed) nucleus**. Motor behavior is controlled by this area, and damage can cause twitching or shaking.
    e. The largest part of the forebrain is the **cerebral cortex** which contains over 80% of the neurons in the CNS. Reasoning and creative skills are derived from this brain area. The cerebral cortex is divided into two near-symmetrical hemispheres: the left hemisphere appears to be responsible for verbal and cognitive processes, whereas the right hemisphere appears more responsible for spatial abilities.
    f. Each hemisphere of the cerebral cortex consists of four separate areas of lobes. The **temporal lobe** is associated with the recognition of sights and sounds and long-term memory storage. The **parietal lobe** is associated with touch recognition. The **occipital lobe** integrates visual input. The **frontal lobe** is most interesting from the standpoint of psychopathology and is largely responsible for thinking and reasoning abilities, memory; it enables one to relate to people and events in the world and to behave as social animals.

D. The **peripheral nervous system** works in coordination with the brain stem to ensure proper bodily functioning and consists of the (1) **somatic nervous system,** which controls muscles and movement, and (2) **autonomic nervous system (ANS)**, which is divided into the **sympathetic** and **parasympathetic nervous systems**. The ANS regulates the cardiovascular system, endocrine system (e.g., pituitary, adrenal, thyroid, and gonadal glands) and aids in digestion and regulation of body temperature.

1. The **endocrine system** produces its own chemical messengers (i.e., **hormones)** and releases them directly into the bloodstream. **Adrenal glands** produce epinephrine (also called adrenaline) in response to stress, including salt-regulating hormones; the **thyroid** produces thyroxine, which facilitates energy metabolism and growth; the **pituitary** is the master gland that produces several regulatory hormones; and the gonads produce sex hormones (e.g., testosterone and estrogen). The endocrine system is closely related to the immune system and is implicated in anxiety, stress-related, and sexual disorders.
2. The sympathetic and parasympathetic branches of the ANS operate in a complementary fashion. The **sympathetic** nervous system mobilizes the body (e.g., increases heart rate) during periods of stress or danger and is part of the emergency or alarm response; the **parasympathetic** nervous system renormalizes arousal and facilitates digestion.
3. The **hypothalamic-pituitary-adrenalcortical axis** (HPA axis) illustrates the connection between the nervous and endocrine systems and is implicated in several forms of psychopathology.

E. Neurotransmitters

1. Brain circuits are pathways of neurotranmitters. Neuroscientists have identified several brain circuits that appear to play a role in psychological disorders. Drug therapies function by either increasing or decreasing the flow of specific neurotransmitters. After a neurotransmitter is released it is quickly drawn back from the synaptic cleft into the same neuron via a process known as **reuptake**. **Agonists** increase the activity of a neurotransmitter by mimicking its effects. Some drugs, known as **antagonists**, function to inhibit or block the production of neurotransmitter or function indirectly to prevent the chemical from reaching the next neuron by closing or occupying the receptors; other drugs increase production of competing biochemicals that deactivate the neurotransmitter or produce effects opposite those produced by the neurotransmitter **(inverse agonists)**. Most drugs are either agnostic or antagonistic.
2. Types of neurotransmitters include:
   a. **Serotonin** (5HT) is concentrated in the midbrain and connected to the cortex, thus producing widespread effects on behavior, mood, and thought processes. Extremely low levels of serotonin are associated with less inhibition, instability, impulsivity, and tendencies to overreact to situations (e.g., aggression, suicide, impulsive overeating, excessive sexual behavior. Tricyclic antidepressants (e.g.,

imipramine), and new classes of serotonin specific reuptake inhibitors (SSRIs; e.g., Prozac) affect the serotonergic system (see also St. John's-wort).

b. **Gamma aminobutyric acid (GABA)** reduces postsynaptic activity which, in turn, inhibits several behaviors and emotions, particularly anxiety. **Benzodiazepines**, or mild tranquilizers, make it easier for GABA to attach to specialized receptors. Effect is not specific to anxiety. The benzodiazepine-GABA system reduces overall arousal and tempers anger, hostility, aggression, and possibly excessive anticipation and even positive emotional states.

c. **Norepinephrine** (also known as noradrenaline) is also part of the endocrine system and important in psychopathology. Norepinephrine stimulates at least alpha-adrenergic and beta-adrenergic receptors. **Beta-blockers** for hypertension reduce the surge in norepinephrine and keep heart rate and blood pressure down. You may ask students to think about what might happen to someone who over does it when they are taking beta-blockers.

d. **Dopamine (also classified as a catecholamine)** has been implicated in schizophrenia and may act by "switching on" various brain circuits that inhibit or facilitate emotions or behavior. Reserpine (from Chapter 1) blocks specific dopamine receptors, thus lowering dopamine activity. Dopamine and serotonin circuits cross at many points and seem to balance one another. An agonist for dopamine is L-DOPA, which has been shown to be effective for treating Parkinson's disease by increasing levels of dopamine. Illustrate to students what happens when Parkinson's patients are given too much dopamine – they begin to show signs and symptoms of schizophrenia, whereas when the levels of dopamine are lower to the extreme schizophrenic patients show behaviors associated with Parkinson's disease.

F. Implications for psychopathology

1. Methods for studying brain images have been applied to psychopathology. For example, persons with obsessive-compulsive disorder show increased activity in the orbital surface of the cerebral cortex, the cingulate gyrus, and to a lesser extent the caudate nucleus. One of the strongest concentrations of neurotransmitters in these areas is serotonin, which is related to over reactive or compulsive behavior. Damage to this brain circuit is related to an inability to ignore irrelevant cues, making the organism over reactive.
2. The work of neuroscience is only beginning and one cannot be certain about the relation between the orbital surface and OCD. It is possible that overactivity in this region of the brain is a consequence, not a cause, of OCD.

G. Psychosocial influences on brain structure and function

1. In addition to potential biological interventions, psychological treatments may be powerful enough to modify brain circuits; for example, the treatment of

OCD via exposure and response prevention can result in the normalization of brain function.

2. Interactions of Psychosocial Factors with Brain Structure and Function
    a. Several recent experiments illustrate the interaction of psychosocial factors and brain function at the level of neurotransmitter activity. Experiments on early effects of controllability over life events in Rhesus monkeys have shown psychosocial factors can exert powerful effects on the action of neurotransmitters over subsequent behavior. Learning and experience can also affect the structure of neurons, including the number of receptors on a cell and how they respond to subsequent experience. One explanation is that learning and experience produces more plastic and rich neural connections in the brain, and that such experience can determine vulnerability to psychological disorders later in life.
    b. Also, psychosocial factors may directly affect levels of neurotransmitters (animal studies indicate that certain neurochemical substances have very different effects depending on the psychological histories of the animals).

IV. Behavioral and Cognitive Science

A. Conditioning and Cognitive Processes

1. Robert Rescorla and others' experiments indicate that basic classical and operant conditioning paradigms *facilitate* the learning of the relations among events in the environment. This learning involves complex cognitive and emotional processing in humans and lower animals.
2. Martin Seligman described the concept of **learned helplessness**, or the lack of behavior shown by an organism when it encounters conditions over which no control is possible. People may make certain attributions about their environment when they believe they have little control over stress in their lives. People may become depressed if they decide or think they can do little about the stress in their lives (i.e., attribution of no control), even if others think there is something that could be done.
3. Albert Bandura observed that organisms can learn simply by watching others in their environment (**modeling or observational learning**). This type of learning requires a symbolic integration of the experiences of others with judgments of what might happen to the observer. Bandura also specified the importance of social context in learning and maintained that much of what we learn depends on our interactions with other people around us.
4. **Prepared learning** reflects the recognition that biology and genetics influence what we learn and how readily we do so. This view is based on the observation that we learn to associate fears and phobias with certain types of objects or situations that have some evolutionary basis in promoting survival (e.g., snakes or spiders. Over the course of evolution certain unconditioned and conditional stimuli become more readily associated for their survival value and this preparedness is passed on via genetics.

B. Cognitive Science and the Unconscious

1. Advances in cognitive science have revolutionized our conceptions of the unconscious. Examples include the concepts of **blind sight** (unconscious vision), dissociation between behavior and unconsciousness (hypnotism), and **implicit memory** (i.e., acting on the basis of things that have happened in the past but being unable to remember the past events).
2. One method for exploring the unconscious (or black box) is the **Stroop color naming paradigm**, where subjects are shown a variety of words printed in different color inks. Delays in color naming occur when the meaning of the word attracts the subject's attention despite efforts to concentrate on the color of the word.

V. Emotions

A. **Emotion** plays an important role in our lives and can contribute in significant ways to the development of psychopathology. The alarm reaction that activates during potentially life-threatening emergencies is called the **flight or fight response**.

B. The Physiology and purpose of fear

1. The physiologist Walter Cannon speculated that **fear** activates the cardiovascular system, blood vessels constrict, arterial pressure rises while blood flow is decreased to the extremities, breathing becomes faster, increased amounts of sugar are released from the liver into the bloodstream, hearing becomes more acute, digestive activity is suspended, shivering and piloerection also occur.
2. Fear is the subjective feeling of terror, a strong motivation for behavior (escape or fighting), and a complex physiological arousal response. This fight or flight reaction was fundamentally important in the course of evolution and is very much with us today in normal behavior and in several forms of psychopathology.

C. Emotional phenomena

1. Emotion is comprised of three components that are often considered in isolation from the others: behavior, physiology, and cognition. Walter Cannon viewed emotion as primarily a brain function, whereas Richard S. Lazarus emphasizes the cognitive aspects of emotion. Many theorists believe that the cognitive and emotional systems interact and overlap, but are fundamentally separate.
2. Defining emotion is difficult, but most agree that it is an **action tendency** to behave in a certain way that is elicited by an external event, a feeling state, and one accompanied by a possibly characteristic physiological response. Emotions function to ensure that we pass our genes on to subsequent generations.

3. Emotions are usually short-lived, temporary states lasting several minutes to several hours. **Mood** is a more persistent period of affect or emotionality. **Affect** usually refers to the momentary emotional tone that accompanies what we say or do, but can also be used generically to summarize commonalities among emotional states that are characteristic of an individual.

D. Anger and emotion in psychopathology

1. Sustained anger and hostility appear closely related to the development of heart disease. This may occur because the ability of the heart to efficiently pump blood throughout the body drops significantly when one is angry (placing the person at increased risk of disturbances in heart rhythm) but not during stress or exercise.
2. Suppressing almost any kind of emotional response (e.g., anger or fear) increases sympathetic nervous system activity and can even help produce the unwanted emotional state and related thoughts. Emotions affect cognitive processes, and many basic emotions (e.g., fear, anger, sadness or distress, excitement) seem to play a direct role in psychological disorders (e.g., anxiety, depression, mania) and may even define them.

VI. Cultural, social, and interpersonal factors

A. In many cultures, individuals may suffer from fright disorders, exaggerated startle responses, and other observable fear reactions (e.g., voodoo, the evil eye). Although fear and phobias are universal, what we fear is strongly influenced by our social environment.

B. **Gender** exerts a strong and puzzling effect on psychopathology. Females are at higher risk for developing particular kinds of phobias (e.g., insect, small animal phobias) and eating disorders, whereas social phobias affect men and women equally. The difference may have to do with cultural expectations of men and women and gender roles.

C. The number and frequency of **social relationships** and contacts is strongly related to mortality. Social relationships seem to protect individuals against high blood pressure, depression, alcoholism, arthritis, progression of AIDS, low birth weight in newborns, and susceptibility to catching a cold and infection. Animal studies also indicate that (1) social instability may lead to suppressed immune responses, and (2) biological factors such as drugs can produce different psychological effects depending on social context.

D. Older persons with few meaningful contacts and little social support report high levels of depression and unsatisfactory quality of life. If they became physically ill, they often receive more substantial family support which serves to reestablish their social bonds and makes life worth living.

E. Psychological disorders carry a substantial **social stigma** in our society.

F. **Global incidence** of psychological disorders

1. Approximately 10 – 20% of all primary medical services in poor countries are sought by patients with psychological disorders; record numbers of men are committing suicide in Micronesia; alcoholism levels among adults in Latin America have risen to 20%. Treatments for disorders that are successful in the United States often cannot be administered in countries where mental health services are limited (e.g., China). Social and cultural factors maintain disorders as most societies do not have the means of alleviating and preventing them.

VII. Development

A. To completely understand psychopathology, one must appreciate how disorders change with time. Persons are not their disorders and are often not disordered at all times and particularly over time.

B. Just like a fever, clinicians and researchers recognize that a particular behavior or disorder may have multiple causes. For example, the **principle of equifinality** is used in developmental psychopathology to indicate that there may be a number of paths to a given outcome. These different paths may result from psychological factors that interact with biological components during various stages of development.

OVERALL SUMMARY

This chapter outlines the primary components of a multidimensional model of psychopathology. The multidimensional model considers genetic contributions, the role of the nervous system, behavioral and cognitive processes, emotional influences, social and interpersonal influences, and developmental factors in explaining the causes, and even the factors that maintain, psychological disorders. This chapter describes these areas of influence as well as their interaction in producing mental disorder.

KEY TERMS

Affect (p. 58)
Agonist (p. 47)
Antagonist (p. 47)
Brain circuits (p. 46)
Cognitive science (p. 54)
Diathesis-stress model (p. 36)
Dopamine (p. 49)
Emotion (p. 57)
Equifinality (p. 64)

Flight or fight response (p. 57)
Gamma aminobutyric acid (GABA) (p. 48)
Genes (dominant, recessive)/chromosomes (sex; X, Y) (p. 34)
Hormone (p. 45)
Implicit memory (p. 56)
Inverse agonist (p. 47)
Learned helplessness (p. 55)
Modeling (also observational learning) (p. 55)
Mood (p. 58)
Multidimensional integrative approach (p. 31)
Neurons (p. 41)
Neuroscience (p. 41)
Neurotransmitters (p. 42)
Norepinephrine (also noradrenaline) (p. 49)
Prepared learning (p. 55)
Reciprocal gene-environment model (p. 38)
Reuptake (p. 46)
Serotonin (5-hydroxytryptamine) (p. 47)
Synaptic cleft (p. 42)
Vulnerability (p. 36)

INFOTRAC KEY TERM EXERCISES

Each exercise is linked to key terms from the Wadsworth InfoTrac on-line searchable database. Key terms must be entered exactly as written.

Exercise 1: **Is Ecstasy the Rave?**
Article: A62266508
Citation: (MDMA [Ecstasy] neurotoxicity: assessing and communicating the risks**)**.
Brendon P Boot; Iain S McGregor; Wayne Hall
The Lancet, May 20, 2000 v355 i9217 p1818

Ecstasy is a synthetic drug that can produce profound effects of behavior, emotion, and cognition. Review this InfoTrac article on the drug ecstasy and describe what is known about how this drug operates at the neurotransmitter level in both primates and humans. How does the drug affect neurotransmitter function? How does the drug affect brain structure? Address the psychological and neurological consequences of Ecstasy use, including the implications of this research for health education. Limit your answer to 3-5 typed double-spaced pages.

Exercise 2: **Nature vs. Nurture: Can and Should We Genetically Engineer Mental Health?**
Key Term: *Nature and Nurture, Periodicals*

Geneticists have shown that cloning is possible and many researchers are scrambling to be the first to clone a human being. Cloning itself raises a host of ethical, legal, moral, and scientific questions. The fundamental premise of cloning humans is the potential to reproduce a person that would be somehow better off – smarter, stronger, more attractive, and physically and psychologically more healthy – than the uncloned. Another premise behind this move is that genes (i.e., nature) are more important than experience (i.e., nurture). Your textbook authors, however, present a different view. Review the InfoTrac article(s) on this topic and outline evidence supporting your position in the context of the following scenario: You are the director of a large behavioral genetics research facility with a federal mandate and blank check to eradicate mental illness in society via genetic engineering. How do you respond? Do you go ahead? How successful will your mission be (assuming you decide to go through with it) in light of what you have read? What is the evidence that this program will achieve its goals of genetically engineering mental health and should it be done? Limit your answer to 3-5 typed double-spaced pages.

Exercise 3 (Future Trend): Brain Cell Regeneration

Neuroscientists have long believed that we are born with a relatively fixed number of brain cells – about 100 billion – and that the adult brain is incapable to growing new cells. The idea that the brain may grow new cells was thought impossible until recently. The web links below provide an overview of this exciting work. Describe and relate these new findings with the neuroscience material covered in Chapter 2 of the text. In so doing, outline regions of the brain where brain cell regeneration has been demonstrated, and for what species. Then offer implications for this work for the treatment of psychiatric conditions that involve brain insult or cell damage.

http://www.brainlightning.com/regen.html

This site provides an overview of research in the area of brain cell regeneration. A good starting point.

http://www.dsrf.co.uk/Reading_material/New_braincells/newbrain1.htm

This site describes the implications of brain cell re-growth into adulthood, with particular attention to the implications of this research for neurological disease.

CLASSROOM ACTIVITIES, DEMONSTRATIONS, AND LECTURE TOPICS

1. **Activity: Brain Areas & Their Function.** To teach your students neuroanatomy and the contributions of neuroscience to psychopathology, prepare two sets of index cards. On one set you should write the brain structures discussed in the text. The second set of cards should list the functions of these structures. For example, your cards would include:

STRUCTURE	**FUNCTION**
Central nervous system	Consists of the brain and spinal cord
Medulla and pons	Breathing, pumping of heart, digestion
Cerebellum	Motor coordination
Midbrain	Coordinate movement with sensory input
Reticular activating system	Processes of arousal and tension
Limbic system	Emotional experiences/basic drives of sex, aggression, hunger, and thirst
Caudate nucleus	Controls motor behavior
Cerebral cortex	Contains over 80% of neurons in the central nervous system

Left hemisphere	Verbal and other cognitive processes
Right hemisphere	Perceiving surrounding events and creating images
Temporal lobe	Recognizing various sights and sounds
Parietal lobe	Recognizing various sensations of touch
Occipital lobe	Integrates various visual input
Frontal lobe	Thinking and reasoning abilities
Peripheral nervous system	Coordination with brain stem to ensure body is working properly
Somatic nervous system	Controls our muscles
Autonomic nervous system	Regulates the cardiovascular system and endocrine system
Endocrine system	Releases hormones into the bloodstream
Sympathetic nervous system	Mobilizes body during times of stress
Parasympathetic nervous system	Renormalizes body after arousal states
Pituitary gland	Master or coordinator of endocrine system

The goal of this quick activity is to have students match various structures of the brain with their respective functions. Divide the class in half and distribute one set of index cards to each group of students. Each student should receive one card. Instruct students to find the match for their structure/ function, and tell them to do the activity without talking.

2. **Activity: Eliminating Test Anxiety through Behavior Therapy**. Eison (1987) has developed a way for students to eliminate their test anxiety with the use of popular behavioral techniques. To eliminate test anxiety through the use of systematic desensitization, allow students to first become familiar with relaxation training; then, while relaxed, ask students to imagine an anxiety-provoking situation involving tests. To demonstrate the effectiveness of rational emotive therapy, ask students to comprise two lists (rational versus irrational) regarding common beliefs about tests (things they say to themselves during exams). Try to encourage students to examine each belief critically; soon they should be able to realize why many fears regarding tests are irrational.

   Source Information. Eison, J.A. (1987) Using systematic desensitization and rational emotive therapy to treat test anxiety. Activities handbook for the teaching of psychology, vol. 2. Washington, DC: American Psychological Association.

3. **Activity: Mental Illness in Social Context: Being Sane in Insane Places**. In 1973 sociologist David Rosenhan sought to examine how difficult it would be for people to shed the "mentally ill" label. He was particularly interested in how psychiatric hospital staff process information about patients. Rosenhan and seven associates had themselves committed to different mental hospitals by complaining that they were hearing voices (a symptom commonly believed to be characteristic of schizophrenia). The staff did not know the "pseudopatients" were actually part an experiment. Beyond the alleged symptoms and falsification of names and occupations, the important events of the pseudopatients' life histories were factually presented to hospital staff as they had occurred. The pseudopatients were instructed to act completely normal upon admission

into the hospital. In fact, Rosenhan told them that acting normal was the only way they could get out. Despite the fact that they did nothing out of the ordinary, the pseudopatients remained hospitalized for an average of 19 days (range 9 to 52 days). Ironically, their sanity was not detected by hospital staff, but it was detected by the actual patients in the hospitals. All of Rosenhan's associates retained the deviant label even after being discharged. Their schizophrenia was said to be "in remission," implying that it was dormant and could possibly resurface. At no time during their stay in the hospital was the legitimacy of their schizophrenic label questioned. It was simply assumed that they were schizophrenic, and everything the pseudopatients did and said while in the mental institutions was understood from this premise. Normal behaviors were overlooked entirely or were profoundly misinterpreted. Minor disagreements became deep-seated indicators of emotional instability. Boredom was interpreted as nervousness or anxiety. Even the act of writing on a notepad was seen by the staff as a sign of some deeper psychological disturbance. Furthermore, even though there was nothing "pathological" about the pseudopatients' past histories, these records were reinterpreted to be consistent with the schizophrenic label. Rosenhan concluded that the staff were doing their jobs as designed and made no conscious effort to misconstrue the evidence. The moral is that psychiatric labels are so powerful that they can profoundly affect the way information is processed and perceived. Had the same behaviors been observed in a different context, they no doubt would have been interpreted in an entirely different fashion. You may use this study and others like it to discuss the role of context in influencing our interpretations of abnormal behavior. Alternatively, this is a great springboard for discussion about the stigma of mental illness, and even the dangers of one-dimensional models. You may also ask students if they can come up with other behaviors that would have been misinterpreted in this situation.

Source Information. Rosenhan, D. (1973). On being sane in insane places. Science, 179, 250-258.

4. **Activity: The Ubiquity of Emotion & Conditioning.** Conditioning is so ubiquitous in everyday experience that it is often hard to see. Have students come up with examples of classically conditioned emotional/evaluative responses and use such examples to illustrate that most conditioning is quite adaptive. If students have trouble coming up with examples, you may start with conditioned taste aversions, objects or events that students fear, or words/images that elicit an emotional response (e.g., fear, anger, disgust; seeing flashing blue lights in your rearview mirror and getting caught for speeding while driving on the highway). Have students talk about the dimensions that are involved in the conditioned responses in keeping with the text description of emotion as involving cognition, behavior, and physiology. As a trick, you may ask students whether they have ever felt that an exam they had taken was unfair. Don't ask for a show of hands. Most students will raise their hands. You can then ask, "Why did you all raise your hands?" Use this example to illustrate the role of experience and socialization in learning and behavior (in this case, automatically raising one's hand in response to a question in the classroom without being asked to do so).

5. **Activity: Susan Mineka's Work on Vicarious Learning of Fear in Primates.** Susan Mineka and her colleagues have performed some interesting experiments demonstrating vicarious learning of fear in lab-reared monkeys. Her work to date represents the most compelling evidence for observational learning of fear. Many students find the description of her classic studies interesting in itself.

SUPPLEMENTARY READING MATERIAL FOR CHAPTER TWO

(= These sources can be found on "*Infotrac, the online library*" provided by Wadsworth and Brooks/Cole Publishing.)

Blows, W. T. (2000). Neurotransmitters of the brain: Serotonin, noradrenaline (norepinephrine), and dopamine. Journal of Neuroscience Nursing, 32, 234-238.

Damasio, A. R. (1995). Descartes' error: Emotion, reason, and the human brain. New York: Avon Books.

Ellis, A., & Harper, R. A. (1976). A guide to rational living. North Hollywood, CA: Wilshire Book Company.

Gross, C. G. (1998). Brain, vision, memory: Tales in the history of neuroscience. Cambridge: MIT Press.

Hundert, E. (1991). A synthetic approach to psychiatry's nature-nurture debate. Integrative Psychiatry, 7, 76-83.

Kolb, B., & Whishaw, I. Q. (1998). Brain plasticity and behavior. Annual Review of Psychology, 49, 1-13.

Kihlstrom, J. F. (1987). The cognitive unconscious. Science, 237, 1445-1452.

Marshall, L. H., & Magoun, H. W . (Eds) (1998). Discoveries in the human brain: Neuroscience prehistory, brain structure, and function. Totowa, NJ: Humana Press.

Mineka, S., Davidson, M., Cook, M., & Keir, R. (1984). Observational conditioning of snake fear in rhesus monkeys. Journal of Abnormal Psychology, 93, 355-372.

Radford, B. (1999). The ten-percent myth (people's use of only 10% of their brains). Skeptical Inquirer, 23, 1-3.

Ramachandran, V. S., & Blakeslee, S. (1998). Phantoms in the brain: Probing the histories of the human mind. New York: William Morrow & Company.

Sacks, O. (1985). The man who mistook his wife for a hat and other clinical tales. New York: Summit Books.

SUPPLEMENTARY VIDEO RESOURCES FOR CHAPTER TWO

CNN today: Abnormal psychology 2000, vol. 1. (*Available through your International Thomson Learning representative)*. The segment titled "An Integrative Approach to Psychopathology: Emotions and Their Influences on the Body" focuses on the emotion of anger in men and what can be done to alleviate it. A brief mention is also made of depression and how it can impact ones health (e.g. high blood pressure, heart attacks). Presents a view that emotions can be dangerous. (2 min, 5 sec)

Deficits of mind and brain. (McDonnell Summer Institute of Cognitive Neuroscience, Eugene, Oregon; *available through your International Thomson Learning representative*). Part one of this videotape provides an overview of neuroimaging techniques and the neuropsychology of cognitive impairments (particularly neglect syndrome) that result from strokes; part two provides a neuropsychological view of schizophrenia. (60 min)

Discovering psychology: The responsive brain. (Annenburg/CPB Collection). Examines the interaction of the brain, behavior, and the environment. Also shows how brain structure and function are influenced by behavioral and environmental factors. (30 min)

Inside information: The brain and how it works. (Films for the Humanities and Sciences: P.O. Box 2053, Princeton, NJ 08543-2053/ (800)-257-5126). This videotape describes how the many areas of the brain function and includes interviews with researchers in the field of neuroscience. (58 min)

The brain, mind, and behavior. (PBS Video Catalog, 1-800-344-3337). This series focuses on the nature and function of the human brain, consciousness, and the effects of the brain and hormones on behavior. (8 parts, 60 min each)

The enchanted loom: Processing sensory information. (Films for the Humanities and Sciences: P.O. Box 2053, Princeton, NJ 08543-2053/ (800)-257-5126). Discusses how the brain is capable of sorting through vast sensory information and interpreting it on the basis of past experience and expectations. (60 min)

The human brain. (Insight Media: 2162 Broadway, New York, NY 10024/ (800)-233-9910). Investigators discuss how the brain's abilities can be enhanced through the proper environmental. Also presents the case of a man who improves his condition after a serious brain injury. (25 min)

The mind. (PBS Video Catalog, 1-800-344-3337). This PBS series focuses on mental development in the context of normal and abnormal development.

The nervous system. (Insight Media: 2162 Broadway, New York, NY 10024/ (800)-233-9910). Explores the function of neurons as well as the central, peripheral and autonomic nervous systems. (25 min)

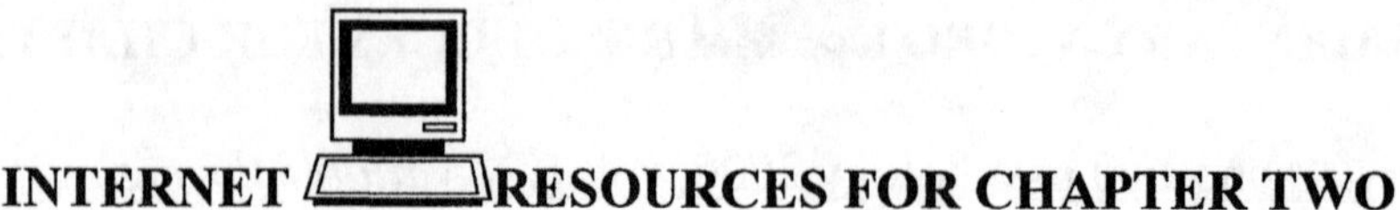

INTERNET RESOURCES FOR CHAPTER TWO

Albert Bandura
http://www.ship.edu/~cgboeree/bandura.html
A web page devoted to the man who discovered observational learning and modeling therapy.

Biochemistry of Neurotransmitters
http://web.indstate.edu/thcme/mwking/nerves.html
Describes the nature and function of several neurotransmitters.

History of Neuroscience
http://faculty.washington.edu/chudler/hist.html
Lists some of the most important events that occurred in neuroscience and psychology in chronological order, dating back to 4000 B.C.

Neuropsychology Central
http://www.neuropsychologycentral.com/index.html
Links to online sources on neuropsychological assessment, treatments, software, and newsgroups just to name a few.

Neurosciences on the Internet
http://ivory.lm.com/~nab/
This site has links to other neuroscience related web pages; also contains information on the biological basis of psychiatric disorders such as Attention Deficit Disorder, Panic Anxiety Disorder, and Alzheimer's Disease.

The Whole Brain Atlas
http://www.med.harvard.edu/AANLIB/home.html
An excellent cite reviewing the structure and function of the human brain.

Anatomic Features of the Human Spinal Cord

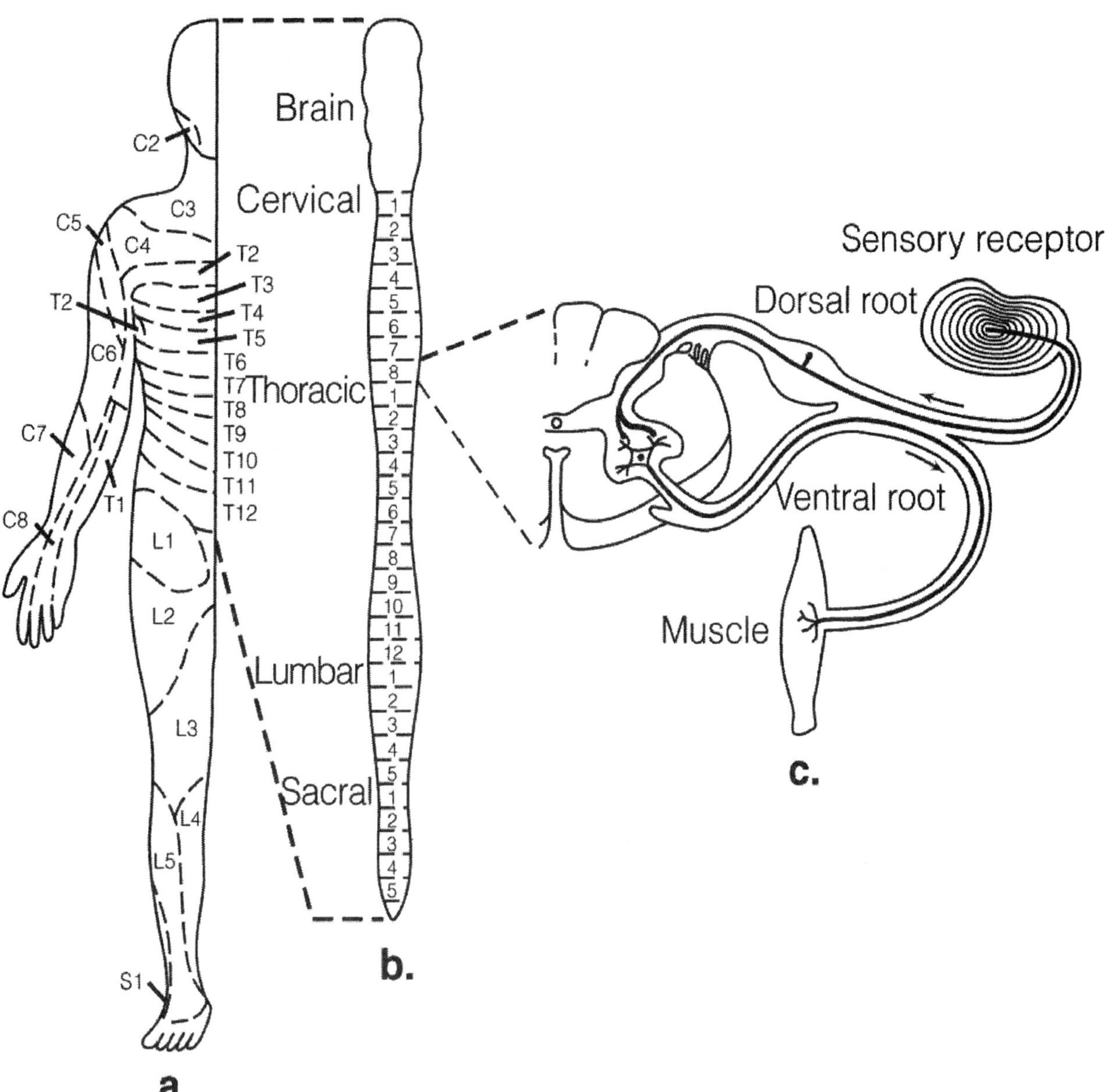

Anatomic Features: Spinal nerves and internal organization of the spinal cord (gray and white matter)

Function: Relays information to and from the brain; responsible for simple reflexive behavior.

Anatomic Features of the Human skull

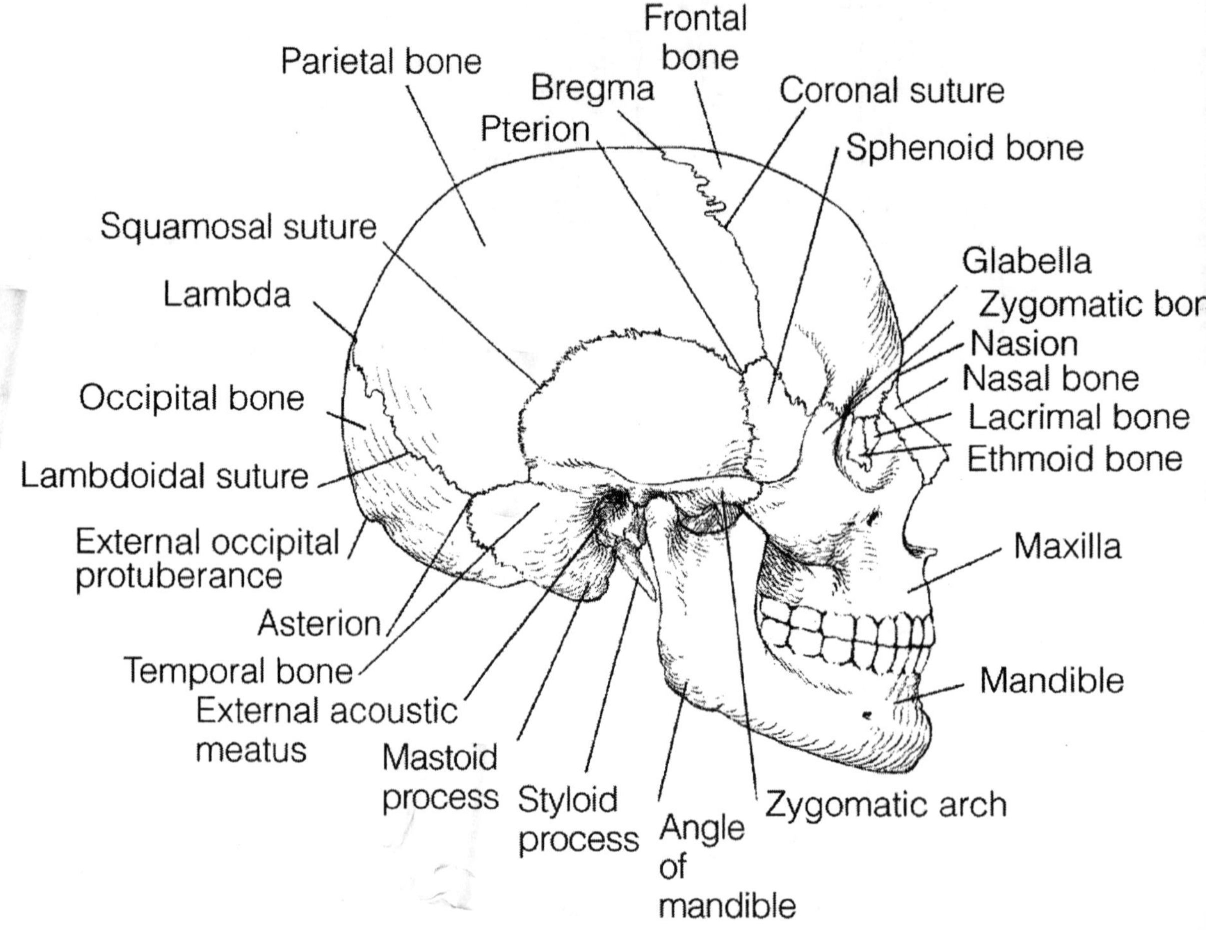

Anatomic Features: A fused connection of bony plates covering the brain

Function: Protection of the brain

Anatomic Features Protective Meninges of the CNS

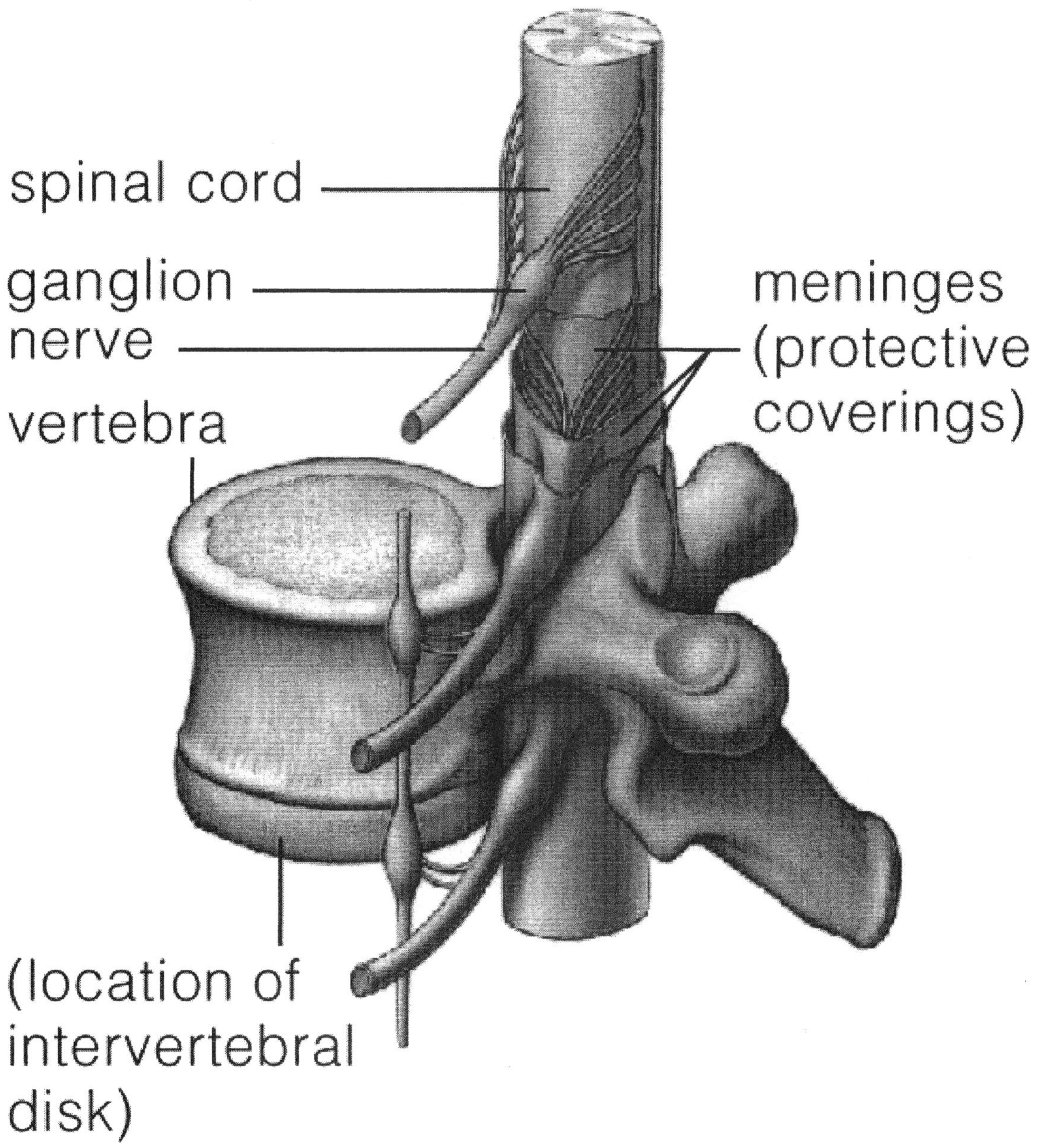

Anatomic Features: Dura mater, arachnoid membrane, and pia mater

Function: Protective covering of the central nervous system (CNS), location of venous drainage, and cerebrospinal fluid absorption

Anatomic Features of the Ventricular System

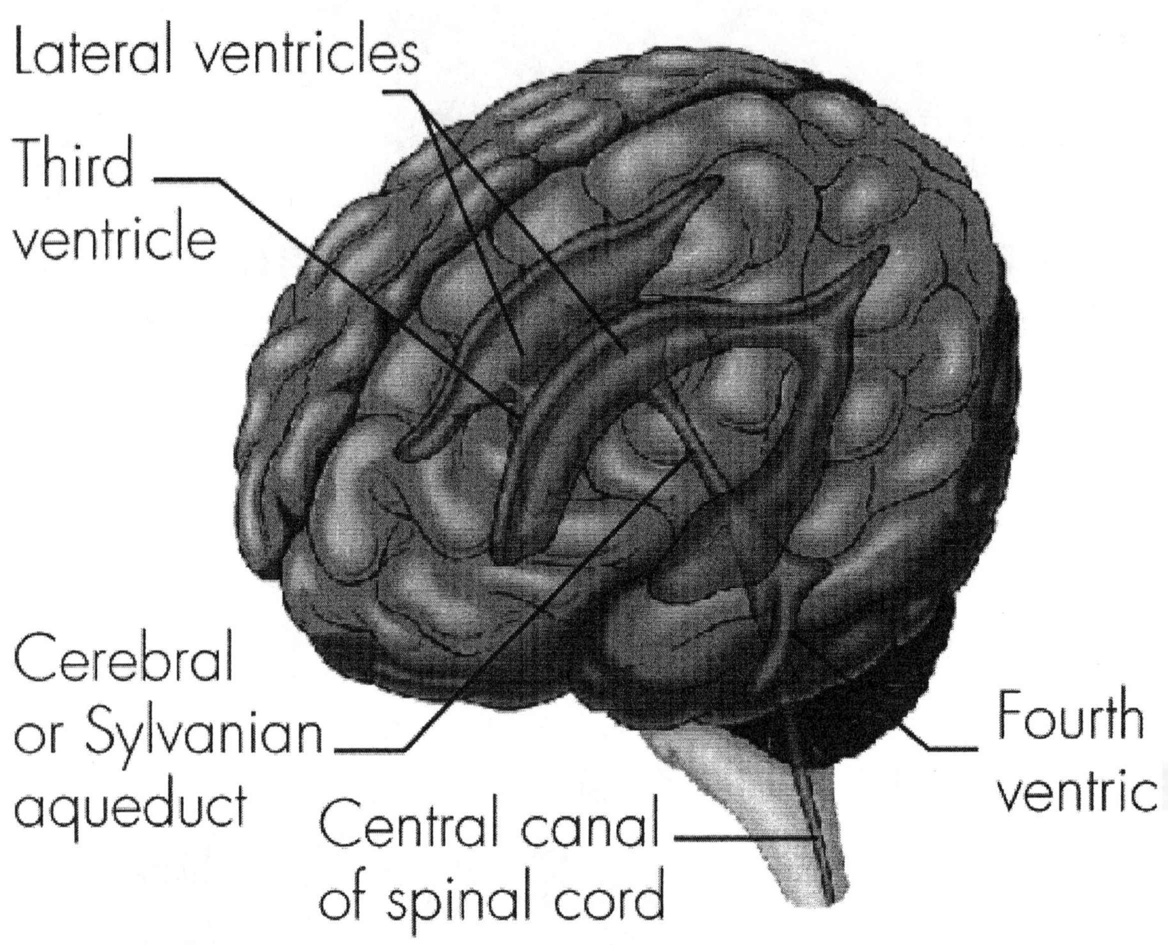

Anatomic Features: Lateral (1st and 2nd), 3rd, and 4th ventricles, choroids plexus, cerebral aqueduct, and arachnoid granulations

Function: Balancing intracranial pressure, cerebrospinal fluid production, and circulation

Anatomic Features of the Brain's Vascular System

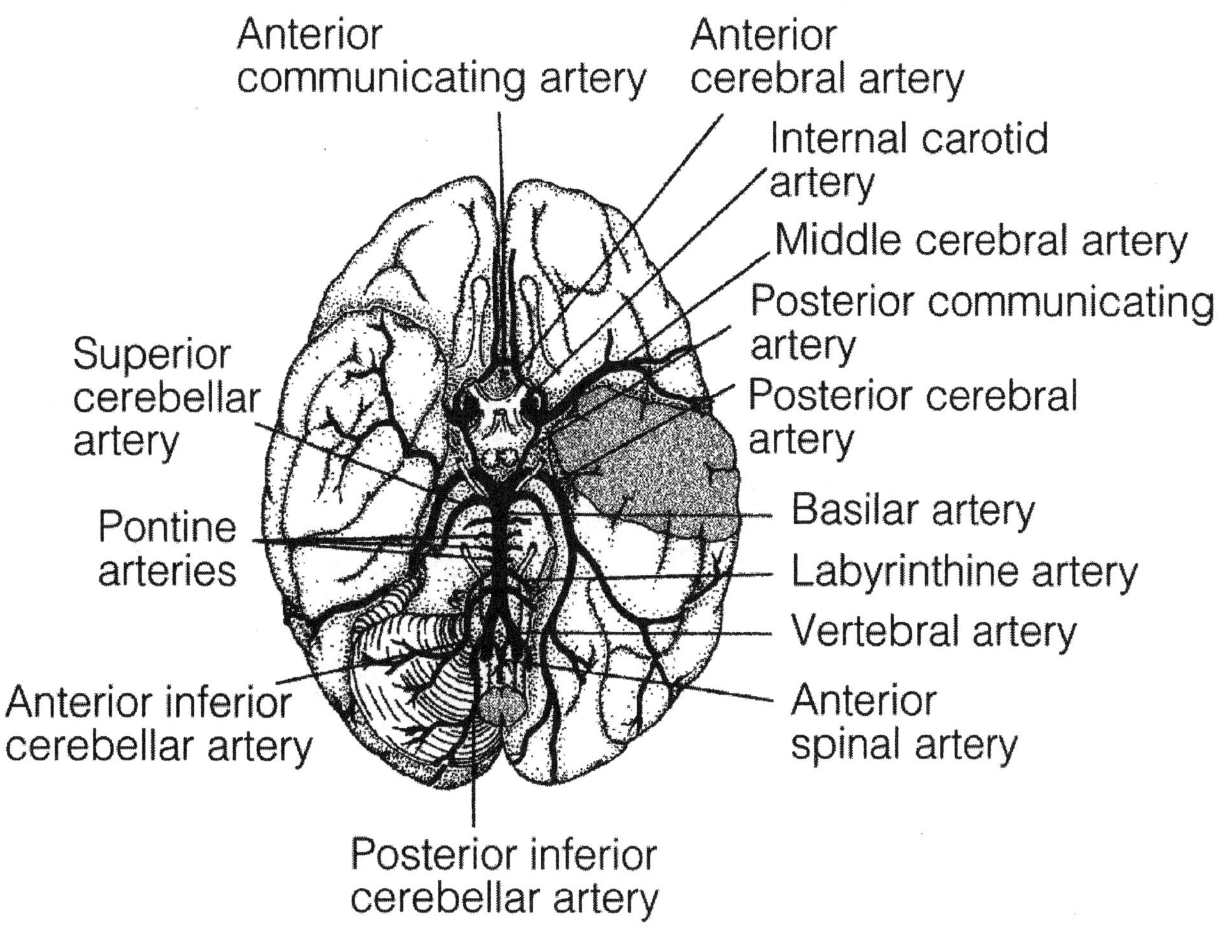

Anatomic Features: Arteries, veins, circle of Willis

Function: Arteries provide nourishment, oxygen, and other nutrients to the brain' the veins carry away waste products

Anatomic Features of the Lower Brain Stem

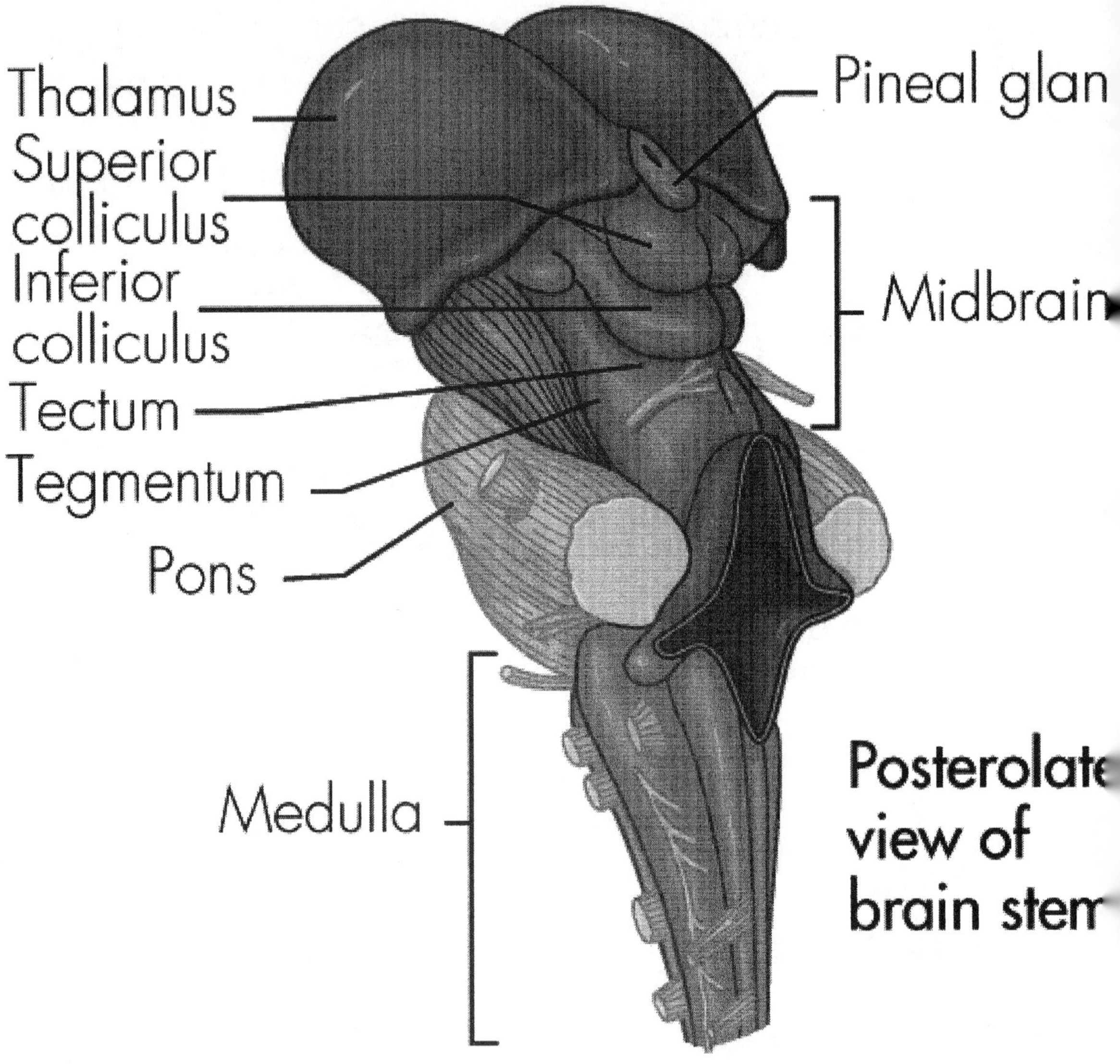

Anatomic Features: Hindbrain contains the medulla oblongata (myelencephalo and pons (metencephalon); Midbrain contains the tectum and tegmentum, cranial nerves, reticular activating system

Function: Relays information to and from the brain; responsible for simple reflexive behavior

Anatomic Features of the Cranial Nerves

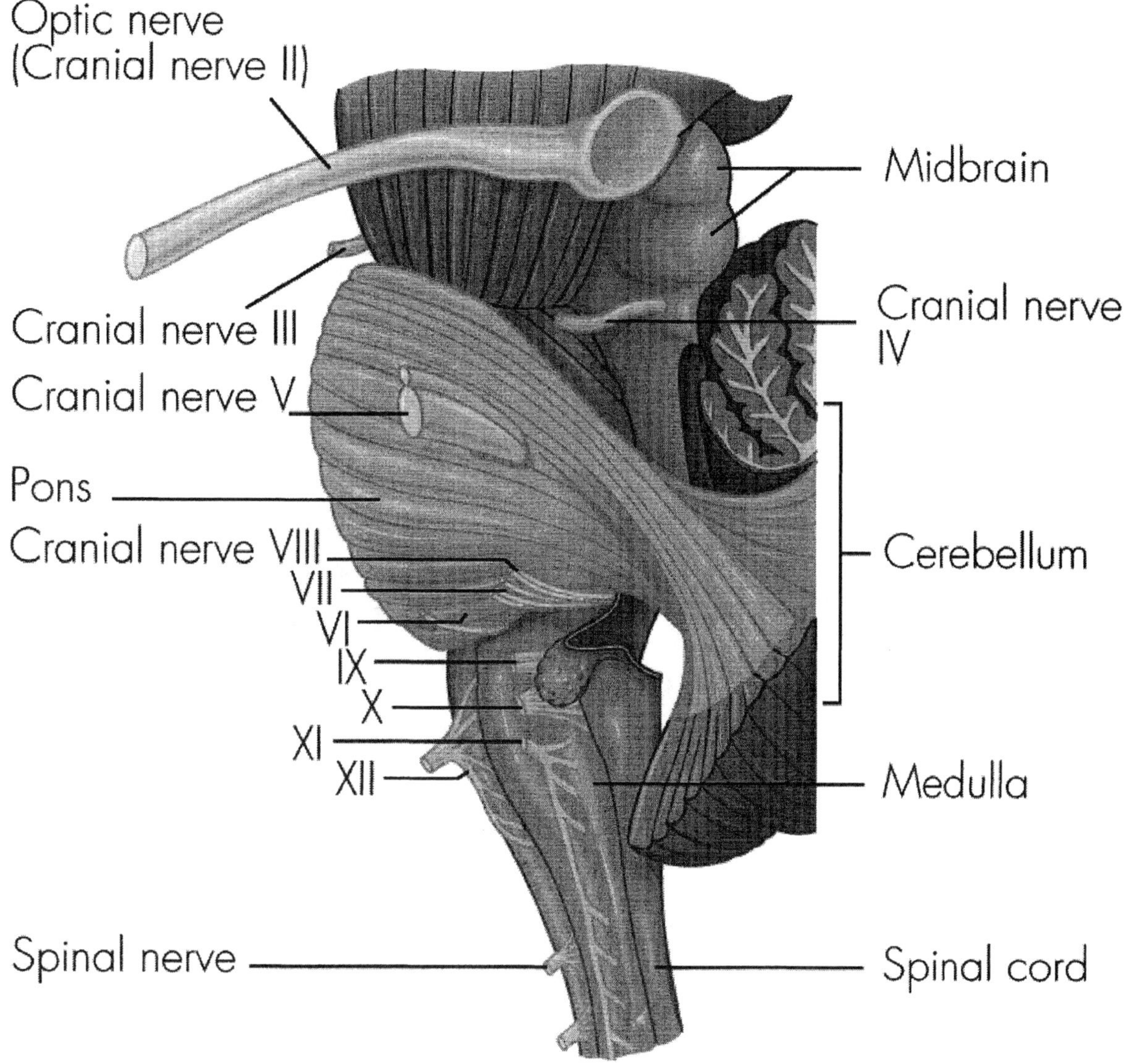

Anatomic Features: Located within the brain stem

Function: Conducting specific motor and sensory information

Anatomic Features of the Reticular Formation

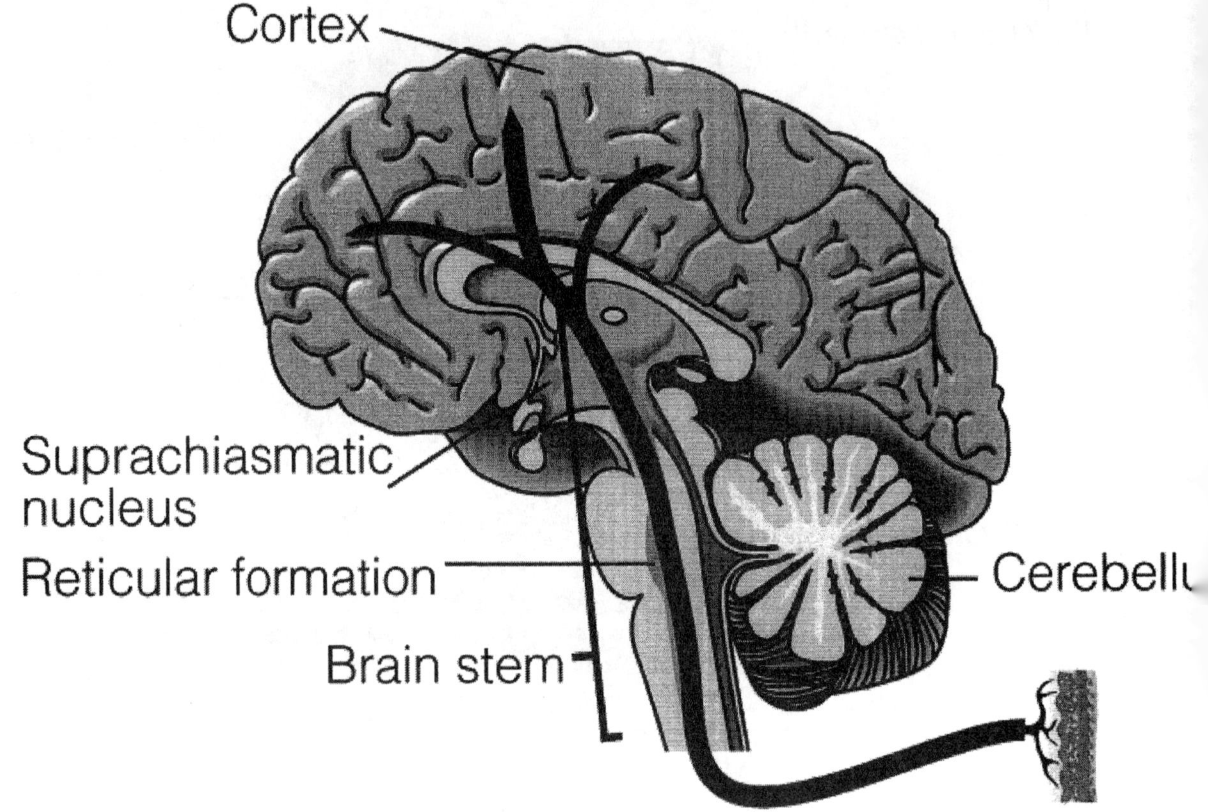

Anatomic Features: Neural network within the lower brain stem connecting the medulla and the midbrain

Function: Nonspecific arousal and activation, sleep and wakefulness

Anatomic Features of the Hypothalamus

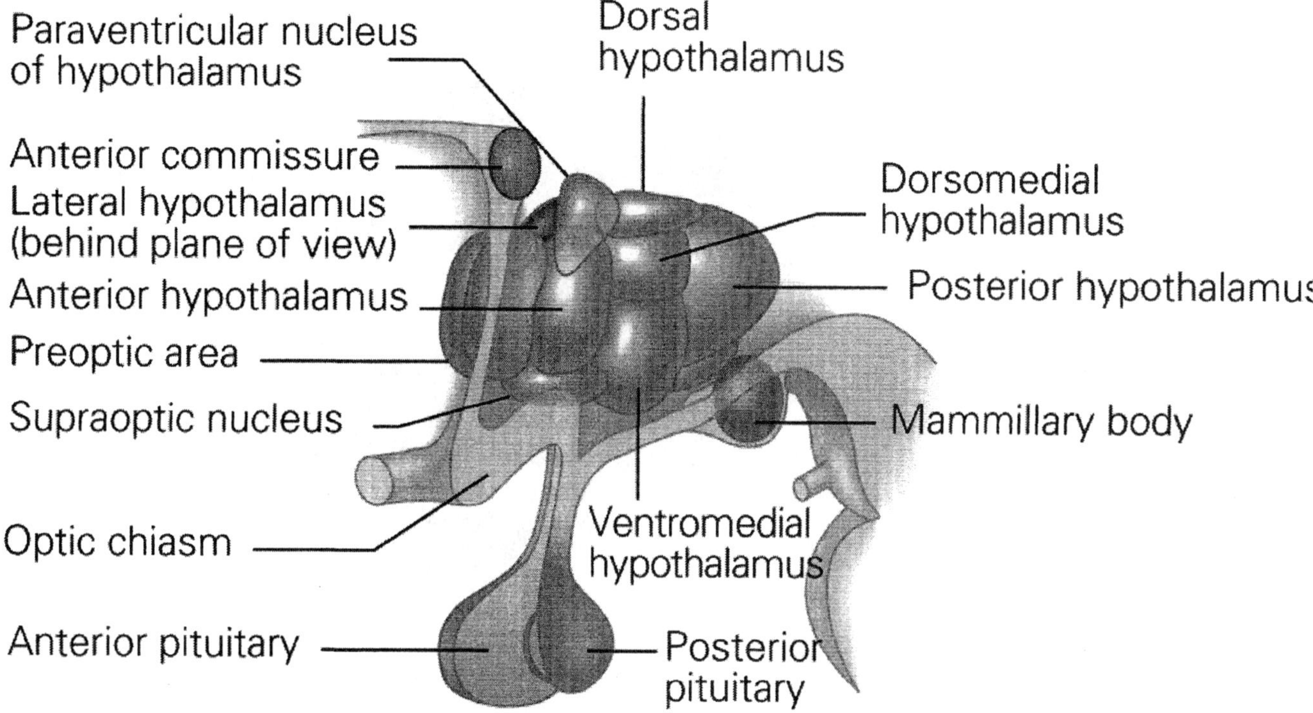

Anatomic Features: Hypothalamic nuclei, major fiber systems, and third ventricle

Function: Activates, controls, and integrates the peripheral autonomic mechanisms, endocrine activity, and somatic functions, including body temperature, food intake, and the development of secondary sexual characteristics

Anatomic Features of the Basal Ganglia

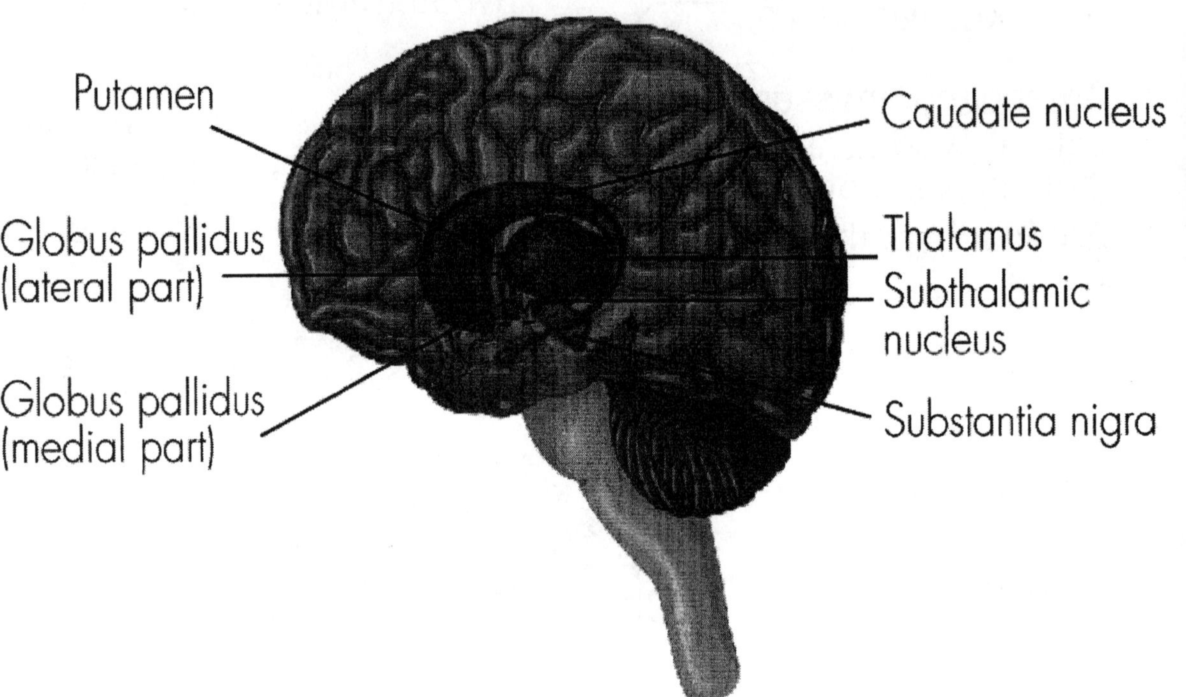

Anatomic Features: Structures of the caudate nucleus, putamen, globus pallidus, substantia nigra, and subthalamic nuclei

Function: Important relay stations in motor behavior (such as the striato-pallido-thalamic loop); connections from part of the extrapyramidal motor system (including cerebral cortex, basal nuclei, thalamus, and midbrain) and coordinate stereotyped postural and reflexive motor activity

Anatomic Features of the Limbic System

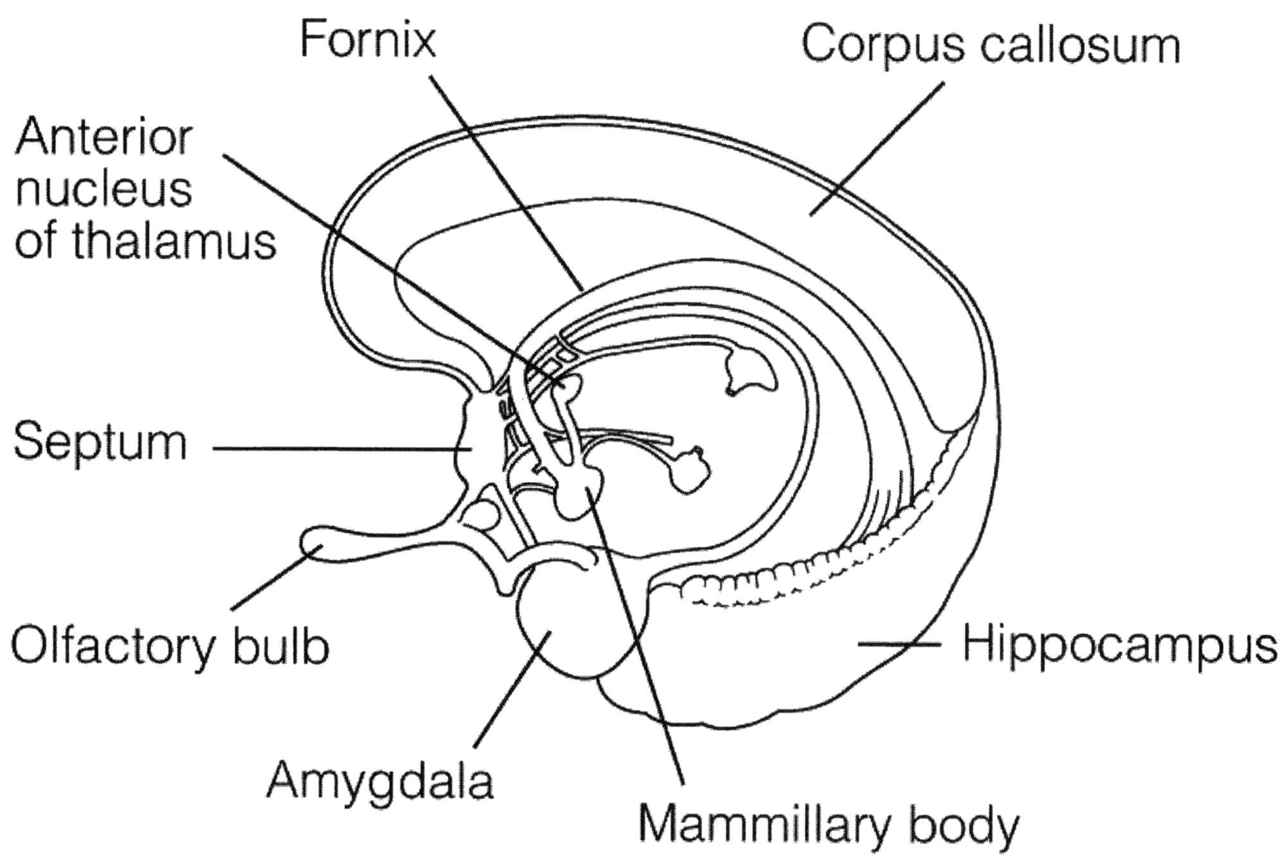

Anatomic Features: Structures of the amygdala, hippocampus, parahippocampal gyrus, cingulate gyrus, fornix, septum, and olfactory bulbs

Function: Closely involved in the expression of emotional behavior and the integration of olfactory information with visceral and somatic information

Anatomic features of the cerebral hemispheres

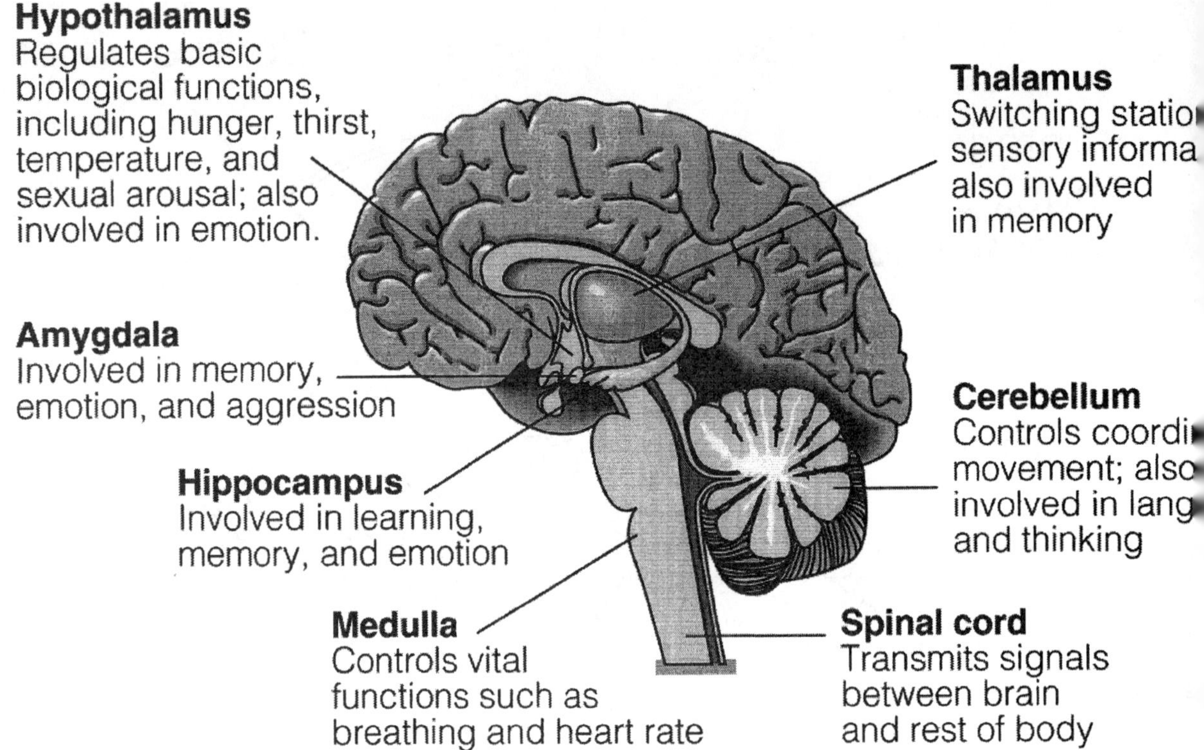
Hypothalamus
Regulates basic biological functions, including hunger, thirst, temperature, and sexual arousal; also involved in emotion.
Thalamus
Switching statio
sensory informa
also involved
in memory
Amygdala
Involved in memory, emotion, and aggression
Cerebellum
Controls coordi
movement; also
involved in lang
and thinking
Hippocampus
Involved in learning, memory, and emotion
Medulla
Controls vital functions such as breathing and heart rate
Spinal cord
Transmits signals between brain and rest of body

Anatomic Features: Structures of the frontal, parietal, occipital, and temporal lobes

Function: Higher cognitive functioning, cerebral specialization, and cortical localization

CHAPTER 3

CLINICAL ASSESSMENT AND DIAGNOSIS

LEARNING OBJECTIVES

1. Describe the nature and function of clinical assessment and the concepts that determine the value of assessment (reliability, validity, and standardization)
2. Describe the purpose of the clinical interview, physical examination, and formal behavioral assessment in the evaluation process.
3. Compare and contrast projective tests, personality inventories, and neuropsychological tests for the purpose of psychological evaluation.
4. Explain how medical techniques such as PET, CAT and MRI scans are appropriate tools for assessing psychological disorders, including limitations of such methods.
5. Explain the nature and purposes of psychiatric diagnosis and how the DSM is used to help therapists and counselors make an accurate psychiatric diagnosis.

OUTLINE

I. Assessing Psychological Disorders

A. **Clinical assessment** is the systematic evaluation and measurement of psychological, biological, and social factors in an individual presenting with a possible psychological disorder. Clinical assessment exemplifies a multidimensional, integrative approach to gathering information about a client in order to make informed and accurate decisions. **Diagnosis** is the process of determining whether a person's problem(s) meets all the criteria for a psychological disorder according to the DSM-IV-TR.

B. The case of Frank

1. Use the textbook case of Frank or another clinical case of your choosing to illustrate the process of clinical assessment below.

C. The process of clinical assessment is **analogous to a funnel** in that it is initially broad in scope and then becomes more specific. For instance, to assess psychological disorders, the clinician first collects a broad range of information and then narrows the focus by ruling out problems in some areas and concentrating more specifically on other areas where problems seem to exist.

D. Key concepts in assessment

1. **Reliability** is the most important requirement of assessment procedures and is the degree to which a measure is consistent. Consistency across two or more raters is called **interrater reliability,** whereas consistency across time is referred to as **test-retest reliability**.
2. **Validity** is the degree to which a technique measures what it is designed to measure. Comparing the results of one assessment measure with the results of

others helps determine **concurrent** or **descriptive validity**. **Predictive validity** is how well the assessment predicts what will happen in the future. Whether the test items look reasonable and valid at first glance is called **face validity**.

3. One can have high reliability without validity, but not validity without reliability. For instance, two independent raters may agree perfectly in how they coded some behaviors (i.e., high reliability), but show low validity because they both coded the wrong behaviors systematically. Seethe in class activity and handout "Paris in the Spring" to help illustrate this concept.
4. **Standardization** is process by which a set of standards or norms is established for a technique to ensure its consistency across different measurements. Such standardization may refer to administrative procedures, scoring, and evaluation of data, and/or demographic factors. A good example to illustrate this concept for students is the SAT.

II. Procedures and Strategies of Clinical Assessment

A. The **clinical interview** is the core of most clinical work and is used primarily to gather information about past and present behavior, attitudes, emotions, and a history of the person's problem(s) and life circumstances. Other important points to cover include precipitating events, family composition and history, sexual development, religious beliefs, cultural concerns, educational achievement, and social-interpersonal history.

1. To organize information obtained during an interview, many clinicians will use a **mental status exam;** an exam that involves the systematic observation of a client's behavior across five domains:
    a. Appearance and behavior
    b. Thought processes (e.g., rate and flow of speech, clarity, and content of speech and ideas)
    c. Mood and affect (e.g., is affect and mood appropriate of inappropriate?)
    d. Intellectual functioning (e.g., does the client have a reasonable vocabulary and memory?)
    e. Sensorium (i.e., general awareness of surroundings such as date, place, time, knowledge of self).
2. The Case of Frank
    a. Use the case of Frank or another clinical case of your choosing to illustrate the process of mental status exam.
3. It is important to conduct the clinical interview in a way that elicits the patient's trust and empathy in order to facilitate communication. Information provided by patients to psychologists and psychiatrists is protected by laws of **confidentiality.**
4. **Unstructured clinical interviews** are not standardized with respect to procedure and content and follow no systematic format. **Semistructured clinical interviews** contain questions that have been carefully phrased and tested to elicit useful information in a consistent manner, but also allow room

for clinicians to depart from the format with additional questions of interest (e.g., Anxiety Disorders Interview Schedule, 4th ed., or the Structured Clinical Interview for DSM).

B. Clinicians often recommend a **physical examination**, particularly if the patient has not been seen by a medical doctor in the past year. The reason for the physical exam is to rule out medical conditions that are associated with psychological disorders and those that may masquerade as psychological disorders. Examples of physical conditions that may lead to psychological problems include toxic states, hyperthyroidism (anxiety), hypothyroidism (depression), brain tumor, and drug ingestion.

C. **Behavioral assessment** takes the mental status exam a step further by using direct observation to formally assess an individual's thoughts, feelings, and overt behaviors in specific situations or contexts. This information is used to explain the maintenance of present problems in the here and now. Observations may occur in the therapy context, in the home, schools, the workplace, or in other real life situations. The purpose of behavioral assessment is to identify **target behaviors** (problematic behaviors) and environmental events that may become targets of therapeutic intervention. This is accomplished via a functional analysis of antecedents, behaviors, and consequences (i.e., the **ABCs of observation**) following the behavior.

1. Behavioral observation may be either formal or informal. In **formal observation**, the observation procedures are usually structured and systematic, and involve behavior rating scales or checklists and clear **operational definitions** of target behaviors. **Informal observation** is less standardized and systematic.
2. People may also be asked to observe their own behavior using a technique called **self-monitoring** or self-observation (e.g., recording the number of cigarettes smoked per day). Self-monitoring may be formal (e.g., using scales, coding sheets, checklists) or informal (e.g., recording overall mood each day).
3. **Reactivity** can distort observational data, and refers to changes in behavior as a result of knowing that one is being observed. Reactivity can occur while being observed by others or when self-monitoring. Behaviors tend to shift in the desired direction with reactivity.

D. **Psychological tests** must be reliable and valid, and cover several specific tests designed to determine cognitive, emotional, or behavioral responses that may be associated with a specific disorder or personality features.

1. **Projective tests** arose out of the psychoanalytic tradition and cover methods in which ambiguous stimuli are presented to a person who is asked to state what s/he sees. The theory is that people will project their own true personality, **unconscious thoughts** and fears onto ambiguous test stimuli and will reveal their hidden unconscious thoughts to the therapist. Though such tests remain controversial due to their origins and weak psychometric properties, they are commonly used. Examples include:

a. The **Rorschach Inkblot test** that was developed by Hermann Rorschach to study perceptual processes and to diagnose psychological disorders. Currently, the Rorschach contains ten inkblot pictures that serve as ambiguous stimuli. **John Exner** developed a standardized version of the Rorschach Inkblot test called the **Comprehensive System.**
b. The **Thematic Apperception Test (TAT)** is the best known projective test, developed in 1935 by Morgan and Murray. The TAT consists of 31 cards depicting less ambiguous pictures. The test taker is asked to tell a dramatic story about what they see in the picture. The TAT is based on the notion that people will reveal their unconscious mental processes in their stories about the pictures. TAT has limited reliability, validity, and standardization procedures.

2. **Personality inventories** are generally more empirically-based than projective tests but often require a substantial amount of time to complete. The most widely used personality inventory is the **Minnesota Multiphasic Personality Inventory (MMPI and MMPI-2)**. MMPI and MMPI-2 contain over 549 questions that are responded to as either true or false. Individual responses to items are not examined. What matters is the pattern of responses and how the pattern relates to people who have known psychological disorders (i.e., empirical criterion keying). The MMPI also includes scales to help determine whether the test-taker was responding to the questions in an open and valid manner (e.g., lie scale, infrequency scale, defensiveness scale, and the cannot-say scale). An MMPI profile from a pseudopatient James S. is presented in the textbook. The MMPI has extensive reliability, validity, standardization, and normative data to back it up.

3 **Intelligence tests** were initially developed to predict how well persons would do in school (e.g., Alfred Binet and Theodore Simon's work with the French government in 1904). The **Binet-Simon test** was revised and translated by Lewis Terman of Stanford University in 1916 and became known as the **Stanford-Binet** in the United States.

   a. The test provided an **intelligence quotient** (i.e., IQ) that was derived by taking the child's mental age based on the IQ test, dividing it by his or her chronological age, and multiplying by 100. Problems with this method concerned the lack of comparability in scores across age groups (e.g., a 4-year old needed to score on 1 year above his or her chronological age to received an IQ score of 125, whereas an 8-year old had to score 2 years above his or her chronological age to receive the same IQ score).
   b. These and other problems led to the current use of the **deviation IQ,** where a person's score is compared only to scores of others of the same age. Other intelligence tests include the Wechsler tests for adults (i.e., Wechsler Adult Intelligence Scale-III; WASI-III), children (i.e., Wechsler Intelligence Scale for Children; WISC-III), and for young children (Wechsler Preschool and Primary Scale of Intelligence-Revised; WPPSI-R). All tests contain verbal and

performance scales and full-scale IQ. All tests contain **verbal** and **performance scales**.

E. **Neuropsychological tests** are used to assess a person's abilities in areas such as receptive and expressive language, attention and concentration, memory, motor skills, perceptual abilities, and learning and abstraction.

1. The purpose of such tests is to help the clinicians to make educated guesses about the person's performance and the possible existence of brain impairment. A secondary aim is to determine s person's assets and liabilities given the potential for neurological problems.
2. Examples of neuropsychological tests include screening devices such as the **Bender Visual-Motor Gestalt** (test involves copying lines and shapes seen on a series of cards), and more sophisticated batteries that can provide precise determinations of organic brain damage such as the **Luria-Nebraska Neuropsychological Battery** and the **Halstead-Reitan Neuropsychological Battery**.
3. There is much overlap between intelligence and neuropsychological testing.
4. Problems of neuropsychological testing, however, include the presence of **false positives** (i.e., test shows a problem where none exists) and **false negatives** (i.e., test fails to detect a problem where one exists) as well as long administration time.

F. **Neuroimaging** is a name for a set of procedures that allow a window on brain structure (i.e., parts of the brain) and function (i.e., what the brain does via blood flow and metabolic activity).

1. **Brain structure** can be assessed using computerized axial tomography (CAT or CT scan) and/or magnetic resonance imaging (MRI):
   a. The **CAT scan** was developed in the early 1970s and uses multiple X-ray exposures of the brain at different angles. CAT scans are noninvasive and depict various slices of the brain. The image of structure is particularly useful for identifying and locating abnormalities in the structure or shape of the brain, including the location of brain tumors, injuries, and other structural abnormalities.
   b. **MRI** provides better resolution than the CAT scan and does not involve X-rays. The technique is called nuclear magnetic resonance imaging, whereby a person's head is placed in a high-strength magnetic field through which radio frequency signals are transmitted. These signals excite the brain tissue, altering protons and hydrogen atoms. A disadvantage is that a person is required to be totally enclosed inside a narrow tube with a magnetic coil around the head.
2. **Brain function** can be assessed using positron emission tomography (PET) or single photon emission computed tomography (SPECT).
   a. The **PET** procedure involves injection of a tracer substance containing radioactive isotopes (i.e., groups of atoms that react distinctively). This substances interacts with blood, oxygen, or glucose in the regions of the brain that are active.

b. **SPECT** works much like PET, though a different tracer substance is used and SPECT is somewhat less accurate than PET. SPECT is less expensive than PET and for this reason is used more frequently.
c. **Functional MRI** (fMRI) takes only milliseconds and allows for examination of immediate responses of the brain to a brief event.

G. **Psychophysiology** refers to measurable changes in the nervous system reflecting emotional or psychological events, whereas **psychophysiological assessment** refers to methods of assessing brain structure and function specifically, and nervous system activity more generally.Psychophysiological Assessment

1. An **Electroencephalogram (EEG)** is a peripheral measure of electrical activity in the head related to the firing of a specific group of neurons, which yields a measure of brain wave activity (i.e., low-voltage current usually associated with the cortex of the brain). Used to assess brain activity associated with waking and sleep states. **Event-related or evoke potentials (ERPs)** refer to EEG activity in response to specific events. Alpha EEG waves are typically associated with waking and calmness and involve a regular pattern. During the deepest most relaxed stage of sleep, EEGs reveal a pattern known as delta waves (i.e., waves that are slower and more irregular than alpha waves).
2. Other typically assessed responses during a psychophysiological evaluation include: (a) heart rate and respiration, (b) electrodermal responding, and (c) EMG (i.e., muscle tension).
3. Psychophysiological assessment is used routinely in the assessment of disorders involving a strong emotional component such as posttraumatic stress disorder, sexual dysfunctions, sleep disorders, headache and hypertension.

III. Diagnosing Psychological Disorders

A. **Assessment** helps to understand what is unique about an individual (i.e., an **idiographic strategy**) so as to tailor a treatment appropriately, whereas **diagnosis** concerns the general class of problems that the person is presenting with and how best to classify such problems based on information about others with similar kinds of problems (i.e., a **nomothetic strategy**). Diagnosis, or identifying a general class of problems that hang together, is useful for obtaining information about psychological profiles, etiology, and treatment. The clinician may be able to use psychiatric diagnosis to help establish a **prognosis**, or likely future course of a disorder under certain conditions.

B. **Classification** is an integral part of science and refers to any effort to construct groups or categories and to assign objects or people to these categories on the basis of their shared attributes or relations (i.e., a nomothetic strategy).

1. The word **taxonomy** refers to classification in a scientific context, and usually takes the form of describing entities for scientific purposes (e.g., rocks, insects, or in psychology behaviors). The word **nosology** refers to the *application* of a taxonomic system to psychological or medical phenomena.

2. **Nomenclature** refers to the names or labels of the disorders that make up the nosology (e.g., anxiety or mood disorders).
3. The nosological system used by most mental health professionals is the *Diagnostic and Statistical Manual of Mental Disorders, Fourth Edition Text Revision* (DSM-IV-TR). The DSM-IV-TR is used world-wide and clinicians refer to the DSM to identify whether a person meets criteria for a specific psychological disorder in the process of making a diagnosis.
4. Classification of behavior disorders is often in categorical or dimensional form.
   a. The **classical (or pure) categorical approach** to classification originated with **Emil Kraepelin** and the biological tradition and assumes that each disorder is unique (i.e., different) with its own unique underlying pathophysiological cause. Only one set of criteria is needed for a given disorder and all must meet all of the criteria to receive a diagnosis. This approach is common in medicine, but not in psychopathology.
   b. A **dimensional approach** to classification seeks to place symptoms on several dimensional ratings; a view that is problematic when theorists cannot agree on the number and types of required dimensions.
   c. A **prototypical approach** is offered as an alternative to the categorical and dimensional approaches. This approach is a categorical approach that combines, in part, the features of the other approaches. The prototypical approach identifies essential features of a psychological disorder so that it can be classified, but allows for nonessential variations that do not necessarily change the classification (e.g., there are several ways one could meet criteria for major depression or panic disorder, but still get the diagnosis). The DSM-IV-TR is based on this approach.
   d. A system of nosology must be reliable and valid (i.e., content, construct, discriminant, and predictive validity). The DSM-IV-TR is a sophisticated attempt to improve on both domains.

C. Evolution of psychiatric diagnosis and the DSM
1. **Diagnosis before 1980** owed much to the biological tradition and the work of Emil Kraepelin. Kraepelin identified schizophrenia under the term dementia praecox. Kraepelin's theorizing about psychological disorders as biological disturbances was influential and led to an early emphasis on classical categorical strategies of abnormal behavior.
   a. In 1948 the **World Health Organization (WHO)** added a section on classification of mental disorders to the *International Classification of Diseases and Health Related Problems* **(ICD)**
   b. The *Diagnostic and Statistical Manual* **(DSM-I)** was published in 1952 by the American Psychiatric Association, however, this system, including the ICD did not have much influence.
   c. **The DSM-II**, published in 1968, greatly influenced the behavior of mental health professionals, but it lacked precision and relied on

unproven theories of the etiology that were not universally accepted (e.g., psychoanalytic theory). The DSM-II was also unreliable.

2. **The DSM-III**, published in 1980, departed radically from its predecessors. Three changes were unique to the DSM-III. First, it took an *atheoretical approach* to diagnosis, relying on precise descriptions of disorders. Second, the specificity of diagnostic criteria made possible studies of diagnostic reliability and validity. Third, the DSM-III contained ratings on five axes.
   a. Axis I: Contained main diagnosis of psychological disorders (e.g., schizophrenia or mood disorder).
   b. Axis II: Was used for more enduring (chronic) disorders of personality.
   c. Axis III: Comprised physical disorders or conditions.
   d. Axis IV: Was used by clinicians to provide dimensional ratings of the amount of psychosocial stress experienced by the individual.
   e. Axis V: Is where clinicians rated the individuals current level of adaptive functioning.
3. **Problems with the DSM-III and DSM-III-R** included (a) unacceptably low reliability for some diagnostic categories (e.g., somatoform and personality disorders), and (b) inclusion of diagnostic criteria were established by committee consensus and that lacked a solid empirical base.
4. The **DSM-IV** emerged in the context of recognition of the need for a consistent worldwide system of nosology; one consistent with the 1993 edition of the ICD-10. DSM-IV relied little on expert consensus. The diagnostic system was to be based on scientific data. The most substantial change in the DSM-IV was the elimination of the distinction between organically-based and psychologically-based disorders. The text revision, **DSM-IV-TR**, included minor modifications, most notably the diagostic criteria for tourette's disorder, dementia of the alzheimer's type, dementia due to other general medical conditions, personality change due to a general medical condition, exhibitionism, frotteurism, pedophilia, sexual sadism, voyeurism.
   a. The **multiaxial system** is retained in the DSM-IV, but only personality disorders and mental retardation are coded on Axis II; pervasive developmental disorders, learning disorders, motor skills disorders, and communication disorders, previously coded on Axis II, are now coded on Axis I; the new Axis IV is used to report psychosocial and environmental problems that might have an impact on the disorder; Axis V was left unchanged. Optional axes are also included (e.g., defense mechanisms, coping styles, social and occupational function, and relational functioning). Some new disorders appear in the DSM-IV, whereas other disorders in previous DSMs were either deleted or subsumed into other DSM-IV categories.
   b. Use the case of Frank or another clinical case of your choosing to illustrate the process of making a psychiatric diagnosis.
   d. DSM-IV allows for integration of important **social and cultural influences** in relation to diagnosis (e.g., what are the person's beliefs,

cultural values, and what is extent to which the person is Westernized into the mainstream culture?).

5. **Criticisms of DSM-IV** include the following:
   a. The boundaries between disorders are often fuzzy, and diagnostic **comorbidity** is quite often the rule, not the exception. This means that either psychopathologists are not as precise in distinguishing amongst disorders, or that there are more similarities among the presumably different diagnostic categories that we would like to believe.
   b. Emphasis on reliability at the expense of validity.
   c. As with any diagnostic system, there is the danger of misuse, and particularly the tendency to **reify** diagnostic categories (i.e., treat them as "things" that exist) and the problem of **labeling** and its negative connotations.

D. Creating a diagnosis

1. Several new diagnoses were considered for inclusion into DSM-IV-TR.
   a. **Mixed anxiety-depression**, for example, is common in persons who present first in primary care settings, but neither the anxiety or depression is frequent or severe enough to meet criteria for an existing anxiety or mood disorder. Mixed anxious and depressive complaints illustrates an important issue with regard to the creation of a classification system; namely concern over adequate thresholds, or the minimum number of criteria required to meet the definition of the disorder. This serves to lessen the health care burden by identifying those with "true" disorders. Several research studies have shown the persons presenting with mixed anxiety-depression are substantially impaired in their social and occupational functioning and do experience distress. Thus, the mixed anxiety-depression diagnosis appears in an appendix in the DSM-IV as a disorder under study.
   b. **Premenstrual dysphoric disorder** (PMDD) brings up the problems of bias and stigmatization; problems that must be considered in the creation of any diagnostic category. This diagnosis concerns a small group of women who present with severe and sometimes incapacitating emotional reactions associated with the late luteal phase of their menstrual period. PMDD was considered for inclusion in the DSM-III-R, but failed due to insufficient data and concerns over making normal endocrinological changes disordered. PMDD was renamed late luteal phase dysphoric disorder (LLPDD) and sparked several studies. Upon review, the DSM-IV Task Force determined that the name late luteal phase dysphoric disorder was not entirely accurate in that the symptoms may not be exclusively related to the endocrine state of the luteal phase. Therefore, LLPDD was changed to PMDD and PMDD appears in an appendix in the DSM-IV as a disorder warranting further study.

OVERALL SUMMARY

This chapter outlines the processes of clinical assessment and diagnosis. Both domains are central to the study of psychopathology. Clinical assessment refers to a systematic evaluation and measurement of psychological, biological, and social factors in persons with psychiatric disorders to provide idiographic information that may be helpful in treatment planning. Diagnosis is a nomothetic process of determining whether a particular problem that distresses a person meets criteria for a psychological disorder. This chapter covers assessment techniques, psychometric issues related to assessment and diagnosis (e.g., reliability, validity, standardization), the nature of the DSM system, and issues surrounding diagnosis and classification (e.g., categorical, dimensional, and prototypic approaches; reliability vs. validity). Throughout the chapter the issues are illustrated with the case of Frank (young, serious, and anxious).

KEY TERMS

Behavioral assessment (p. 74)
Classical categorical approach (p. 87)
Classification (p. 86)
Clinical assessment (p. 69)
Comorbidity (p. 91)
Diagnosis (p. 69)
Dimensional approach (p. 87)
Electroencephalogram (EEG) (p. 84)
False negatives (p. 83)
False positives (p. 83)
Idiographic strategy (p. 86)
Intelligence quotient (p. 81)
Labeling (p. 92)
Mental status exam (p. 72)
Neuroimaging (p. 83)
Neuropsychological testing (p. 82)
Nomenclature (p. 86)
Nomothetic strategy (p. 86)
Nosology (p. 86)
Personality inventories (p. 79)
Projective tests (p. 78)
Prototypical approach (p. 87)
Psychophysiological assessment (p. 84)
Reliability (p. 71)
Standardization (p. 71)
Taxonomy (p. 86)
Validity (p. 71)

INFOTRAC KEY TERM EXERCISES

Each exercise is linked to key terms from the Wadsworth InfoTrac on-line searchable database. Key terms must be entered exactly as written.

Exercise 1: **The Utility of Projective Tests**
Article: A55683969
Citation: (Projective measures of personality and psychopathology: How well do they work?). Scott O. Lilienfeld.
Skeptical Inquirer, Sept-Oct 1999 v23 i5 p32(8)

Projective tests are a class of assessment measures that are enormously popular in mental health care. Such tests also are becoming more and more controversial with the development of more objective assessment devices. Review this InfoTrac article on six of the more commonly used projective tests and answer the following questions: What is the rationale underlying the use of projective tests?; How did such tests develop over time?; How well do projective tests work?; and, What are some of the reasons for their continued popularity in mental health circles. Limit your answer to 3-5 typed double-spaced pages.

Exercise 2: **Public Opinion and Misunderstandings About Psychological Disorders**
Key Term: *Mental Illness, Public Opinion*

Despite advances in our scientific understanding of psychiatric disorders, including diagnostic classification, general public misunderstanding about mental illness persists. Review the InfoTrac article(s) on this topic and evaluate what the general public believes about mental illness in relation to the stigma that often occurs with diagnostic labeling. What are some of the proposed solutions to change public misunderstanding and stigmatization of the mentally ill and how does labeling relate to the concept of reification as described in the textbook? Include ideas of your own that you see may help reduce the stigma of mental illness, but also increase public understanding about psychological disorders. Limit your answer to 3-5 typed double-spaced pages.

Exercise 3 (Future Trend): Prescription Privileges for Psychologists

Several states (e.g., New Mexico, Hawaii) have granted prescription authority for psychologists and others are likely to follow. Nonetheless, the move toward prescription privileges by psychologists remains controversial. This topic is one that students will likely find interesting to discuss in class, and lends itself quite nicely to a pro vs. con debate format. Integrate into the discussion ways in which prescription privileges might impact the assessment and diagnosis of abnormal behavior. The suggested readings and web links provided below should serve as useful starting points.

Hayes, S. C., & Heiby, E. (Eds.) (1998). Prescription privileges for psychologists: A critical appraisal. Reno, NV: Context Press. http://www.contextpress.com/ presprivforp.html.

http://www.apa.org/apags/profdev/reconsiderrxp.html
http://www.mspp.net/SSCPscriptpriv.htm
http://goinside.com/98/3/oppose.html

CLASSROOM ACTIVITIES, DEMONSTRATIONS, AND LECTURE TOPICS

1. **Activity: An Introduction to Assessment Methods.** To help familiarize students with the various clinical assessment tools, begin by introducing a partial case history of a client. Your students may work in groups or individually, but ask them to evaluate what tests and methods they would use with each client to determine a diagnosis. For example, you may present the following cases:

    a. Jack was brought into the rehabilitation unit last week. Three weeks ago he suffered a head injury in a car accident. He has been referred to your office to determine the extent of his cognitive damage. What tests and methods of assessment should you use in your evaluation? *The Answer?*: referral for medical exam/neuroimaging, mental status, behavioral observation, intelligence tests, neuropsychological tests, including perhaps interviews with other sources).

    b. Carla reports feeling very depressed. She has isolated herself from friends and family, and has been unable to work. Carla's family is concerned that she might try to commit suicide. They have approached you for help and advice. What tests and methods of assessment should you use in your evaluation? *The Answer?*: clinical/structured interview, physical examination, checklist or rating scales (e.g., Beck Depression Inventory, projective and/or objective psychological tests).

    c. Norman performs poorly in school compared to his classmates. He is fidgety and aggressive and has great difficulty completing his homework assignments. His teachers are considering holding him back a year and want your advice. What tests and methods of assessment should you use in your evaluation? *The Answer?*: clinical interview, behavioral assessment and observation in therapy and in the school, physical examination, teacher and parent checklists or rating scales, intelligence and achievement tests.

    d. A man shows up at the emergency room at a hospital. You are called to consult on this case. The man does not know his own name. He is unable to identify what city he lives in, and is not sure how he got to the hospital. What tests and methods of assessment would you want to administer at this point? *The Answer?*: physical and mental status examinations.

    Note. You may want to draw from additional cases from the DSM-IV-TR Casebook. This exercise helps students learn about the assessment tools and learn that the assessment process entails choosing assessment devices and methods that appropriately address individual clients' needs.

2. **Activity: Reliability, Validity, and Perceptual Bias in Clinical Assessment**. A neat and simple exercise that can readily illustrate the relation between reliability and validity and the problem of personal bias is to do the following. First, tell students that you are about to put something up on the screen and that you want them all to watch carefully. As soon as the image disappears, they are to write down exactly what they saw. After

these opening remarks, select the Transparency Master with the text "Paris in the the spring" and flash it up on a projection screen briefly (i.e., no longer than 5 seconds). Then, take it away and ask students to write down what they saw. You can then poll the students and tally responses on the board. What usually happens is that the majority of the class will report seeing "*Paris in the Spring*." Indeed, you could go ahead and calculate the inter-observer reliability for the class and you would likely find it to be quite high. You can then go on to point out that while most of the class was in agreement, most of the class was also wrong. You can then put up the overhead for a closer examination and point out that what was flashed on the screen were the words "*Paris in the the Spring*." This is also a good time to point out the relation between reliability and validity and the issue of how our own experiences and preconceptions can bias what we see and how we interpret and respond to sense data during clinical assessment.

3. **Activity: Disclosing Highly Personal Information: Secrets and Resistance in Psychotherapy**. The following is an exercise that can be used as a way to help students understand what it is like for clients in psychotherapy to reveal personal information about themselves, why they may keep secrets, and the reasons for showing "resistance" to the therapeutic process. Start by telling the class that anyone can choose not to participate in the exercise. Then instruct students to write down on a small piece of paper something important and personal about themselves that they have NEVER told anyone else - a secret wish, fantasy, feeling, belief, or something from their past. If they can't think of anything, suggest that they write down something they have told maybe only one or two people who are close to them. As the instructor, you should make a promise to the students that NO ONE will see what they have written. When they are finished, tell them to fold the paper up several times, very tightly, in a tiny ball. Then walk around the room and ask some students, one at a time, if they will hand you the paper. A few will do so with little worry, a few will refuse, but most will comply, albeit with some hesitation. For those who do agree, I take the paper and do the following, usually in a humorous way:
   a. ask them if you can open it (but never actually open it)
   b. hold it up to the light as if you can see into it (which everyone can see is impossible)
   c. hold it to your head and pretend you can mind-read it, and like Carnac "carelessly" toss it into the air
   d. ask if you can give it to someone else (but never do so)
   e. stick it into your pocket and pretend to forget it's there (but always give it back)
   f. take one person's paper in your right hand, another in your left, wave your arms back and forth over each other, and pretend that you have then become confused as to whose secret belongs to whom

Once you have finished and have handed each paper back to its owner, talk about the reactions to the exercise. Discuss how the students would have felt if the paper was read by someone (e.g., anxiety, anger, embarrassment, shame, helplessness) and point out that clients often struggle with the same feelings in psychotherapy, and this struggle may account for their "resistance." Ask students how they think a therapist might react to them revealing such information. Point out that while what they wrote on the paper was a conscious secret, clients in psychotherapy also must contend with deep seated "secrets" that may be even MORE sensitive. You may then open up the discussion to broader issues related to your handling of the papers as real or fantasized situations in psychotherapy. For example, do clients sometimes think that therapists can see right into them, or read their minds?; might a client worry that the therapist might treat lightly or carelessly something personal that the client reveals?; what if the therapist told someone else about the client's disclosures (this raises the practical and ethical issues about confidentiality)?; what if the therapist forgot something important the client told him/her, or confused that information with another client?

Source Information. This activity was developed by J. Suler, Secrets and resistance in psychotherapy, and can be found at http://www.rider.edu/users/suler/resist.html.

4. **Activity: Personality and Somatotypes**. In the 1940s, Sheldon proposed a theory about how there are certain body types ("somatotypes") that are associated with certain personality characteristics. He claimed that there are three such somatotypes: endomorphy, mesomorphy, and ectomorphy. Using Handout 3.1, ask students to rate themselves on each of these three dimensions using a scale from 1 (low) to 7 (high) with a mean of 4 (average). According to Sheldon, a person who is a pure mesomorph would have a score of 1-7-1. A pure endomorph would be 7-1-1. A pure ectomorph would score a 1-1-7. A mostly average person who has some endomorphic tendencies would have a score of 6-4-4 ... etc. After having students rate their body type according to the handout, ask them to walk around and find other students who have a similar rating. I suggest that they talk about whether the somatotype theory seems accurate (i.e., valid). This exercise often leads to interesting discussions about the possible biological basis of temperament and personality and the more general issue of validity when it comes to personality assessment. Because some people are sensitive about their body image, make sure the students know that this exercise is optional.

Source Information. This activity was developed by J. Suler, Somatotypes, and can be found at http://www.rider.edu/users/suler/somato.html.

5. **Activity: Self-Monitoring, Reactivity, and Behavior Change.** To illustrate the demands of self-monitoring, including reactivity, you can have students select some specific behavior, thought, emotion that they would like to change (either increase in frequency or decrease in frequency). Examples might include the number of times they say "um" during a conversation, the number of cigarettes they smoke, the amount of time they spend studying, number of pages of text they read each day, the amount of food or drink they consume daily, the number of steps walked each day. Then, have students record the occurrence of the behavior immediately after it occurs for a period of one week. Students can then be asked to plot their data by day (i.e., "y axis" = frequency of the behavior, "x axis" day). Reactivity should produce changes in the behavior in the desired direction. Encourage students to select a behavior that they would like to change, but also one that they would be comfortable discussing in class. It should be noted, however, that the point of the exercise could be illustrated without knowledge of the behavior in question. Use this exercise to talk about reactivity, the demands of self-

monitoring more generally, and the importance of accurate (reliable and valid) self-monitoring in clinical assessment. Most students will find it hard to regularly monitor the frequency of each occurrence of the selected behavior.

Paris in the the spring

HANDOUT 3.1
Somatotypes

In the space provided, rate the degree to which you think you possess each of the three body types using a scale from 1 (low) to 7 (high) with a mean of 4 (average).

- **Endomorphic Body Type:**
  Soft body; underdeveloped muscles; round shaped; over-developed digestive system

  Associated personality traits: love of food; tolerant; evenness of emotions; love of comfort; sociable; good humored; relaxed; need for affection.

  Your Rating: ______

- **Mesomorphic Body Type:**
  Hard, muscular body; overly mature appearance; rectangular shaped; thick skin; upright posture

  Associated personality traits: adventurous; desire for power and dominance; courageous; indifference to what others think or want; assertive, bold; zest for physical activity; competitive; love of risk and chance.

  Your Rating: ______

- **Ectomorphic Body Type:**
  Thin; flat chest; delicate build; young appearance; tall; lightly muscled; stoop-shouldered; large brain

  Associated personality traits: self-conscious; preference for privacy; introverted; inhibited; socially anxious; artistic; mentally intense; emotionally restrained.

  Your Rating: ______

Questions to Consider:

1. Do the personality traits associated with your ratings seem accurate (i.e., valid)?
2. Do you think this somatotype theory is generally accurate for most people?
3. Do you know any people for whom this theory works or doesn't work?
4. What might be some problems with this theory and test?

SUPPLEMENTARY READING MATERIAL FOR CHAPTER THREE

(i = These sources can be found on *"Infotrac, the online library"* provided by Wadsworth and Brooks/Cole Publishing.)

American Psychiatric Association. (1994). Diagnostic and statistical manual of mental disorders (4th ed.). Washington, DC: Author.

i Bird, H. R., Davies, M., Fisher, P., Narrow, W. E., Jensen, P. S., Hoven, C., Cohen, P., & Dulcan, M. K. (2000). How specific is specific impairment? Journal of the American Academy of Child and Adolescent Psychiatry, 39, 1182-1189.

Danna, R. H. (1993). Multicultural assessment perspectives for professional psychology. Boston: Allyn & Bacon.

Golden, C. J. (1990). Clinical interpretation of objective psychological tests. Boston: Allyn and Bacon.

Halleck, S. L. (1991). Evaluation of the psychiatric patient: A primer. New York: Plenum.

Kellerman, H. (1991). Handbook of psychodiagnostic testing: An analysis of personality in the psychological report. Boston: Allyn and Bacon.

Lukas, S. R. (1993). Where to start and what to ask: An assessment handbook. New York: Norton.

Mash, E. J., & Terdal, L. G. (Eds.) (1988). Behavioral assessment of childhood disorders (2nd ed.). New York: Guilford.

Morrison, J. (1995). DSM-IV made easy: The clinician's guide to diagnosis. New York: Guilford.

i Nathan, P. E., & Langenbucher, J. W. (1999). Psychopathology: Description and classification. Annual Review of Psychology, 79, 1-13.

Trzepacz, P. T. (1993). The psychiatric mental status examination. New York: Oxford University Press.

SUPPLEMENTARY VIDEO RESOURCES FOR CHAPTER THREE

Abnormal behavior: Fact and fiction. (Insight Media: 2162 Broadway, New York, NY 10024/ (800)-233-9910). This video examines both historical and current misconceptions and stereotypes regarding mental illness. Showing clips of two survivors of mental illness discussing their experiences, the video addresses the difficulties faced by these individuals in such everyday tasks as finding jobs and maintaining families. The video concludes by offering different approaches to viewing mental illness, advocating a more compassionate and humane understanding. (60 min)

Basic interviewing skills. (Insight Media: 2162 Broadway, New York, NY 10024/ (800)-233-9910). This video presents vignettes that focus on techniques for interviewing clients. The five basic skills — listening, reflecting, questioning, expressing, and interpreting — are taught in separate segments that progress from basic to complex situations. The video concludes with a session in which all of these skills are integrated. (51 min)

Behavioral interviewing with couples. (Research Press, PO Box 3177, Department J, Champaign, IL, 61821). Shows the six basic stages of an initial marriage counseling interview. (14 min).

Comprehensive clinical assessment. (Insight Media: 2162 Broadway, New York, NY 10024/ (800)-233-9910). This video discusses the range of skills that exemplify the art of social work practice and that are critical for effective intervention. (30 min)

CNN today: Abnormal psychology 2000, vol. 1. (*Available through your International Thomson Learning representative)*. The segment titled "Clinical Assessment and Diagnosis: Unabomber Mental Test" discusses competency criteria to stand trial within the context of the unabomber case. (2 min)

Deficits of mind and brain. (McDonnell Summer Institute of Cognitive Neuroscience, Eugene, Oregon; *available through your International Thomson Learning representative*). The segment in part one of this videotape, titled "Neuroimaging," introduces the methodological techniques for investigating cerebral physiology and structure as it relates to behavior. Illustrations of CAT and MRI imaging are provided, along with their respective strengths and shortcomings.

Deficits of mind and brain. (McDonnell Summer Institute of Cognitive Neuroscience, Eugene, Oregon; *available through your International Thomson Learning representative*). The segment in part one of this videotape, titled "Patient Examinations," begins with a discussion of the interpersonal treatment of patients prior to examination, stressing the importance of appropriately addressing patient's fears and mental status, speaking slowly when necessary, and providing rationales for testing prior to testing. Examples of determining visual acuity (e.g., bilateral visual testing) prior to testing and its importance to testing are discussed. Useful to illustrate the nature of neuropsychological assessment (see also segments titled "Cognitive Analysis" and "Pattern Recognition").

Emotional intelligence. (Insight Media: 2162 Broadway, New York, NY 10024/ (800)-233-9910). Emotional intelligence describes a person's comfort level with emotions and fluency with such social skills as listening, sharing, and being kind. This video presents research showing that school-aged children who cope better with daily social stresses stay healthier and learn more effectively. (30 min)

Intelligence. (Insight Media: 2162 Broadway, New York, NY 10024/ (800)-233-9910). This video explains what IQ tests are designed to measure, describing their origins, their uses, and some of their failures. It addresses the debates on whether IQ tests measure aptitude or achievement and whether intelligence is fixed or changeable. (30 min)

Intelligence testing. (Insight Media: 2162 Broadway, New York, NY 10024/ (800)-233-9910). This three-volume set features noted experts discussing aspects of intelligence testing. Arthur Jensen defends his contention that intelligence is a genetic fact of nature that correlates with certain physical attributes, Jonathan Baron offers a more social definition of intelligence, and Richard Burian responds to each contention. (3 Volumes / 114 min total)

Multiple intelligences: Intelligence, understanding, and the mind. (Insight Media: 2162 Broadway, New York, NY 10024/ (800)-233-9910). The first part of this set presents Howard Gardner's theory of multiple intelligences. It discusses naturalist intelligence, recent work on performance-based assessments, new ideas about education for understanding, myths and applications of multiple intelligence theory, and teaching for understanding. The second presents Gardner fielding questions from educators about his theory. (2 Volumes / 90 min total)

Personality. (CRM/McGraw-Hill). Depicts a college student undergoing a thorough assessment by a clinical psychologist that includes self-report, report from collateral sources, and the use of intelligence and projective tests. (30 min)

The assessment/therapy connection. (Research Press, Champaign, IL). Arnold Lazarus performs a multi-modal assessment of a 45-year old depressed woman. (29 min)

The clinical psychologist. (Insight Media: 2162 Broadway, New York, NY 10024/ (800)-233-9910). Depicts an initial assessment using formal and informal methods of assessment. (24 min)

Violence risk assessment. (Insight Media: 2162 Broadway, New York, NY 10024/ (800)-233-9910). While clinicians can never predict violence or incidences of repeat violence with certainty, there are social, psychological, and biological risk factors that can be examined as part of a thorough assessment. This video uses a case dramatization to present a model for violence risk assessment. (37 min)

What is normal? (Insight Media: 2162 Broadway, New York, NY 10024/ (800)-233-9910). This video shows how mental disorders are classified through DSM-III-R and considers related controversies. It analyzes case studies of depression and panic attack. (30 min)

INTERNET 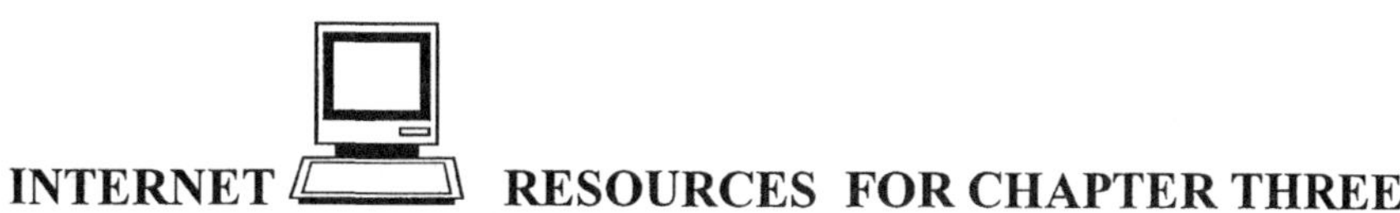 RESOURCES FOR CHAPTER THREE

Diagnostic and Statistical Manual of Mental Disorders, 4th ed. (DSM-IV)
http://www.behavenet.com/capsules/disorders/dsm4classification.htm
This site provides diagnostic criteria and information relevant to the DSM-IV-TR.

Diagnostic and Statistical Manual of Mental Disorders, 4th ed., Text Revision (DSM-IV-TR-TR)
http://www.behavenet.com/capsules/disorders/dsm4tr.htm
This site provides information about the recent text revision to DSM-IV-TR, including information about diagnostic criteria.

Glossary of Terms
http://www.cityscape.co.uk/users/ad88/gloss.htm#affect
This web site provides a glossary of terms and definitions of DSM criteria.

History of Influences on the Development of Intelligence Theory and Testing
http://www.indiana.edu/~intell/map.html
An excellent resource of historical information related to intelligence testing.

Mental Disorders: Symptoms and Treatments
http://www.cmhc.com/sxlist.htm
This web site includes a list of pages on psychological disorders broken down into three categories: adult disorders, childhood disorders, and personality disorders. A self-help questionnaire is also provided for those who feel they may need professional mental health assistance.

Neuroimaging Links
http://www.neuropsychologycentral.com/interface/content/links/page_material/imaging/imaging_links.html#a
This site contains a series of excellent links to resources related to neuroimaging, neuroanatomy, and their relation to psychopathology.

Neuropsychology Central
http://www.neuropsychologycentral.com/index.html
This site contains information and links about neuropsychology and neuropsychological assessment.

Psychological Testing
http://www.apa.org/science/testing.html
This APA web site contains information and useful links related to psychological testing, including the ethics of testing.

The Bell Curve Workbook
http://webusers.anet-stl.com/~civil/bellcurveillustration2.html

A site containing scholarly links to contrasting views about Herrnstein and Murray's *The Bell Curve: Intelligence and Class Structure in American Life*

Two Views of the Bell Curve
http://www.apa.org/journals/bell.html

This site provides two contrasting reviews of Richard J. Herrnstein and Charles Murray's *The Bell Curve: Intelligence and Class Structure in American Life*

Two Views of the DSM-IV
http://www.apa.org/journals/nietzel.html

Two contrasting views on the DSM-IV manual are provided by Michael T. Nietzel (pro) and Jerome C. Wakefield (con).

Research Criteria for Premenstrual Dysphoric Disorder

A. During most of her menstrual cycles for the past year, a woman has experienced at least five of the following symptoms for most of the time one week before, and possibly during menstruation. The symptoms were not present approximately one week after menstruation, and at least one of the symptoms was 1-4.

1. Substantially depressed mood, feeling hopeless, or negative thoughts about oneself.
2. Increased anxiety or agitation.
3. Sudden changes in mood or greater emotional sensitivity.
4. Increased anger or irritability, or more frequent conflicts in relationships.
5. A loss of interest in regular activities.
6. Problems with concentration.
7. Being easily tired, loss of energy.
8. A substantial change in appetite, overeating, or cravings for certain foods.
9. Getting too little sleep (insomnia) or too much sleep (hypersomnia).
10. A sense of being out of control or overwhelmed.
11. Physical symptoms including headaches, bloating, weight gain, swelling or tenderness of the breasts, pain in muscles or joints.

B. The person's symptoms cause difficulty within relationships, social activities, work, school, etc.

C. The symptoms are not just the result of a complication of another mental health condition.

D. The above criteria must be validated by daily recordings made during a minimum of two consecutive menstrual cycles in which the symptoms are present.

Transparency 3-2

Research Criteria for Mixed Anxiety-Depressive Disorder

A. Persistent or recurrent dysphoric mood lasting at least 1 month.

B. The dysphoric mood is accompanied by at least 1 month of four (or more) of the following symptoms.

1. Difficulty concentrating or mind going blank.
2. Sleep disturbance (difficulty falling or staying asleep, or restless unsatisfying sleep).
3. Fatigue or low energy.
4. Irritability.
5. Worry.
6. Being easily moved to tears.
7. Hypervigilance.
8. Anticipating the worst.
9. Hopelessness (pervasive pessimism about the future).
10. Low self-esteem or feelings of worthlessness.

C. The symptoms cause clinically significant distress or impairment in social, occupational, or other important areas of functioning.

D. The symptoms are not due to the direct physiological effects of a substance (e.g., drug abuse, a medication) or a general medical condition.

E. All of the following:

1. Criteria have never been met for Major Depressive Disorder, Dysthymic Disorder, Panic Disorder, or Generalized Anxiety Disorder.

2. Criteria are not currently met for any other Anxiety or Mood Disorder (including an Anxiety or Mood Disorder, In Partial Remission).

3. The symptoms are not better accounted for by any other mental disorder.

Proposed DSM Axes for Further Study

Three additional axes have been placed in the appendix of DSM-IV-TR for further study for possible inclusion in subsequent editions of the DSM. Research on the usefulness of these axes will continue for the next several years.

Defensive Functioning Scale

With this axis clinicians use up to seven specific defense mechanisms, starting with the most prominent—meaning the coping style used most frequently—and then indicate whether the defenses are adaptive or unadaptive.

Social and Occupational Functioning Assessment Scale (SOFAS)

Social and occupational functioning is rated by the clinician on a 0-100 scale, where a score of 100 indicates superior functioning in a wide range of activities while a score of 1 would reflect an inability to maintain even minimal personal hygiene.

Global Assessment of Relational Functioning (GARF) Scale

In this scale, the clinician rates, also on a 0-100 scale, the degree to which the family or other personal relationships provide the necessary social and emotional support for the individual.

CHAPTER FOUR

RESEARCH METHODS

LEARNING OBJECTIVES

1. Describe the basic components of research, including the distinction between a hypothesis and a testable hypothesis, independent and dependent variables, internal and external validity, and statistical and clinical significance.
2. Compare and contrast different research designs (e.g., case study, correlational, group and single-case experimental designs), including the types of questions that are appropriate/inappropriate for each.
3. Explain the aims and purposes of behavioral genetics, including the advantages and disadvantages of family, adoption, twin, and genetic linkage analysis and association studies.
4. Compare and contrast the assets and liabilities of cross-sectional designs versus longitudinal designs.
5. Explain the general place of cultural and ethical principles in the research process.
6. Explain how studying behavior over time and across cultures fits within research design and the research process more generally.
7. Describe the nature and function of replication in research, and distinguish a program of research from research that is not programmatic.

OUTLINE

I. Examining Abnormal Behavior
   A. The following research questions are addressed throughout the textbook and specifically, in terms of research design and methodology:
      1. *What problems cause distress and impair functioning?* (i.e., address the nature of abnormal behavior)
      2. *Why do people behave in unusual ways?* (i.e., address the causes or etiology of abnormal behavior)
      3. *How do we help people behave in more adaptive ways?* (i.e., develop better and more effective treatments and better treatment outcomes).

   B. The basic components of a research study include:
      1. A **hypothesis**, or educated guess, about what is to be studied and what one expects to find. The research design is the method used to evaluate and test the hypothesis. Not all hypotheses are testable, but those used in science must be formulated so that they are **testable**.
      2. When you want to test the hypothesis, you formulate a **research design** that includes specifying the **independent variable(s)** that you believe will influence aspects of the person's behavior you are interested in (the **dependent variable[s]**). That is, you want to know what factors influence what the person does, thinks, feels, talks about, including biological factors, and you want to test for such relations in a more convincing and systematic

way. Though most of us continually formulate hypotheses for events in the world, including our own behavior and the actions of others, we rarely test our hunches empirically to see if they are correct. This is what science is for.

3. When developing a research design to test a hypothesis, researchers attempt to balance internal and external validity.
    a. **Internal validity** refers to the extent to which we are confident that the independent variable caused the dependent variable to change.
    b. **External validity** refers to how well the results of the study relate to the aspects of the real world beyond the study, or how do the findings generalize to people who were not part of the research study.
4. **Confounds** are contaminating factors in a research study, or uncontrolled alternative explanations for the changes observed in our dependent variable. Confounds represent threats to internal validity. When they are present, we cannot be confident that the independent variable was responsible for producing changes in the dependent variable.
5. Three strategies are used by researchers to avoid confounds and to ensure that a study retains a high degree of internal validity.
    a. A **control group** is a group of people who are similar to the **experimental group** in every way, but are not exposed to the independent variable. For example, one group may be given an active treatment (i.e., the independent variable) while the control group never gets the treatment and is simply placed on a waiting list. Control groups help rule out alternative explanations for changes in behavior that have nothing to do with the independent variable under study.
    b. **Randomization** is another strategy that helps bolster the internal validity of a study, and is defined as a process of randomly assigning people to different experimental conditions in such a way that each person has an equal chance of being placed in any condition (e.g., random numbers, coin toss). For example, whether a person would be assigned to your active treatment condition or a wait list control condition (no treatment) would depend on the flip of a coin (heads = treatment, tails = wait list control). Randomization helps to distribute differences evenly amongst participants and across experimental conditions, and thus reduces systematic bias in study conditions that could confound interpretation of the results.
    c. A third way to improve internal validity is to use **analog models**, which involve recreating aspects of real world phenomena in the laboratory so that they closely approximate the real world. Analog models could be thought of as creating a close replica of facets of the real world in the laboratory so that those facets can be studied more systematically.
6. **External validity** or **generalizability** refers to the degree to which a study's results may be applied to other people or settings. That is, researchers want to be able to generalize their findings to real world phenomena. The rub, of

course, is that if the experimental situation is so tightly controlled and artificial, the results may be compelling, but have very little meaning beyond the research setting. In general, as internal validity increases, external validity decreases.

C. Researchers rely on data to support their inferences and often use statistics as a means to test whether their inferences are, in fact, correct. The use of **statistics**, a branch of mathematics that addresses the gathering, analyzing, and interpretation of data, has helped move the discipline of psychology from prescientific to scientific status.

1. **Statistical significance** in psychological research means that the probability of obtaining an observed effect by chance is small. Whether that difference is important and meaningful is another matter.
2. Although results may be statistically significant, they may not be **clinically significant**. In other words, one may detect a significant difference between experimental and control conditions, but the **size of the effect** (i.e., the difference or change) is clinically meaningless. This is particularly important in treatment research. For example, a treatment that is shown to produce statistically significant reductions in anxiety (say by 5 points on a 100 point scale) is probably clinically insignificant in terms of producing clinically meaningful changes that would warrant recommending this treatment for routine use in patient populations. Assessing **social validity**, or the degree to which the person being treated (including significant others), feels that the changes that have occurred are important and meaningful is another way to address clinical significance.

D. A problem with psychopathology research is that individual differences are often de-emphasized. The tendency to view all participants as homogeneous (e.g., persons meeting DSM criteria for major depression) in a group study is the **patient uniformity myth**. This myth leads researchers to make broad and perhaps inaccurate generalizations about disorders and treatment from groups of treated patients to individuals who may later undergo the treatment. The problem is that the average gains in the treatment group contain persons who got worse or did not improve at all. There is no way to know whether an individual client represents the part of the group that improved, remained the same, or got worse in response to treatment. You may also illustrate this concept by relating the concept of patient uniformity to categorical vs. prototypic forms of classification.

II. Types of Research Methods

A. Studying individual cases

1. One way to intensively examine an individual with unique behavioral and physical patterns is the **case study** method. This method involves extensive observation and clinical description of a person and can provide important information about a particular disorder, its causes, and treatment.
2. Case studies have been important in the history of psychology (e.g., Sigmund Freud's development of psychoanalytic theory was based on intensive

observations from several single cases). Free association emerged out of this approach. Masters and Johnson debunked several myths about sexual behavior based on case studies.

3. The case study method is used less frequently in abnormal psychology for the following reasons:
    a. It does not use the scientific method.
    b. Few efforts are made to ensure internal validity, and most case studies contain several confounds that interfere with conclusions.
    c. Uncontrolled extraneous factors may operate alone, or in combination with other unknown factors, to produce the observed effects.

B. Research by correlation

1. Any statistical relation between two variables is called a **correlation**. Unlike experimental designs, correlational designs do not involve the manipulation of an independent variable. Rather, data are sampled from phenomena just as they occur and are then examined to see how the variables relate with one another. That is, correlation involves relations among dependent variables.
2. The results of a correlational study simply indicate that two or more dependent variables co-vary together or they do not. As such, correlation **does not imply causation**. The reason is the problem of **directionality** with regard to causes and effects (e.g., does A cause B, B cause A, or a third variable C that causes A and B?).
3. The statistical values for correlational coefficients range from –1.0 to +1.0.
    a. A **positive correlation** means that the strength of one variable is associated with the strength of another variable. That is, one variable is large, the other is large; when one variable is small, the other variable also tends to be small. A perfect positive correlation is denoted by a correlation coefficient of +1.00; a virtual rarity in science.
    b. A **negative correlation** is represented by a negative sign, and means that as one variable increases in size or strength, the other variable tends to decrease in size or strength. A perfect negative correlation is denoted by a correlation coefficient of –1.00; another virtual rarity in science.
    c. **No correlation** (meaning no relation among variables) is indicated by correlation coefficients that hover around 0.
4. **Epidemiology** is the study of incidence, distribution, and consequences of a problem or set of problems in a population. The primary goal of epidemiologists is to determine the extent of a problem or disorder in a group of people and to find important clues as to why a disorder exists, extent of the problem in the general population at a particular time point (i.e., **prevalence**), why a disorder or problem may be increasing or decreasing in the general population (i.e., **incidence**), and even the **course** of a disorder. **Epidemiological research** relies largely on correlational methods to address such issues. Examples include effects of stress following a natural disaster, and AIDS.

C. Research by experiment

1. An **experiment** involves the *manipulation* of an independent variable and the observation of its effects of the dependent variable(s) of interest. The independent variable is manipulated systematically to address the question of **causality**.
2. In **group experimental designs**, researchers introduce, change, and/or withdraw an independent variable to assess how that change influences the behavior of individual members of different groups. To ensure internal validity in an experiment, control groups are typically employed. Types of control groups include:
   a. **Placebo control groups** control for the possibility that the changes observed in the study may have been due simply to the expectation of getting better (e.g., people getting the active treatment may believe it will help them, whereas those in the control group may be disappointed). A placebo in medicine is an inactive medication, but in psychology having a true placebo control group is more difficult. Use of a placebo control group helps to distinguish effects due to positive expectations from effects resulting from the actual treatment.
   b. A **double-blind control** is a variant of the placebo control group procedure, where both the participants and researchers or therapists are blind (i.e., unaware) of what group they are in or what treatment they are given, including in some cases the diagnostic status of the patient. The double-blind procedure is used to control for subject expectations, but also researcher and therapist bias, particularly bias related to allegiance or belief in the superiority of a particular form of treatment (i.e., **the allegiance effect**). The double blind procedure is not perfect, however.
   c. A **comparative treatment design** is an alternative to use of no-treatment control groups. In this design, two or more comparable groups of people with a particular disorder are selected and provided with different forms of treatment. The process and outcome of treatment are two important issues that can be addressed with this particular design.
      i. With regard to **treatment process**, the questions is *"Why does the treatment work?"* The answer may be found by addressing therapist, therapy (i.e., active ingredients), and client variables that may operate alone or in combination to produce beneficial outcome. Addressing such questions can lead the way to more powerful interventions.
      ii. **Outcome research** focuses on the positive and/or negative consequences of treatment. The questions addressed here are *"Does the treatment work?"* and *"Do the positive benefits of therapy outweigh the potential negative consequences and risks?"* Unlike process research that focuses on change during therapy, outcome research focuses on changes resulting from treatment.

Successful outcome will depend on how it is defined and where one looks for it.

D. **Single-case experimental designs,** owing much to the methodological innovations of B. F. Skinner, involve the systematic study of an individual under a variety of experimental conditions and over time. Single-case experimental designs differ from case studies in their use of several strategies to improve internal validity, while reducing the number of confounding variables. Single-case experimental designs are experiments, but with a focus on the individual, not an overall group average. Most often such experiments contain data from several individuals (really $N = 1+$ design, not $N = 1$ design). Such experiments have the following unique features:

1. One of the more important strategies used in single-case experimental design is **repeated measurement**, in which behavior is measured several times instead of only once before and after you change the independent variable. Changes in behavior are evaluated for changes in **variability, level, and trend** as a function of time and changing conditions (i.e., independent variables) across time. This allows determination of whether observed changes are due to treatment effects.
2. **Withdrawal designs** are commonly used to determine whether the independent variable is truly responsible for changes in behavior. A simple withdrawal design **has three parts**: First, a person's condition is evaluated before treatment to establish a baseline; second, a change in the independent variable is introduced and its effects on behavior assessed; and last, treatment is withdrawn (i.e., return to baseline) and behavior is assessed to examine whether it tracks the withdrawal of the independent variable. Withdrawal designs are not always appropriate, and ethically suspect when the withdrawal involves an obviously effective treatment, or in cases where the treatment cannot be removed (e.g., changes in thoughts, acquired skills). It should be noted, however, that natural withdrawals occur routinely throughout the course of therapy (e.g., patient goes on vacation, misses an appointment, and drug holidays in the case of medications).
3. **Multiple baseline designs** provide an alternative to withdrawal designs, in that the effects of the intervention can be evaluated in the controlled systematic fashion across settings, behaviors, and persons. For example, three behaviors could be selected for treatment. All behaviors would first undergo baseline, and then the first behavior would be targeted while the remaining behaviors are assessed in baseline. Once the first behavior shows stable response to the intervention, the second behavior would be targeted, while the third behavior still remains in an extended baseline, and so on. Multiple baseline designs resemble the way treatment is naturally implemented, whether with a single client, or across clients seeking treatment.

III. Genetics and Research Across Time and Cultures

A. Studying genetics

1. We know that there is an interaction between our genetic makeup and our experiences. This interaction determines, in part, how we will develop. The goal of **behavioral geneticists** (i.e., people who study the genetics of behavior) is to identify the role of genetics in these interactions.
2. Genetic researchers examine **phenotypes** (i.e., the observable characteristics or behaviors of an individual) and **genotypes** (i.e., the genetic composition of an individual). For example, persons with Down syndrome have some level of mental retardation and several other physical characteristics (i.e., phenotypes), but the genotype that causes Down syndrome is an extra 21st chromosome. Knowledge of phenotype of psychological disorders far exceeds our knowledge of the genotypes of psychological disorders.
3. **Four main research strategies** used by scientists to study the interaction between environment and genetics in psychological disorders include: family studies, adoption studies, twin studies, and genetic linkage analysis.
    a. In **family studies**, scientists examine a behavioral pattern or emotional trait in the context of family members. The family member with the trait singled out for study is called the **proband**. The role of genetics is supported, in part, if the trait occurs more often in first-degree relatives (i.e., parents, siblings, or offspring) than in second-degree or more distant relatives. Blood-injury-injection phobia is an example of a disorder that tends to run in families.
        i. The problem with family studies is that it is difficult to separate the contribution of shared environment from the contribution of genetics.
    b. **Adoption studies** begin to allow one to separate environmental from genetic contributions to psychopathology. In **adoption studies**, scientists identify adoptees that have a particular behavioral pattern or psychological disorder and attempt to locate first-degree relatives who were raised in different family settings. If persons raised in different families display the disorder more frequently than expected by chance, then the inference may be made that genetic factors were influential in the development of the disorder.
    c. **Twin studies** give behavioral geneticists their closest possible look at the role of genes in development. Identical (monozygotic) twins look identical and have identical genes, whereas fraternal (dizygotic) twins come from different eggs and have about 50% of their genes in common (i.e., same as siblings). The main focus is on whether identical twins share a trait of disorder more often than fraternal twins. Still, the problem of shared environment vs. genetic contribution is difficult to separate unless one combines the adoption study with a twin study.
    d. Family, twin, and adoption studies may suggest that a disorder has a genetic component, but only **genetic linkage analysis** and **association studies** can locate the site of the defective gene.
        i. The principle of **genetic linkage analysis** is simple. When a family disorder is studied, other inherited characteristics are also

assessed. The other characteristics (called **genetic markers**) are selected because we know their exact location. If a match of link is discovered between the inheritance of the disorder and inheritance of a genetic marker, the genes for the disorder and the genetic marker are probably close together on the same chromosome. This analysis occurs in a large group of people with a particular disorder.

ii. **Association studies** also use genetic markers but compare markers in people with and without the disorder. If certain markers occur significantly more often in people with the disorder, it is assumed that the markers are close to the genes involved in the disorder. Association studies are better able to identify genes that may only be weakly associated with a disorder.

B. Studying behavior over time

1. Here the research question is *"How does a disorder or behavior pattern change across time (if at all)?"* This is important in determining whether to bother treating someone, particularly if you know that the problem will likely improve on its own. This knowledge is also important with regard to understanding developmental changes in abnormal behavior (e.g., people who are at risk). Finally, if we understand how a disorder manifests over time, we may be able to design interventions and services to prevent such problems from becoming problems in the first place.
    a. **Prevention research** includes the study of biological, psychological, and environmental risk factors for developing later problems (called **pre-intervention research**), treatment interventions to help prevent later problems (called **prevention intervention research**), and more widespread structural issues such as governmental policies that could assist with prevention efforts (called **preventive service systems research**).
2. Research strategies used in prevention research for examining psychopathology across time combine individual and group methods, including correlational and experimental designs. Two of the most frequently used designs are cross-sectional and longitudinal designs.
    a. **Cross-sectional designs** represent a variation of correlational research involving comparisons of different people at different age groups on some characteristic. The participants in each age group are called **cohorts**. Confounding of age and experience is known as the **cohort effect** and represents a limitation of cross-sectional designs. Such designs do not address how problems develop in individuals.
    b. **Longitudinal designs** evaluate the same persons over time and assess changes directly. The cohort effect is not an issue. Such research is costly and time-consuming, and there is the danger that the original research question will become irrelevant by the time the study is complete. Longitudinal designs suffer from a problem similar to the cohort effect; namely the **cross-generational effect** (i.e., trying to

generalize findings to groups whose experiences are very different from those of the study participants). An example of this problem is attempting to generalize about drug use from a sample followed from the early 1960s and 1970s to a sample now in the 1990s.

c. **Sequential designs** combine longitudinal and cross-sectional designs.

C. Studying behavior across cultures

1. Although studying the differences between cultural behaviors can provide substantial knowledge about the etiology and treatment of mental illness, much of the psychopathological research literature originates in Western cultures and may be **ethnocentric** in nature.
2. Researchers do use culture as an independent variable in studying abnormal behavior, but problems may arise. For example, no random assignment to groups is made and differences in genetic backgrounds may not be considered. Moreover, standard definitions of psychological disorders may not apply equally well across cultures. An additional complicating factor is varying tolerances or thresholds for abnormal behavior across cultures. Finally, treatment research is complicated by cross-cultural differences, particularly as cultures have their own treatment models that reflect their unique values.

D. The power of a program of research

1. Research designs must be evaluated in the context of the kinds of questions one wishes to answer; designs are, therefore, not comparatively better or worse out of context.
2. A **program of research** comprises a series of inter-related questions, which often draw upon a series of research designs in order to find answers to them. You can think of a program of research as a large tree, with the trunk representing the core questions or general area, and the limbs representing related sub-questions, and the branches more fine grained specific questions. Programs of research are conducted in stages, and entail using multiple perspectives to derive a complete picture of a behavioral problem. All perspectives are part of the same tree, and some limbs and branches will die and fall off (i.e., a subarea of the program leads to a dead end), but the hope is that many more will grow over time. The tree metaphor also illustrates that a program of research takes time to evolve, much like a tree takes time to grow.

E. Replication

1. **Replication** is the credo of science (show me, show me again, and better yet, have someone else show me what you found). Replication increases confidence that findings are not due to chance or coincidence. Programs of research replicate findings in different ways, with different designs and methods, and hence build confidence in the results.

F. Research ethics

1. **Informed consent** involves a research participant's or therapy client's agreement to cooperate in a study or therapy with full understanding and

disclosure of the nature of the research or treatment, the person's role in it, and the expected benefits and or negative consequences.

2. The concept of informed consent emerged following the war trials after WWII.
3. True informed consent is often elusive. The basic components are **competence** (i.e., capable of consenting), **voluntarism** (i.e., not coerced), **full information** (i.e., have necessary information to make an informed decision), and **comprehension** (i.e., understand what they are getting into) on the part of the person.
4. Research in university and medical settings must be approved by **institutional review boards**; committees that have as their main goal the protection of the rights, welfare, and dignity of research participants.
5. The **American Psychological Association's code of ethics** stress protecting research participants and therapy clients from harm, and place the burden of responsibility for such protection of the shoulders of the researcher or therapist.
6. The **Society for Research in Child Development** has developed ethical guidelines for conducting research with children. Specifically, these guidelines require informed consent from children's caregivers and from children themselves if they are age 7 or older.
7. Ethics often extend beyond protection of research participants and clients, and include how researchers deal with their data, fraud in science, giving publication credit to others.
8. A current development in the field of psychological research is to involve consumers of research in the design, running and interpretation of research projects, in order to improve the relevance of the research and the treatment of the participants.

OVERALL SUMMARY

This chapter outlines components of the research process in abnormal psychology. These components include the establishment of a testable hypothesis, protection of internal validity, types of research design (i.e., case study, correlational, group and single-case experimental design, genetic linkage and analysis, cross-sectional and longitudinal designs), the role of cultural factors that impinge upon research, and research ethics. This chapter examines methods developed to discover what behaviors constitute problems, why people engage in behavioral disorders (etiology), and what constitutes effective treatments and beneficial treatment outcome.

KEY TERMS

Adoption studies (p. 112)
Allegiance effect (p. 107)
Analog model (p. 102)
Association studies (p. 112)
Baseline (p. 109)
Case study method (p. 103)

Clinical significance (p. 102)
Cohort (p. 113)
Cohort effect (p. 113)
Comparative treatment research (p. 107)
Confound (p. 101)
Control group (p. 101)
Correlation (p. 104)
Correlation coefficient (p. 104)
Cross-generational effect (p. 114)
Cross-sectional design (p. 113)
Dependent variable (p. 100)
Directionality (p. 105)
Double-blind control (p. 107)
Effect size (p. 102)
Epidemiology (p. 105)
Etiology (p. 100)
Experiment (p. 106)
External validity (p. 100)
Family aggregation (p. 111)
Family studies (p. 111)
Generalizability (p. 102)
Genetic linkage analysis (p. 112)
Genetic markers (p. 112)
Genotype (p. 111)
Human genome project (p. 111)
Hypothesis (p. 100)
Incidence (p. 105)
Independent variable (p. 100)
Informed consent (p. 117)
Internal validity (p. 100)
Level (p. 108)
Longitudinal design (p. 114)
Manipulating a variable (p. 106)
Multiple baseline (p. 109)
Negative correlation (p. 105)
Patient Uniformity Myth (p. 103)
Phenotype (p. 111)
Placebo control group (p. 107)
Placebo effect (p. 107)
Positive correlation (p. 104)
Preintervention (p. 113)
Prevalence (p. 105)
Prevention intervention (p. 113)
Preventive service systems (p. 113)
Proband (p. 111)
Repeated measurement (p. 108)

Research design (p. 100)
Retrospective information (p. 114)
Randomization (p. 101)
Sequential design (p. 114)
Single-case experimental design (p. 108)
Statistical significance (p. 102)
Testability (p. 101)
Treatment outcome research (p. 116)
Trend (p. 108)
Twin studies (p. 112)
Variability (p. 108)
Withdrawal design (p. 108)

INFOTRAC KEY TERM EXERCISES

Each exercise is linked to key terms from the Wadsworth InfoTrac on-line searchable database. Key terms must be entered exactly as written.

Exercise 1: **Tapping Our Problems Away: The Science of Thought-Field Psychotherapy**
Article: A63693004
Citation: (Can we really tap our problems away?: A critical analysis of Thought Field Therapy). Brandon A. Gaudiano & James D. Herbert. Skeptical Inquirer, July 2000 v24 i4 p29

Proponents of thought field therapy claim that psychological problems can be treated with a sequence of movements and taps on various body parts that correspond to meridians used in acupuncture therapy. Review the InfoTrac article on this topic and evaluate the scientific merits of thought field therapy. What is thought field therapy and what research evidence is there to support its effectiveness? Do we know whether tapping is an important process variable in outcome? What are the potential confounds or threats to internal validity related to thought field therapy? And, what are some of the criticisms of this new brand of therapy, including the ethical issues involved? In formulating your response, it may be helpful for you to consider whether you would seek out such therapy, or recommend it to a friend. Limit your answer to 3-5 typed double-spaced pages.

Exercise 2: **What do We Know About Placebos and Their Role in Psychotherapy Research?**
Key Term: *Placebo Effect*

The placebo effect (i.e., people getting better because they expect to get better) is quite commonly cited in medicine and psychotherapy. Yet, we know surprising little as to why people get better or heal on the basis of belief alone. The placebo effect raises a host of issues relevant to medication and psychotherapy treatment, particularly how much of treatment is really due to the treatment itself vs. a patient believing that undergoing treatment will make them well, regardless of what is actually done in therapy. Review the InfoTrac article(s) on this topic and evaluate the role of placebos in psychiatric and psychological practice. What do we know about placebos? How do researchers attempt to control for the placebo effect in their research? Are there medications or psychotherapies that are really nothing more than a sugar pill? Limit your answer to 3-5 typed double-spaced pages.

Exercise 3 (Future Trend): Is Psychotherapy Research Relevant to Clinical Practice?

In the early 1950s Hans Eysenck noted the lack of reliable evidence that psychotherapy was more helpful than doing nothing and waiting for recovery. Now, this is no longer the case. Hundreds of studies show that psychotherapy is better than doing nothing at all. Nonetheless, there remains a long-standing debate between researchers and front-line practitioners about the relevance of controlled outcome studies in more naturalistic clinical settings. The Division 12 Task Force on the Promotion and Dissemination of Psychological Procedures has been instrumental in helping to set criteria to determine whether psychotherapies have empirical support. Practitioners, however, are quick to point out that the highly controlled conditions used in Randomized Clinical Trials are quite unlike the less controlled conditions they face in naturalistic clinical settings. This is the classic effectiveness vs. efficacy debate. As an instructor, you can use this topic to address several interesting issues. For instance, you might introduce students to the criteria used to determine whether a psychosocial intervention has empirical support and relate such criteria with research design issues. Alternatively, you could use this topic to address the science vs. practice debate in mental health care, including perhaps how such issues relate with managed behavioral health care. More broadly, you could ask students to consider whether psychology needs to adopt a system to regulate psychotherapies much like the FDA with medications. Below are some relevant web links that should be helpful in this regard.

http://www.apa.org/divisions/div12/rev_est/
http://pantheon.yale.edu/~tat22//
http://www.apa.org/journals/seligman.html
http://www.apa.org/practice/peff.html
http://www.psych.org/psych_pract/ispe_efficacy.cfm
http://www3.oup.co.uk/jnls/list/clipsy/scope/

CLASSROOM ACTIVITIES, DEMONSTRATIONS, AND LECTURE TOPICS

1. **Activity: Finding Meaning in the Method.** Dr. Philip Zimbardo developed an excellent in-class activity to teach students about the importance of conducting formal experiments in the field of psychology. The activity involves measuring reaction times in male or female students (after proposing a hypothesis that one sex is slower than the opposite sex). Zimbardo provides a "reaction time meter" which is held above a student's fingers; the student must then catch the "meter" as quickly as possible before hitting the floor. The instructor must remember to give those students who are believed to be faster a *warning* as to when you will drop the meter; do *not* give the "slower" students any warning and be sure to hold the meter at a level even with the student's fingers! Upon completion of this task, students will have the opportunity to discuss the importance of relevant vs. irrelevant variables (relevant variables are those that could affect the outcome or dependent variable).

   Source Information. Zimbardo, P.G. (1981). Finding Meaning in the Method. Activities handbook for the teaching of psychology (Vol. 1). Washington, DC: American Psychological Association.

2. **Activity: The Case Study Method.** To demonstrate the advantages and disadvantages of case study methodology, encourage students to conduct a case study of their own. They may look for a person who is willing to discuss a disorder they have (e.g., alcoholism, insomnia, eating disorder, etc.) or they can conduct a case study on a person's experience of a phenomenon (e.g., divorce, war, loss, etc.), including some aspect of their own life and experience. Discuss the advantages of using this methodology and the drawbacks.

3. **Activity: The Correlational Method.** Have your students look through popular literature to find claims about new and newsworthy psychological findings (see below under the heading *Internet Resources* for an online resource to *Abnormal Psychology in the News*). Most of the time, the popular literature is utilizing correlational data. Assist students in learning how to critically evaluate data that is presented in the popular literature. You may want to illustrate how easy it is to make false assumptions about correlational data. For example, if you tell your class that obesity and the number of hours children watch television is positively correlated, may students will surmise that those results are due to the fact that watching television prohibits children from exercising. However, an alternative explanation is that obese children choose to watch television because it is more difficult for them to exercise. Caution students about directionality problems and the possibility of a third factor being responsible for correlations. Again, correlation does not imply causation.

4. **Activity: Establishing Empirically Support Treatments.** Use the transparency master titled "Criteria for Empirically-Supported Treatments" to illustrate how research design and research criteria translate into the science of psychotherapy (note that the current terminology has changed from "empirically-validated" to "empirically-supported," to dissuade psychologists from thinking that treatments making this efficacy list are there to stay). The criteria for empirically-supported treatments contains a rich source of information about research design, and the process of developing efficacious treatments. You may also use this topic as a spring board to discuss the current controversies surrounding empirically-supported psychotherapies, the highlight the distinction between efficacy vs. effectiveness research, and to discuss whether psychologists should move toward having a model like the Food and Drug Administration (FDA) in sanctioning psychotherapies, and what empirically-supported treatments mean for consumers of psychological services. Note that this transparency is also relevant to material covered in Chapter 16.

   Source Information. You may find on-line reports regarding empirically supported treatments, including manualized treatments, at the following web site: http://www.wpic.pitt.edu/research/sscp/ empirically_supported_treatments.htm.

5. **Activity: Random Assignment and Expectations Regarding Psychotherapy.** The following activity is designed to illustrate random selection and random assignment and also the role of expectations and feelings regarding treatment. To illustrate random selection, tell students that you are going to perform a little experiment in class that may involve the possibility of earning extra credit. Also explain that everyone should pretend

that the class represents the population as a whole. Begin by stating that your study has two conditions: a treatment and a wait-list control and that persons in the treatment condition will receive extra credit, but the others will not but may at some point in the future. Using your roster, begin by randomly selecting 10 students from the class and ask them to come forward one at a time (do this slowly). Now, pull out a coin, and flip it as each student comes forward (illustrates the process of random assignment). If the coin comes up heads for the first student, then place him or her in the treatment group off to your right. If the coin comes up tails for the next student, then place him or her off to your left in the wait list control group. You will want to make this part dramatic, so again handle each student one at a time (i.e., randomly select 1 student, then go through the process of random assignment, and then move on). Continue until all 10 students are separated into groups (you should end up with about 4-5 students in each group). This is a good time to discuss how students felt being selected for the Extra Credit Treatment study and how they felt immediately after they learned that they were being assigned to either the Wait List Control or Extra Credit Treatment. Relate their feelings to what patients may experience (but on a much larger scale) when enrolling in treatment research. You may want to go ahead and offer extra credit to all students who participated, or perhaps a small prize, cheers, applause, etc.

SUPPLEMENTARY READING MATERIAL FOR CHAPTER FOUR

(I = These sources can be found on "*Infotrac, the online library*" provided by Wadsworth and Brooks/Cole Publishing.)

Bersoff, D. N. (1995). Ethical conflicts in psychology. Washington, DC: American Psychological Association.

Bromley, D. B. (1986). The case-study method in psychology and related disciplines. New York: Wiley.

I Chambless, D. L., & Ollendick, T. H. (2001). Empirically supported psychological interventions: Controversies and evidence. Annual Review of Psychology, 52, 685-716.

Estes, W. K. (1991). Statistical models in behavioral research. Hillsdale, NJ: Erlbaum.

Greenberg, L. S., & Pinsof, W. M. (1994). Reassessing psychotherapy research. New York: Guilford.

Hayes, S. C., Barlow, D. H., & Nelson-Gray, R. O. (1999). The scientist practitioner: Research and accountability in the age of managed care, 2nd ed. Boston, MA: Allyn & Bacon.

Hayes, S. C., Follette, V. M., Dawes, R. M., & Grady, K. E. (1995). Scientific standards of psychological practice: Issues and recommendations. Reno, NV: Context Press.

Kazdin, A. E. (Ed.) (1992). Methodological issues and strategies in clinical research. Washington, DC: American Psychological Association.

Kopta, S. M., Lueger, R. J., Saunders, S. M., & Howard, K. I. (1999). Individual psychotherapy outcome and process research: Challenges leading to greater turmoil or a positive transition? Annual Review of Psychology, 441 (1).

Kratochwill, T. R., & Levin, J. R. (Eds.) (1992). Single-case research design and analysis: New directions for psychology and education. Hillsdale, NJ: Erlbaum.

Levine, G. (1994). Experimental methods in psychology. Hillsdale, NJ: Erlbaum.

McGuigan, F. J. (1993). Experimental psychology: Methods of research. Englewood Cliffs, NJ: Prentice-Hall.

Routh, D. K. (1993). Clinical psychology since 1917: Science, practice, and organization. New York: Plenum.

Trierweiler, S. J., & Stricker, G. (1998). The scientific practice of professional psychology. New York: Plenum.

Wahlsten, D. (1999). Single-gene influences on brain and behavior. Annual Review of Psychology, 599(1).

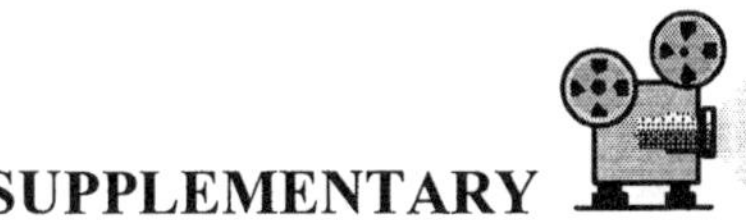

SUPPLEMENTARY VIDEO RESOURCES FOR CHAPTER FOUR

Abnormal psychology inside/out, vol. 3. *(available through your International Thomson Learning representative)*. David H. Barlow of Boston University talks about the research methodology used in studying panic patients, and in studying clients with sexual disorders. He also discusses the ethical issues in selecting subjects and the changes that technology has brought to data collection.

Ethics and scientific research. (Insight Media: 2162 Broadway, New York, NY 10024/ (800)-233-9910). This video addresses ethical issues faced by scientific researchers, focusing on scientific misconduct and its control. It features Robert L. Sprague, recipient of the AAAS Scientific Integrity and Freedom Award, who discusses a case of a scientist who faked research on psychotropic drugs. (30 min)

Experimental design. (Insight Media: 2162 Broadway, New York, NY 10024/ (800)-233-9910). This program distinguishes between observational studies and experiments, teaching basic principles of experimental design. It covers comparison, randomization, and replication, and includes a program that examines the question of causation. (30 min each)

Experiments in human behavior. (Insight Media: 2162 Broadway, New York, NY 10024/ (800)-233-9910). This still-image video shows how psychological experiments are designed, using examples from research on prisoner/guard relationships, obedience to authority, cult behavior, and alcohol consumption. It also discusses experimenter bias and examines when to use field studies, observational studies, and questionnaires. (35 min)

How numbers lie: Media truth or fiction. (Insight Media: 2162 Broadway, New York, NY 10024/ (800)-233-9910). Numbers are powerful persuasion tools that can be twisted to support a particular point of view. This program teaches viewers how to think critically and analyze statistics disguised as facts. "Provides excellent examples…thought-provoking." (23 min)

Nature and nurture interwoven. (Insight Media: 2162 Broadway, New York, NY 10024/ (800)-233-9910). Using research in behavior genetics, ideas of heritability, and data from twin studies, this video questions the extent to which parents can alter their children's futures by changing the circumstances of their lives. It profiles the Oliveira children from urban São Paulo, showing their visit to the rural region where their parents grew up and their encounter with their country cousins. (30 min)

The mystery of twins. (Insight Media: 2162 Broadway, New York, NY 10024/ (800)-233-9910). Presenting the findings of a range of current research projects on the links between identical twins, this video explores what twins may be able to reveal about the different impacts of nature and nurture. It questions the importance of genes to behavioral choices, considers the evolutionary significance of naturally occurring clones, and addresses the possibility of ESP between people with matching genetic material. (52 min)

The scientific method. (Insight Media: 2162 Broadway, New York, NY 10024/ (800)-233-9910). Tracing the evolution of the scientific method, this program shows the three-step process of observing, developing a hypothesis, and testing it through experimentation. It presents examples of how the scientific method is applied in the classroom and in professional research. Blue Ribbon, American Film & Video Festival. (23 min)

INTERNET 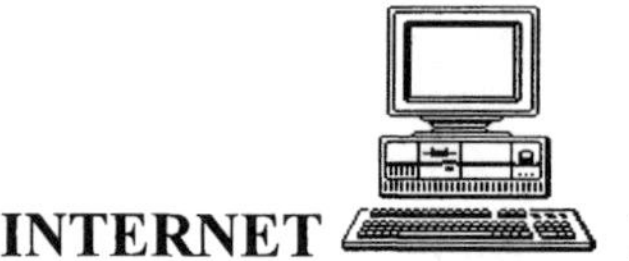 RESOURCES FOR CHAPTER FOUR

Abnormal Psychology News
http://taxa.psyc.missouri.edu/abnormal/

This is a collection of articles, primarily newspaper articles, relevant to abnormal psychology. They are highly variable in quality, but nearly all come from top news sources and journals. This site is one that you will likely want to refer to time again throughout your teaching!

APA Ethical Principles and Code of Conduct
http://www.apa.org/ethics/code.html

This is the online version of the American Psychological Association's Ethical Principles of Psychologists and Code of Conduct.

Encyclopedia of Psychology: Pseudoscience
http://www.psychology.org/links/Resources/Pseudoscience/

This site contains several links to pseudoscientific issues in psychology, and abnormal psychology in particular.

Internal Validity Tutorial
http://psych.athabascau.ca/html/Validity/

A tutorial on validity that is part of an experimental design course.

Library Research
http://www.apa.org/science/lib.html

This APA web site is designed for students and explains how to find library resources about psychology by searching journals, books, newspapers, etc.

On Being A Scientist: Responsible Conduct In Research
http://www.nap.edu/readingroom/books/obas/

A formal introduction to research ethics and the responsibilities that these commitments imply.

Preparing Your Laboratory Report
http://www.psywww.com/tipsheet/labrep.htm

A "tipsheet" web page devoted to writing a psychological report based on the publication manual of the American Psychological Association.

Psychotherapists and FDA Standards
http://www.successfulschizophrenia.com/articles/fda.html

The possibility of imposing standards for psychotherapy that are comparable to the standards the FDA has established for drugs and drug therapy, raises major issues about psychotherapy, including the possibility that some psychotherapies and the treatment of schizophrenia could be banned.

Research Design Explained
http://spsp.clarion.edu/mm/RDE3/start/

Aids for teaching research methods in psychology.

Criteria for Empirically-Supported Treatments

Well-Established Treatments

I. At least two good between group design experiments demonstrating efficacy in one or more of the following ways:

A. Superior to pill or psychological placebo or to another treatment.

B. Equivalent to an already established treatment in experiments with adequate statistical power (about 30 per group; cf. Kazdin & Bass, 1989).

OR

II. A large series of single case design experiments (n ³ 9) demonstrating efficacy. *These experiments must have:*

A. Used good experimental designs and

B. Compared the intervention to another treatment as in I.A.

FURTHER CRITERIA FOR BOTH I AND II:

III. Experiments must be conducted with treatment manuals.

IV. Characteristics of the client samples must be clearly specified.

V. Effects must have been demonstrated by at least two different investigators or investigatory teams.

Probably Efficacious Treatments

I. Two experiments showing the treatment is more effective than a waiting-list control group.

OR

II. One or more experiments meeting the Well-Established Treatment Criteria I, III, and IV, but not V.

OR

III. A small series of single case design experiments ($n \geq 3$) otherwise meeting Well-Established Treatment Criteria II, III, and IV.

CHAPTER FIVE

ANXIETY DISORDERS

LEARNING OBJECTIVES

1. Describe psychological and biological similarities and differences between anxiety, fear, and a panic attack.
2. Describe the essential features of panic disorder, including the differences between the three DSM-IV-TR subtypes of panic attack.
3. Describe the essential features of generalized anxiety disorder, proposed causal and maintaining factors, and available treatment approaches.
4. Compare and contrast generalized anxiety disorder, agoraphobia, specific phobia, and social phobia in terms of etiology, symptom presentation, and core identifying features.
5. Describe the essential features of posttraumatic stress disorder, its proposed causal factors, and available treatment approaches.
6. Describe the essential features of obsessive-compulsive disorder (i.e., obsessions and compulsions) and why they are considered maladaptive.
7. Be able to discuss genetic and biological vulnerability factors that are known to influence the development of certain anxiety disorders, including the role of neurotransmitter systems in the experience of fear and anxiety.
8. Describe biological and psychological approaches that have been successful in treating anxiety-related disorders.

OUTLINE

I. Anxiety, Fear, and Panic: Some Definitions

A. **Anxiety** is a mood state characterized by marked negative affect and somatic symptoms of tension in which a person apprehensively anticipates future danger or misfortune. In humans, anxiety may be expressed as subjective unease, worried behaviors, and/or physiological responses.

1. Anxiety is a normal emotion that is adaptive when experienced in moderate amounts. It is a future-oriented mood state that prepares humans to take action.
2. The emotion of anxiety becomes problematic (psychologically speaking) when it is experienced in excessive amounts and interferences with important areas of life functioning.

B. **Fear** is an immediate alarm reaction to dangerous or life threatening situations (fight or flight response; emergency or defensive reaction fear). Fear is a present-oriented mood state characterized by strong avoidance and activation of the sympathetic nervous system. Much evidence suggests that fear differs psychologically and biologically from anxiety.

1. Fear is also a normal emotional response that is adaptive when experienced in response to real danger or threat. Fear is accompanied by strong urge to escape and a surge of the sympathetic branch of the autonomic nervous system.
2. The emotion fear becomes problematic (psychological speaking) when it is experienced in excessive amounts in the absence of real threat or danger and interferes with important areas of life functioning.
3. Textbook case of Gretchen illustrates excessive fear in the absence of real threat or danger.

C. A **panic attack** is an abrupt experience of intense fear or discomfort accompanied by physical symptoms such as heart palpitations, chest pain, shortness of breath, and dizziness. The word **panic** derives from Pan, the Greek god of nature.

1. Three types of panic attacks are described in the DSM-IV-TR:
    a. **Situationally bound (cued) panic attack** is one that is expected in a given situation and is bound to some situations and not others. This type of panic attack is common in persons suffering from specific phobias and social phobia.
    b. **Unexpected (uncued) panic attack** is completely unanticipated in nature, and often occurs without warning. This form of panic attack is common in persons suffering from panic disorder.
    c. **Situationally predisposed panic attack** falls between situationally bound and unexpected panic, and is characterized by panic that may or may not occur in a given setting. This form of panic attack is also common in persons suffering from panic disorder.

D. Causes of anxiety disorders

1. **Biological contributions** for anxiety and panic suggest that people *inherit* the tendency to be anxious or highly emotional. This is likely the result of weak contributions from many genes that produce a vulnerability to response with excessive anxiety and panic in response to the right psychological and social factors, particularly under stress. The tendency to panic runs in families and seems to have a genetic component.
    a. Anxiety is associated with specific brain circuits and neurotransmitter systems, particularly low levels of GABA. The noradrenergic system and serotonergic systems are also involved.
    b. Corticotropin releasing factor (CRF) is receiving increasing attention as this system is central to the activation of the HPA axis described in Chapter 2. CRF has wide-ranging effects on the brain, including the limbic system (particularly the hippocampus and amygdala), locus cereleus in the brainstem, prefrontal cortex, and the dopaminergic system. CRF is also related to GABA.
    c. The brain area most associated with anxiety is the limbic system, in particular the septal-hippocampal system innervated by both serotonergic circuits in the raphe nuclei and noradrenergic circuits in the locus coeruleus (i.e., the **behavioral inhibition system, BIS**). The

BIS is activated by brain stem signals of unexpected events or danger signals from the cortex and results in anxiety, whereas the **fight/flight system (FFS)** originates in the brain stem, activates the amygdala, and results in an immediate alarm-and-escape response in animals that looks very much like the emotion of panic.

2. **Psychological contributions** for anxiety and panic originated with Freud, who saw anxiety as a psychic reaction to danger surrounding the reactivation of an infantile fear situation. Behaviorists view anxiety as a product of classical conditioning or modeling. A more integrated psychological model postulates that youngsters initially obtain a perception that events are not always under their control and that this is dangerous. This sense of control emerges via interaction with parents that are encouraging, predictable, and responsive to a child's needs, whereas uncontrollability seems related to parents that fail to provide a secure home and parents that are often overprotective and over intrusive. Such a perception of uncontrollability is a central psychological risk factor that makes persons vulnerable to anxiety later in life.
3. **Social contributions** focus on the relation between stressful life events as triggers for biological and psychological vulnerabilities for anxiety and panic. Many stressors that activate biological and psychological vulnerabilities to anxiety are interpersonal (e.g., marriage, divorce, work problems, death of a loved one, including social pressures related to school, peers). Also, familial influences seem particularly strong in the development of anxiety disorders.

E. **An integrated model** of etiological risk factors considers the complex interaction among biological, psychological, experiential, and social variables. According to the model proposed in the textbook, one may be born with a biological vulnerability to be anxious, but this vulnerability then interacts with socialized beliefs that the world is dangerous and that events are uncontrollable. Such factors, coupled with experience of life stressors and learning experiences, may then activate the diathesis for anxiety and begin a positive spiral that may lead to an anxiety disorder.

F. Anxiety disorders often co-occur, and rates of **comorbidity** among anxiety disorders are high (e.g., a recent study showed that 55% of patients who received a principal diagnosis of an anxiety or depressive disorder had at least one additional anxiety or depressive disorder at the time of assessment). Major depression is often the most common secondary diagnosis in persons suffering from anxiety disorders. This fact emphasizes that anxiety disorders (and depression) share common features, including similar vulnerabilities. Anxiety disorders differ with respect to their foci and pattern.

II. Generalized Anxiety Disorder

A. **Generalized anxiety disorder (GAD)** is often considered the "basic" anxiety disorder because it is characterized by intense unfocused anxiety. Persons with GAD typically worry about minor daily life events, whereas children with GAD worry about academic, athletic, or social competence and physical injury. The elderly tend to focus on health and often report difficulty sleeping. The textbook illustrates the features of GAD with the case of Irene.

B. The **DSM-IV-TR criteria** specify that excessive anxiety and worry (apprehensive expectation) must be ongoing more days than not for a period of a least 6 months. It must also be difficult to turn off or control the worry process; a feature that distinguishes pathological worry from normal worry.

C. The physical symptoms of GAD differ from panic, and include muscle tension, mental agitation, susceptibility to fatigue, irritability, and difficulty sleeping. Focusing attention is often difficult.

D. Approximately 4% of the general population meet criteria for GAD, and GAD is quite common in the elderly. Although this is a common problem, few seek treatment compared to those with panic disorder. The *male to female ratio for GAD is about 2:1*. Onset of the disorder is usually in early adulthood and usually in response to some life stressor, and often progresses more gradually compared with other anxiety disorders.

E. GAD may be caused by several factors, including a genetic contribution as indicated by twin studies. What is inherited appears to be a tendency to be anxious, not GAD itself.

F. Individuals with GAD are less physiologically responsive than persons with anxiety disorders where panic is prominent. For this reason, persons with GAD have been called **autonomic restrictors**. Muscle tension is the only autonomic measures that consistently distinguishes persons with GAD from other nonanxious persons. It is believed that autonomic restriction is the result of automatic bias for threat coupled with an lack of processing the associated imagery and the emotional components of that imagery that would normally elicit strong autonomic responses.

G. **Treatment of GAD** has typically involved benzodiazepine drug treatment, although this has not been empirically supported. Psychological treatments focus on the worry process and avoidance of feelings of anxiety and negative affect and seem to work about as well as drugs. Exposure to worrisome thoughts and anxious images is utilized with coping skills training. Preliminary evidence supports this approach. Recently, a treatment for GAD has been developed that incorporates procedures focusing on acceptance rather than avoidance of distressing thoughts and feelings.

III. Panic Disorder With and Without Agoraphobia

A. To meet criteria for **panic disorder**, a person must experience an unexpected panic attack and develop anxiety about the possibility of another attack or the implications of the attack. **Agoraphobia** is fear and avoidance of "unsafe" situations where a panic attack may occur. Persons with **panic disorder with agoraphobia (PDA)** experience severe unexpected panic attacks during which time they feel a loss of control or endangered. Persons may also experience panic disorder without agoraphobia. The textbook illustrates panic disorder with extreme agoraphobia in the case of Mrs. M.

B. Many persons with panic disorder develop agoraphobia (i.e., fear of the marketplace). Agoraphobic avoidance appears to be one complication of severe unexpected panic attacks. Agoraphobic behavior can become independent of panic attacks. According to the DSM-IV, agoraphobia may be characterized either by avoiding situations or enduring them with marked distress. Some forms of agoraphobia involved interoceptive avoidance, particularly of activities that may increase physical symptoms of arousal.

C. Panic disorder with or without agoraphobia is fairly common, with a 3.5% lifetime prevalence in the general population. Two-thirds are women, and the mean age of onset of panic disorder is between 25 and 29. The higher prevalence of panic in women may be due to socialization and differential alcohol use. Most initial unexpected panic attacks begin after puberty. Panic disorder is generally less pervasive among the elderly; though agoraphobia is quite common.

D. Panic disorder exists worldwide, though how it is expressed varies widely across cultures. Rates of PD are similar across different ethnic groups in the US.

E. Approximately 60% of people with panic disorder experience **nocturnal panic attacks** (i.e., panic during sleep). Nocturnal panic occurs most often between 1:30 am and 3:30 am than at any other time, and such attacks have been shown to occur during delta wave sleep (the deepest stage of sleep, but not dream sleep). In African Americans, isolated sleep paralysis is often associated with nocturnal panic attacks.

F. The **causes of panic disorder** are numerous, and include an interaction of psychological, biological, and social-experiential influences. The textbook suggests that a biologically inherited vulnerability to be overreactive to daily events, coupled with stress, may establish a predisposition to associate the response with internal and external cues (i.e., moving from a false to a learned alarm response). Such factors, coupled with a psychological vulnerability to catastrophically misinterpret such events and the development of anxiety over the possibility of future panic attacks may, in turn, lead to panic disorder.

G. Treatment

1. **Medications** for anxiety and panic largely affect the serotonergic, noradrenergic, and benzodiazepine GABA neurotransmitter systems, such as imipramine, tend to block panic attacks. SSRIs (e.g., Prozac and Paxil) are currently the preferred drug for panic disorder; though sexual dysfunction is a

common side effect. Relapse rates for panic are high once the medication is discontinued.

2. **Psychological interventions**, and particularly cognitive-behavior therapies, are quite effective for panic disorder. Such treatment typically involves gradual exposure exercises combined with anxiety-reducing coping skills, such as relaxation and breathing retraining. As many as 70% of patients undergoing these treatments substantially improve, but very few are cured. Panic Control Treatment (PCT) is a cognitive-behavioral treatment that arranges for mini-exposures to panic sensations in therapy, and includes cognitive therapy to address attitudes and misperceptions about the feared sensations and situational triggers and relaxation and breathing retraining.
3. **New Evidence on combined treatments** (i.e., medications plus cognitive-behavior therapy) suggest that combined treatment was no better than individual treatments in the short term, however in the long term persons receiving CBT alone maintained most of their treatment gains, whereas those taking medication alone or in combination with CBT deteriorated somewhat. This result led to the recommendation that psychological treatment should be offered initially, followed by drug treatment for those patients who do not respond adequately or for whom psychological treatment is not available.

IV. Specific Phobia

A. A **specific phobia** is an extreme and irrational fear of a specific object or situation that markedly interferes with one's ability to function. Most persons with specific phobias recognize that their fears are unreasonable and many go to great lengths to avoid the objects of their fear. There are as many phobias as there are objects and situations. The four major subtypes of specific phobia are as follows:

1. Persons suffering from **blood-injury-injection phobia** differ from all the other phobias in that they experience drops in heart rate and blood pressure and increased urges to faint. This vasovagal reaction occurs in response to blood, injury, or the possibility of an injection and has a strong genetic component. The phobia develops over the possibility of having a vasovagal response. Mean age of onset for this phobia is 9.
2. A **situational phobia** refers to a group of phobias characterized by fear of public transportation or enclosed places (e.g., planes, trains, elevators, small enclosed spaces). Onset of this phobia is in the early to mid 20s. Persons with situational phobias do not experience panic attacks outside their feared situation.
3. **Natural environment phobia** concerns extreme fears of situations or events occurring in nature, such as heights, storms, or water. People may be biologically prepared to fear some of these stimuli; however, to call such fears a phobia requires that the response be persistent and that it interferes with life functioning.
4. **Animal phobia** refers to fears of animals and insects. To be considered a phobia, such otherwise common fears must interfere with functioning. The mean age of onset for these phobias is approximately 7.

5. **Other phobias** is a category that includes phobias that do not neatly fit into one of the other four categories (e.g., fear of choking, vomiting). Other phobias that are frequent and cause substantial problems include:
    a. **Illness phobias**, or fears of contracting a disease or settings where germs could be found.
    b. **Choking phobia**, or fear and avoidance of swallowing pills, food, or fluids, and can result in significant weight loss.

B. **Separation anxiety disorder (SAD)** is an anxiety disorder specific to childhood; SAD is characterized by unrealistic and persistent worry that something terrible will happen to one's parents or oneself. As a result, the child may refuse to attend school or sleep alone because of separation from parents. School phobia, on the other hand, is a fear that is focused on something specific to the school situation and the child can leave parents or other attachment figures to go somewhere other than school. Separation anxiety typically dissipates as the child ages.

C. Specific fears are quite common, and the most common phobias are of *snakes* and *heights.* With the exception of fear of heights, most persons with specific phobia are female. Hispanics are two times more likely to report specific phobias than white Americans. Specific phobias affect about 11% of the population, although people with the disorder are often not referred for treatment. Phobias tend to run a chronic course.

D. The **causes of phobias** are quite complex. Some, but not all, specific phobias are caused by exposure to traumatic events. Persons may also develop a specific phobia by experiencing a false alarm or panic attack (e.g., during driving), observing someone else experience severe fear (e.g., during a dental visit), or being told of some danger (information transmission). In addition, however, a person with specific phobia must develop anxiety *over the possibility of experiencing another traumatic event or false alarm.*

E. The basic **treatment** of specific phobia is straightforward and involves structured and consistent exposure-based exercises in a supervised therapeutic context. In addition, tension and release of muscle groups is utilized to induce relaxation.

V. Social Phobia

A. **Social phobia** refers to individuals who are extremely and painfully shy in almost all social and performance-related situations; however, social phobia is more than shyness. Persons who are extremely and painfully shy in almost all social situations meet DSM-IV-TR criteria for a subtype of **social phobia—generalized type**, occasionally called social anxiety disorder. Social phobia is illustrated in the textbook with the case of Billy.

B. As many as 13.3% of the general population suffer from social phobia at some point in their lives, making social phobia the most prevalent psychological disorder. Females are slightly more represented than males, but males tend to seek help more frequently than females. Social phobia begins during adolescence with a peak age of onset at about 15 years; most are also single.

C. The **causes of social phobia** are complex. It appears that humans may be biologically predisposed or prepared to fear angry, critical, or rejecting people or faces. In addition, some infants are predisposed to agitation and hyperarousal when faced with new stimuli; such infants may also be predisposed to increased inhibition. Three pathways to developing social phobia include:
   1. Biological vulnerability to develop anxiety or to be socially inhibited. This vulnerability may be increased under stress or when events are perceived as uncontrollable.
   2. A persons may also experience an unexpected panic attack (i.e., false alarm) during a social situation or experience a social trauma resulting in conditioning (i.e., a learned alarm). In these scenarios, conditioning may occur and social settings may be avoided.
   3. Finally, modeling of *socially anxious parents* may also play an etiological role in the development of social phobia. Indeed, for a social anxiety disorder to develop an individual with pre-existing vulnerabilities must also have learned growing up that social evaluation is dangerous.

D. Cognitive-behavioral treatment for social phobia includes rehearsal or role-play of feared social situations in a group setting. In addition, intensive cognitive therapy and social support may be employed. Evidence suggests that the exposure component is more important in treatment than the cognitive component. Beta blockers are ineffective. Tricyclic antidepressants and monoamine oxidase inhibitors are drugs which have been found to reduce social anxiety. In 1999, the SSRI Paxil was approved by the FDA for treatment of social anxiety disorder. Relapse is common when medications are discontinued.

VI. Posttraumatic Stress Disorder

A. The emotional disorder that often arises after a trauma such as war, assault, natural disaster, or death of a loved one is **posttraumatic stress disorder(PTSD)**. According to the DSM-IV-TR, a person with PTSD must have been exposed to some event during which he/she feels fear, helplessness, or horror. Then, the person continues to reexperience the event through memories, reenactments, nightmares, or flashbacks. Cues that remind the person of the event are avoided and emotional responsiveness is numbed. Often such individuals are chronically overaroused, easily startled, and quick to anger. PTSD is illustrated in the textbook with the case of The Joneses. The DSM-IV-TR subdivides PTSD in acute and chronic types.
   1. **Acute PTSD** may be diagnosed 1-3 months after the traumatic event, whereas **chronic PTSD** is diagnosed after 3 months. PTSD cannot be diagnosed sooner than 1 month post-trauma.
   2. Chronic PTSD is associated with more long-term avoidance and greater comorbidity than acute PTSD.

3. If a person does not show any symptoms until long after the traumatic event, then a diagnosis of delayed onset PTSD is warranted.

B. **Acute stress disorder** is a new disorder in the DSM-IV, and refers to PTSD occurring within the first month after a trauma. The different name emphasizes the very severe reaction that some people have immediately following a traumatic event. PTSD symptoms are accompanied by severe dissociative symptoms. This disorder was included in the DSM-IV so that people with early severe reactions could receive insurance coverage for immediate treatment.

C. Recent surveys indicate that among the population, approximately 7.8% have experienced PTSD, and that combat and sexual assault are the most common traumas.

D. Key etiological factors of PTSD include close exposure to the trauma and intensity of the traumatic experience, with more severe trauma associated with a higher proportion of PTSD victims. Experience with unpredictable or uncontrollable events in the context of less severe traumas represent important psychological vulnerabilities. Biological /genetic vulnerability to anxiety is also a significant factor, as are possible neurobiological effects and changes in the locus coeruleus. Moreover, trauma may alter brain structure and function, with studies showing damage to the hippocampus (which plays an important role in learning and memory) in groups of patients with combat PTSD and adult survivors of childhood sexual abuse. Finally, social and cultural factors, particularly having strong and supportive people around, seems to lessen the risk of developing PTSD.

E. The psychological **treatment of PTSD** typically focuses on having the person gradually re-experience aspects of the traumatic event within a supportive context to develop effective coping procedures and to produce corrective emotional learning. This is referred to as *catharsis* in psychoanalysis. Because recreating the trauma is not desirable, **imaginal exposure** is usually conducted. Treatment may be complicated, however, by repressed memories of an event that are triggered and flood back to the person in a frightening manner. Some SSRIs (e.g., Prozac, Paxil) may be helpful for PTSD because they relieve the severe anxiety and panic attacks that are so prominent with this disorder.

VII. Obsessive-Compulsive Disorder

A. **Obsessive-compulsive disorder (OCD)** is similar in many respects to the other anxiety disorders, but the dangerous event in OCD is not external but internal (i.e., thoughts, images, impulses). **Obsessions** are intrusive and nonsensical thoughts, images, or urges that one tries to resist or eliminate. **Compulsions** are thoughts or actions designed to suppress the thoughts and provide relief. Compulsions may be behavioral (e.g., hand washing, checking) or mental (e.g., counting, praying), and usually bear no logical relation to the obsession. OCD is illustrated in the textbook with the case of Richard.

1. **Typical obsessions** include thoughts about contamination, aggressive impulses, sexual content, somatic concerns, and the need for symmetry (i.e., keeping things in perfect order or doing something in a very specific way). Most persons with OCD display multiple obsessions.
2. **Typical compulsions** include checking and order and arranging, followed by washing and cleaning. Most persons with OCD present with cleaning and washing or checking rituals. Persons with **washing rituals** often fear contact with contaminating objects and wash to restore their sense of safety and control. **Checking rituals**, however, serve to prevent a future imagined disaster or catastrophe.
3. Aggressive and sexual obsessions seem to lead to checking rituals, whereas obsessions with symmetry often lead to ordering and arranging or repeating rituals. Obsessions with contamination lead to washing rituals. Some persons compulsively hoard things.

B. The lifetime prevalence of OCD is 2.6%, although 10-15% of normal college students engaged in checking behavior substantial enough to score within the range of patients with OCD. Most persons with OCD are female, and mean age of onset is early adolescence to young adulthood. In children, the sex ratio is reversed due, in part, to the tendency for boys to develop OCD earlier than girls. OCD is typically chronic and the symptomatology of OCD appears stable across cultures.

C. The causes of OCD parallel those for other anxiety disorders. However, those with OCD probably have early life experiences with dangerous or unacceptable thoughts. This may be especially true for persons exposed to fundamental religious beliefs, where thoughts and actions are often not distinguished. Persons with OCD equate thoughts with the specific actions or activity represented by the thought, a phenomenon referred to as thought-action fusion (e.g., thinking that the thought of abortion is the moral equivalent of actually having an abortion). Believing that some thoughts are unacceptable and therefore must be suppressed puts one at greater risk for OCD.

D. **Treatment of OCD** includes drug therapy to target the serotonergic neurotransmitter system, exposure and ritual prevention, hospitalization, and psychosurgery (cingulotomy). Clomipramine and other SSRIs seem to benefit up to 60% of patients with OCD; however, relapse is common when medications are discontinued. The most effective psychological treatment is exposure and ritual prevention (ERP). Combined exposure and response prevention treatment with medication does not work as well compared to ERP alone. Psychosurgery is reserved from intractable cases of OCD that fail to respond to other less invasive forms of treatment.

OVERALL SUMMARY

This chapter outlines the concept of anxiety, fear, and its related disorders. Anxiety is a future oriented state characterized by negative affect in which a person focuses on the possibility of uncontrollable danger or misfortune. Fear is a present-oriented mood state characterized by strong urges to escape and a surge of the sympathetic branch of the autonomic nervous system. This chapter provides detailed descriptions of the nature and phenomenology of anxiety and panic attacks, and each of the major anxiety disorders (i.e., generalized anxiety disorder, panic attacks and panic disorder, agoraphobia, specific and social phobia, posttraumatic stress disorder, and obsessive-compulsive disorder). For each, case examples are provided as well as summaries of symptomatology, course, prevalence, and etiological factors. Psychological and drug treatments are also discussed.

KEY TERMS

Agoraphobia (p. 122)
Animal phobia (p. 133)
Anxiety (p. 113)
Behavioral inhibition system (BIS) (p. 115)
Blood-injection-injury phobia (p. 132)
Compulsions (p. 147)
Fear (p. 114)
Fight/flight system (FFS) (p. 116)
Generalized anxiety disorder (p. 118)
Natural environment phobia (p. 133)
Obsessions (p. 147)
Obsessive-compulsive disorder (p. 147)
Panic (p. 114)
Panic attack (p. 114)
Panic control treatment (p. 129)
Panic disorder with agoraphobia (p. 122)
Panic disorder without agoraphobia (p. 123)
Posttraumatic stress disorder (PTSD) (p. 141)
Separation anxiety disorder (p. 133)
Situational phobia (p. 132)
Specific phobia (p. 131)

INFOTRAC KEY TERM EXERCISES

Each exercise is linked to key terms from the Wadsworth InfoTrac on-line searchable database. Key terms must be entered exactly as written.

Exercise 1: **Is Online Sexual Addiction a Form of Obsessive-Compulsive Disorder?**
Article: A99514094
Citation: (A brief summary of assessment and treatment issue for compulsive online sexual activity--Part 2). Gale H. Golden; Alvin Cooper.

Annals of the American Psychotherapy Association, Spring 2003 v6 i1 p28(4)

Many people are being diagnosed with so-called sex addiction; a diagnosis not formally recognized in the DSM-IV. Such persons report obsessions with sex and irresistible compulsions to engage in excessive sexual activity. Review the InfoTrac article on this topic, and provide an overview of assessment and treatment issues related to online sexual activity. Based on what you have learned about obsessive-compulsive disorder, make an argument for or against the claim that compulsive online sexual activity is really obsessive-compulsive disorder in disguise. Limit your answer to 3-5 typed double-spaced pages.

Exercise 2: Recovered Memories for Childhood Trauma: Separating Fact From Fiction
Key Term: *False Memory Syndrome*

Trauma early in life (e.g., sexual assault, physical abuse) can often have lasting effects on behavioral and psychological functioning. Yet, psychologists face challenges when trying to separate fact from fiction with regard to extent of childhood abuse and its relation to present functioning, particularly in adult survivors of alleged child sexual abuse who present with symptoms of post-traumatic stress disorder. Such concerns have received national attention under the headings "False Memory Syndrome" and "Recovered Memory." Review some of the InfoTrac article(s) on this topic, and describe the psychological, ethical, and legal issues involved in the assessment of past history of child trauma. In so doing, evaluate whether therapists can really plant false traumatic memories in their clients?, and whether such memories could result in the symptoms associated with posttraumatic stress disorder. Limit your answer to 3-5 typed double-spaced pages.

Exercise 3 (Future Trend): Using Medications to Minimize the Psychological Impact of Trauma: Is this a Good Thing?

Roger Pitman and colleagues have been investigating the efficacy of several medications as a means to minimize the lasting impact of traumatic events. Such medications, delivered shortly after the trauma, appear to minimize the likelihood of subsequent PTSD symptoms. Nonetheless, some might argue that traumatic events, though undesirable, ought to be processed fully for meaningful recovery. Drugs that interfere with this process are viewed as counter therapeutic, while implicitly conveying that trauma memories are bad and should be minimized. One could envision similar approaches with other forms of human suffering (guilt, shame, regret), raising obvious moral and ethical concerns. This topic could be integrated into the discussion of PTSD and its treatment, and lends itself nicely to an in-class debate format. The links below provide some additional information on this and related topics.

http://www.news.harvard.edu/gazette/2004/03.18/01-ptsd.html
http://www.grailwerk.com/docs/bostonglobe10.htm
http://www.villagevoice.com/issues/0304/baard.php
http://my.webmd.com/content/article/85/98584.htm?printing=true
http://ist-socrates.berkeley.edu/~kihlstrm/trauma.htm

CLASSROOM ACTIVITIES, DEMONSTRATIONS, AND LECTURE TOPICS

1. **Activity: Preparedness and the Pathways to Phobic Fear Acquisition.** Objects of phobic fear are nonrandomly distributed to objects or situations that were threatening to

the survival of the species throughout the course of evolution. This evolutionary perspective is described under the concept of preparedness. That is, we are prepared to more readily associate fear with some objects or situations (e.g., snakes, heights) over others (e.g., pajamas, electrical outlets) even though both may be associated with panic or trauma. Moreover, we know that fears may be acquired via direct conditioning, or indirectly through observational learning or information transmission. To illustrate both concepts, have students write down an object or situation that they are particularly afraid of, including what event(s) they think led to the development of this top fear. Then, collect the sheets and categorize and tally the lists (or a representative sample thereof, particularly for large classes) on the board or via overhead. What you should find is that most students report fearing objects or situations that have some prepared evolutionary basis. You should also be able to illustrate that few student can recall actual direct conditioning events to explain how their fears developed, and that many may simply say "I can't remember how my fear started." This exercise is a good spring board to a discussion of the nature and etiology of phobias, including the relation between phobias and impairment in life functioning.

2. **Activity: Demonstrating What Panic Attacks are Like.** This exercise is designed to help students appreciate what it might be like to have the breathing difficulties and other autonomic symptoms associated with a panic attack. You will need 4" coffee stirring straws with a tiny lumen (obtained from restaurants, grocery stores, or your campus food court/cafeteria). Before beginning this exercise, inform students that this activity may lead to shortness of breath and may not be appropriate for those with respiratory difficulties due to colds, asthma, or other problems. Also inform students that this exercise is entirely voluntary; though participation is encouraged. Distribute one straw to each student. While seated, students should practice breathing only through the straw. They should avoid breathing through their noses or around the straw. Have students stand and, while continuing to breathe only through the straw, run in place for five minutes. Discuss the students' experiences after running. Many find they become so short of breath they cannot continue to exercise as designed. Many will also report feeling light headed, dizzy, tingly, and some may experience increased perspiration. Explore what it might be like to experience shortness of breath and the related sensations, particularly out of the blue in the course of their daily routine (e.g., going to class, when out on a date, at the library, a party, a movie, driving in a car, to name a few). Could they imagine how a panic attack might follow or coincide with the experience of these kinds of physical symptoms? Finally, it is important to have students understand that panic attacks are often very sudden events, and that their physical and psychological experience at the end of the straw exercise would happen much more abruptly during an actual panic attack. I often illustrate the concept of abruptness by asking students whether they have ever been pulled over for speeding. Many students will report yes. I then ask them to imagine how they felt when they looked into their rear view mirror and saw flashing blue lights and a police car riding their tail. Most report feeling gripped by fear, including a sinking feeling in the stomach, nervousness, and the like. The immediacy of this reaction is analogous to a panic attack.

3. **Activity: Demonstration of Graduated Exposure for Phobias or Panic.** Students often appreciate being able to see what treatment might look like. Devise a hypothetical

hierarchy of exposure for a common specific phobia or for panic disorder. Then, ask for a student volunteer and demonstrate how you would proceed to conduct exposure therapy including the therapist-client issues you would consider as you move up the rungs of the fear hierarchy.

4. **Activity: Reliving Trauma in Therapy.** Students often have a difficult time understanding why one would want to have a patient suffering from PTSD relive memories and emotions associated with their trauma in therapy. Most often, students find treatments such as trauma processing and flooding unethical and inhumane. This is a good opportunity to discuss the rationale for reliving the trauma in therapy and why it is believed to be beneficial for the patient.

5. **Activity: Student Debate on the Efficacy of Medications vs. Psychological Interventions in the Treatment of Anxiety-Related Disorders.** Have students select an anxiety disorder of interest. Then, for each anxiety-disorder, have students divide up into debate teams. One team is to take a pro medication perspective for a particular anxiety disorder, and the other a pro psychotherapy perspective. Have the respective teams go to the library and research the evidence and arguments favoring their positions. During class, follow discussion of each anxiety disorder with the corresponding debate. For example, after you cover panic disorder, have the debate teams present their cases for either drug treatment or psychotherapy. Use the debate as a springboard for class discussion about the current state-of-the-art regarding treatment efficacy, including how taking a one-sided position can be problematic when devising treatment.

SUPPLEMENTARY READING MATERIAL FOR CHAPTER FIVE

(I = These sources can be found on "*Infotrac, the online library*" provided by Wadsworth and Brooks/Cole Publishing.)

Barlow, D. H. (2001). Anxiety and its disorders: The nature and treatment of anxiety and panic, 2nd ed. New York: Guilford.

Barlow, D. H. (2000). Unraveling the mysteries of anxiety and its disorders from the perspective of emotion theory. American Psychologist, 55, 1247-1263.

Barlow, D. H., Brown, T. A., & Craske, M. G. (1994). Definitions of panic attacks and panic disorder in the DSM-IV: Implications for research. Journal of Abnormal Psychology, 103, 553-564.

Craske, M. G., & Barlow, D. H. (2000). Mastery of your anxiety and panic, 3rd ed. New York: The Psychological Corporation.

Craske, M. G. (2003). *The origins of phobias and anxiety disorders: Why more women than men?* Amsterdam: Elsevier.

Bouton, M. E., Mineka, S., & Barlow, D. H. (2001). A modern learning theory perspective on the etiology of panic disorder. Psychological Review, 108, 4-32.

Eisen, A. R., Kearney, C. A., & Schaefer, C. E. (Eds.) (1995). Clinical handbook of anxiety disorders in children and adolescents. Northvale, NJ: Jason Aronson.

McCann, I. L., & Pearlman, L. A. (1990). Psychological trauma and the adult survivor: Theory, therapy and transformation. New York: Brunner/Mazel.

Mineka, S., Watson, D., & Clark, L. A. (1998). Comorbidity of anxiety and unipolar mood disorders. Annual Review of Psychology, 49, 377(36).

Ruiz-Caballero, J. A., & Bermudez, J. (1997). Anxiety and attention: Is there an attentional bias for positive emotional stimuli? The Journal of General Psychology, 124, 194(17).

Steketee, G. S. (1996). Treatment of obsessive-compulsive disorder. New York: Guilford.

Tuma, A. H., & Maser, J. D. (Eds.) (1985). Anxiety and the anxiety disorders. Hillsdale, NJ: Erlbaum.

Walker, J. R., Norton, G. R., & Ross, C. A. (Eds.) (1991). Panic disorder and agoraphobia: A comprehensive guide for the practitioner. Pacific Grove, CA: Brooks/Cole.

SUPPLEMENTARY 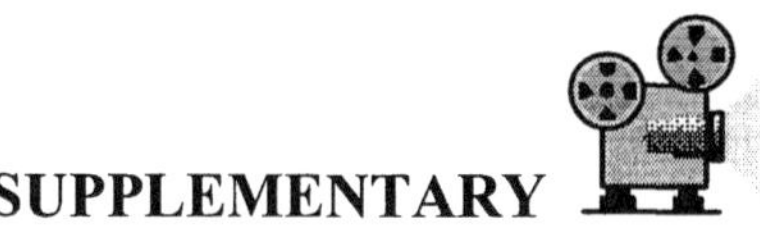 VIDEO RESOURCES FOR CHAPTER FIVE

Abnormal psychology inside/out vol. 1. (*available through your International Thomson Learning representative).* The case of Steve, diagnosed with panic disorder, illustrates panic disorder. Steve reported his first panic attack while driving at the age of 39. At the time, he thought it was a heart attack and felt many of the typical symptoms associated with an attack. He also describes nocturnal panic attacks and has experienced at least 6 months of depression. Steve's panic attacks resulted in agoraphobic tendencies to avoid certain situations, including fear of heights. (2 min 77 sec)

The case of Chuck, diagnosed with obsessive-compulsive disorder, illustrates constant checking and intruding thoughts. He has a long history of depression and the OCD and depression have coexisted since he was a child. When questioned about his current state of depression he humorously stated that seven years of drugs and psychotherapy have helped. (13 min)

As good as it gets. (Hollywood Film; Romance). Jack Nicholson portrays a homophobic, racist novelist with an obsessive compulsive disorder.

Born on the fourth of July. (Hollywood Film; Drama/War/Biography). Tom Cruise depicts a paralyzed Vietnam veteran coping with re-integration into post-war life. The film has particularly compelling scenes of VA hospitals during that time.

Chattahoochee. (Hollywood Film, Drama). Korean war veteran with posttraumatic stress disorder is hospitalized and treated. Dennis Hopper plays a major role as a fellow patient.

CNN today, abnormal psychology, vol 1. (*available through your International Thomson Learning representative).* Different cases of women experiencing panic attacks are presented. This segment discusses prevalence of panic disorder and difficulties regarding correct diagnosis by physicians. Closes with a promise of CBT. (2 min)

A second segment depicts several cases of men with PTSD. Discusses how PTSD affects brain function and suggests a possible physical cause of PTSD. (2 min)

Cognitive therapy for panic disorder. (APA Psychotherapy Videotape Series II: Specific Treatments for Specific Problems, American Psychological Association, 1-800-374-2721). This video illustrates the process of cognitive therapy for panic disorder. (45 min)

Copycat. (Hollywood Film; Suspense/Drama). Sigourney Weaver stars as criminal psychologist Helen Hudson who is involved in unlocking the psyches of her previous subjects— an incurable psychotic (Harry Connick, Jr.)—who almost murdered her. Now she's an agoraphobic, living a terrified existence defined by the walls of her apartment, with her computer modem and her loyal and compassionate assistant, Andy, her only links to the outside world. This films provides an excellent depiction of extreme agoraphobia.

Extending the boundaries of treatment for panic. (Insight Media: 2162 Broadway, New York, NY 10024/ (800)-233-9910). This video explains the clinical goals of treatment of panic disorder, including the alleviation of attacks and relief of such symptoms as agoraphobia, anticipatory anxiety, phobic avoidance, and effective treatment strategies. It assesses the relative benefits of pharmacotherapy, cognitive-behavioral therapy, and combined regimens. (90 min)

Fear and anxiety. (Films for the Humanities and Sciences, Princeton, NJ, 1-800-257-5126). In this program, expert panelists discuss symptoms of anxiety disorders, how anxiety impacts everyday life, the relationship between fear and emotional memory, and new developments in treatment. (56 min)

Fear itself: agoraphobia (Films for the Humanities and Sciences, Princeton, NJ, 1-800-257-5126). Explores the organic causes of phobias as well as possible treatments, focusing on agoraphobia. (26 min)

Obsessive-compulsive disorder: The boy who couldn't stop washing. (Films for the Humanities and Sciences, Princeton, NJ, 1-800-257-5126). Adapted Phil Donahue show with Dr. Judith Rapport, author of the book by the same title. Considers symptoms, diagnosis, and possible cures of OCD. (28 min)

Panic attacks. (Films for the Humanities and Sciences, Princeton, NJ, 1-800-257-5126). Covers the diagnosis and treatment of panic attacks and related disorders. (15 min)

Posttraumatic stress disorder (videotape). Princeton, NJ: Films for the Humanities and Sciences.

Things that go bump: Facing our fears. (Prime Post, Los Angeles, CA, 1-323-878-0782). This multi-part series that aired on the Discovery Health Channel cover the etiology and treatment of specific phobias, social phobia, and panic disorder.

Treatment and assessment of childhood depression and anxiety. (Insight Media: 2162 Broadway, New York, NY 10024/ (800)-233-9910). Focusing on the broadening pharmacological treatment options for childhood depression and anxiety disorders, this video examines diagnostic criteria, epidemiology, and known neurobiological factors. It discusses separation anxiety disorder, selective mutism, post-traumatic stress disorder, and generalized anxiety disorder. Produced by Distance Learning Network. (120 min)

INTERNET 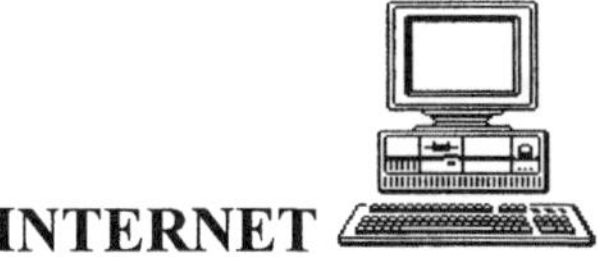 RESOURCES FOR CHAPTER FIVE

Agoraphobia
http://www.mentalhealth.com/fr20.html
Provides a description of agoraphobia and a set of related links.

Anxiety Disorders Association of America (ADAA)
http://www.adaa.org/
This is the official web site of the Anxiety Disorders Association of America (ADAA). The ADAA promotes the prevention and cure of anxiety disorders and works to improve the lives of all people who suffer from them.

Anxiety Disorders Education Program
http://www.nimh.nih.gov/anxiety/
The Anxiety Disorders Education Program is a national education campaign developed by the National Institute of Mental Health (NIMH) to increase awareness among the public and health care professionals that anxiety disorders are real medical illnesses that can be effectively diagnosed and treated. This web site is an excellent resource.

Anxiety Today
http://www.thegrid.net/dakaiser/today/anxiety.htm
Is a huge mega site of current research and resources related to anxiety disorders.

Generalized Anxiety Disorder
http://www.mentalhealth.com/dis/p20-an07.html

This is a page located at the "Internet Mental Health" web site. It provides information specific to generalized anxiety disorder, including treatments, research references, books, magazine articles, and other related links.

Mental Health Net
http://www.cmhc.com/

This site may be the largest mental health site on the world-wide web. Includes links to other mental health-related sites, an online magazine for self-help organizations plus a directory for therapists.

National Anxiety Foundation
http://lexington-on-line.com/naf.html

Information on panic disorder, obsessive-compulsive disorder, and a directory of anxiety health care professionals are available at this site.

Obsessive-Compulsive Foundation (OCF)
http://www.ocfoundation.org/

This web page, developed by the Obsessive-Compulsive Foundation and the Mend Association, includes information on support groups, services, and publications on this disorder.

The Phobia List
http://phobialist.com/

This site provides a comprehensive list of the names of all phobias, including additional links to other phobia sites.

The National Center for PTSD
http://www.ncptsd.org/

This web site provides a wealth of information about PTSD, including current research and available treatments.

WARNING SIGNS FOR GENERALIZED ANXIETY DISORDER

- Continuous worry about major and minor events without just cause
- Headaches and other aches and pains for no apparent reason
- Constant bodily tension, feelings of fatigue, and difficulty relaxing
- Difficulty focusing on one thing or task at a time
- Frequent irritability (i.e., getting crabby or grouchy)
- Trouble falling asleep or staying asleep
- Experience excessive sweatiness or hot flashes
- Feeling of having a lump in throat or feeling the need to vomit when worried

WARNING SIGNS FOR PANIC DISORDER

- Repeated experience of sudden bursts of fear for no reason
- Experience of chest pains or a racing heart
- Feeling dizzy, difficulty breathing, or experiencing excessive sweating
- Frequent stomach problems and the feeling to vomit
- Shaking, trembling, or tingling sensations
- Feeling out of control
- Feeling that one's reactions are unreal
- Fear of dying or going crazy

WARNING SIGNS FOR SPECIFIC PHOBIAS

- Feelings of panic, dread, horror, or terror in response to thoughts, images, or exposure to a specific object or situation (e.g., snakes, heights, planes)
- Recognition that the fear goes beyond normal boundaries and the actual threat of danger
- Reactions that are automatic and uncontrollable, practically taking over the person's thoughts
- Rapid heartbeat, shortness of breath, trembling, and an overwhelming desire to flee the situation—all the physical reactions associated with extreme fear
- Extreme measures taken to avoid the feared object or situation

WARNING SIGNS FOR SEPARATION ANXIETY DISORDER

- Child feels unsafe staying in a room by themselves
- Child displays clinging behavior
- Child displays excessive worry and fear about parents or about harm to themselves
- Child shadows the mother or father around the house
- Child has difficulty going to sleep
- Child has frequent nightmares
- Child has exaggerated, unrealistic fears of animals, monster, burglars, fear being alone in the dark, or has severe tantrums when forced to go to school

WARNING SIGNS FOR SOCIAL PHOBIA

- Feeling afraid or uncomfortable around other people
- Difficulty being in situations where other people are involved
- Intense fear of embarrassment
- Constant fear of making a mistake and being watched and judged by others
- Fear of embarrassment results in avoidance of important social activities
- Excessive worry about upcoming social situations
- Frequent blushing, sweating, trembling, or nausea before or after a social event
- Avoidance of social situations (e.g., school events, making speeches)
- Consumption of alcohol as a means to reduce such social fears

WARNING SIGNS FOR POSTTRAUMATIC STRESS DISORDER

- Recurring thoughts or nightmares about the event
- Having trouble sleeping or changes in appetite
- Experiencing anxiety and fear, especially when exposed to events or situations reminiscent of the trauma
- Being on edge, being easily startled or becoming overly alert
- Feeling depressed, sad and having low energy
- Experiencing memory problems including difficulty in remembering aspec of the trauma
- Feeling "scattered" and unable to focus on work or daily activities
- Having difficulty making decisions
- Feeling irritable, easily agitated, or angry and resentful
- Feeling emotionally "numb," withdrawn, disconnected or different from others
- Spontaneously crying, feeling a sense of despair and hopelessness
- Feeling extremely protective of, or fearful for, the safety of loved ones
- Not being able to face certain aspects of the trauma, and avoiding activities places, or even people that remind you of the event

WARNING SIGNS FOR OBSESSIVE-COMPULSIVE DISORDER

- Feeling of being trapped in a pattern of unwanted and upsetting thoughts
- Feeling a need to repeat thoughts/behaviors over and over for no good reason
- Upsetting thoughts or images repeatedly enter one's mind
- Feeling an inability to stop thoughts or images
- Difficultly stopping oneself from doing things again and again (e.g., counting, checking on things, washing hands, re-arranging objects, doing things until it feels right, collecting useless objects)
- Excessive worry that terrible things will happen if not careful
- Fear that you will harm someone you care about

DSM-IV-TR Criteria for Panic Disorder

A. Recurrent unexpected Panic Attacks

Criteria for Panic Attack: A discrete period of intense fear or discomfort, in which four (or more) of the following symptoms developed abruptly and reached a peak within 10 minutes:

1. palpitations, pounding heart, or accelerated heart rate
2. sweating
3. trembling or shaking
4. sensations of shortness of breath or smothering
5. feeling of choking
6. chest pain or discomfort
7. nausea or abdominal distress
8. feeling dizzy, unsteady, lightheaded, or faint
9. derealization (feelings of unreality) or depersonalization (being detached from oneself)
10. fear of losing control or going crazy
11. fear of dying
12. paresthesias (numbness or tingling sensations)
13. chills or hot flushes

B. At least one of the attacks has been followed by 1 month (or more) of one (or more) of the following:

1. persistent concern about having additional attacks
2. worry about the implications of the attack or its consequences (e.g., losing control, having a heart attack, "going crazy")
3. a significant change in behavior related to the attacks

C. The Panic Attacks are not due to the direct physiological effects of a substance (e.g., a drug of abuse, a medication) or a general medical condition (e.g., hyperthyroidism).

D. The Panic Attacks are not better accounted for by another mental disorder, such as Social Phobia (e.g., occurring on exposure to feared social situations), Specific Phobia (e.g., on exposure to a specific phobic situation), Obsessive-Compulsive Disorder (e.g., on exposure to dirt in someone with an obsession about contamination), Posttraumatic Stress Disorder (e.g., in response to stimuli associated with a severe stressor), or Separation Anxiety Disorder (e.g., in response to being away from home or close relatives).

Transparency 5-2

DSM-IV-TR Criteria for Panic Disorder with Agoraphobia

A. Both 1 and 2:

1. Recurrent unexpected panic attacks are present.

2. At least one of the attacks has been followed by 1 month (or more) of one (or more) of the following: (a) persistent concern about having additional attacks, (b) worry about the implications of the attack or its consequences (e.g., losing control, having a heart attack, 'going crazy'), or (c) a significant change in behavior related to the attacks.

B. The presence of agoraphobia in which the predominant complaint is anxiety about being in places or situations from which escape might be difficult or embarrassing, or in which help may not be available in the event of an unexpected or situationally predisposed panic attack or panic-like symptoms. Agoraphobic fears typically involve characteristic clusters of situations that include being outside the home alone; being in a crowd or standing in a line; being on a bridge; and traveling in a bus, train, or automobile.

C. The panic attacks are not due to the direct physiological effects of a substance (e.g., drug of abuse, medication) or a general medical condition (e.g., hyperthyroidism).

D. The panic attacks are not better accounted for by another mental disorder, such as social phobia (e.g., occurring on exposure to feared social situations), specific phobia (e.g., on exposure to a specific social situation), obsessive-compulsive disorder (e.g., on exposure to dirt, in someone with an obsession about contamination), posttraumatic stress disorder (e.g., in response to stimuli associated with a severe stressor), or separation anxiety disorder (e.g., in response to being away from home or close relatives).

DSM-IV-TR Criteria for Generalized Anxiety Disorder

A. Excessive anxiety and worry (apprehensive expectation), occurring more days than not for at least 6 months, about a number of events or activities (such as work or school performance).

B. The person finds it difficult to control the worry.

C. The anxiety and worry are associated with three (or more) of the following six symptoms (with at least some symptoms present for more days than not for the past 6 months). Note: Only one item is required in children.

1. restlessness or feeling keyed up or on edge
2. being easily fatigued
3. difficulty concentrating or mind going blank
4. irritability
5. muscle tension
6. sleep disturbance (difficulty falling or staying asleep, or restless unsatisfying sleep)

D. The focus of the anxiety and worry is not confined to features of an Axis I disorder, e.g., the anxiety or worry is not about having a Panic Attack (as in Panic Disorder), being embarrassed in public (as in Social Phobia), being contaminated (as in Obsessive-Compulsive Disorder), being away from home or close relatives (as in Separation Anxiety Disorder), gaining weight (as in Anorexia Nervosa), having multiple physical complaints (as in Somatization Disorder), or having a serious illness (as in Hypochondriasis), and the anxiety and worry do not occur exclusively during Posttraumatic Stress Disorder.

E. The anxiety, worry, or physical symptoms cause clinically significant distress or impairment in social, occupational, or other important areas of functioning.

F. The disturbance is not due to the direct physiological effects of a substance (e.g., a drug of abuse, a medication) or a general medical condition (e.g., hyperthyroidism) and does not occur exclusively during a Mood Disorder, a Psychotic Disorder, or a Pervasive Developmental Disorder.

DSM-IV-TR Criteria for Specific Phobias

A. Marked and persistent fear that is excessive or unreasonable, cued by the presence or anticipation of a specific object or situation (e.g., flying, heights, animals, receiving an injection, seeing blood).

B. Exposure to the phobic stimulus almost invariably provokes an immediate anxiety response, which may take the form of a situationally bound or situationally predisposed Panic Attack. Note: In children, the anxiety may be expressed by crying, tantrums, freezing, or clinging.

C. The person recognizes that the fear is excessive or unreasonable. Note: In children, this feature may be absent.

D. The phobic situation(s) is avoided or else is endured with intense anxiety or distress.

E. The avoidance, anxious anticipation, or distress in the feared situation(s) interferes significantly with the person's normal routine, occupational (or academic) functioning, or social activities or relationships, or there is marked distress about having the phobia.

F. In individuals under age 18 years, the duration is at least 6 months.

G. The anxiety, Panic Attacks, or phobic avoidance associated with the specific object or situation are not better accounted for by another mental disorder, such as Obsessive-Compulsive Disorder, Posttraumatic Stress Disorder, Separation Anxiety Disorder, Social Phobia, Panic Disorder With Agoraphobia, or Agoraphobia Without History of Panic Disorder.

Specify type:

Animal Type
Natural Environment Type (e.g., heights, storms, water)
Blood-Injection-Injury Type
Situational Type (e.g., airplanes, elevators, enclosed places)
Other Type (e.g., phobic avoidance of situations that may lead to choking, vomiting, or contracting an illness; in children, avoidance of loud sounds or costumed characters)

Transparency 5-5

DSM-IV-TR Criteria for Social Phobia

A. A marked and persistent fear of one or more social or performance situations in which the person is exposed to unfamiliar people or to possible scrutiny by others. The individual fears that he or she will act in a way (or show anxiety symptoms) that will be humiliating or embarrassing. Note: In children, there must be evidence of the capacity for age-appropriate social relationships with familiar people, and the anxiety must occur in peer settings, not just in interactions with adults.

B. Exposure to the feared social situation almost invariably provokes anxiety, which may take the form of a situationally bound or situationally predisposed panic attack. Note: In children, the anxiety may be expressed by crying, tantrums, freezing, or shrinking from social situations with unfamiliar people.

C. The person recognizes that the fear is excessive or unreasonable. Note: In children, this feature may be absent.

D. The feared social or performance situations are avoided or are endured with intense anxiety or distress.

E. The avoidance, anxious anticipation, or distress in the feared social or performance situations) interferes significantly with the person's normal routine, occupational (academic) functioning, or social activities or relationships, or there is marked distress about having the phobia.

F. In individuals under age 18, duration is at least 6 months.

G. The fear or avoidance is not due to the direct physiological effects of a substance (e.g., a drug of abuse, medication) or a general medical condition, and is not better accounted for by another mental disorder (e.g., panic disorder with or without agoraphobia, separation anxiety disorder, body dysmorphic disorder, a pervasive developmental disorder, or schizoid personality disorder).

H. If a general medical condition or another mental disorder is present, the fear in criterion A is unrelated to it; e.g., the fear is not of stuttering, trembling in Parkinson's disease, or exhibiting abnormal eating behavior in anorexia nervosa or bulimia nervosa.

Specify if:

Generalized: if the fears include most social situations

DSM-IV-TR Criteria for Separation Anxiety Disorder

A. Developmentally inappropriate and excessive anxiety concerning separation from home or from those to whom the individual is attached, as evidenced by three (or more) of the following:

1. recurrent excessive distress when separation from home or major attachment figures occurs or is anticipated
2. persistent and excessive worry about losing, or about possible harm befalling, major attachment figures
3. persistent and excessive worry that an untoward event will lead to separation from a major attachment figure (e.g., getting lost or being kidnapped)
4. persistent reluctance or refusal to go to school or elsewhere because of fear of separation
5. persistently and excessively fearful or reluctant to be alone or without major attachment figures at home or without significant adults in other settings
6. persistent reluctance or refusal to go to sleep without being near a major attachment figure or to sleep away from home
7. repeated nightmares involving the theme of separation
8. repeated complaints of physical symptoms (such as headaches, stomachaches, nausea, or vomiting) when separation from major attachment figures occurs or is anticipated

B. The duration of the disturbance is at least 4 weeks.

C. The onset is before age 18 years.

D. The disturbance causes clinically significant distress or impairment in social, academic (occupational), or other important areas of functioning.

E. The disturbance does not occur exclusively during the course of a Pervasive Developmental Disorder, Schizophrenia, or other Psychotic Disorder and, in adolescents and adults, is not better accounted for by Panic Disorder With Agoraphobia.

Specify if:

Early Onset: if onset occurs before age 6 years

Transparency 5-7

DSM-IV-TR Criteria for Posttraumatic Stress Disorder Criteria A and B

A. The person has been exposed to a traumatic event in which both of the following were present:

1. the person experienced, witnessed, or was confronted with an event or events that involved actual or threatened death or serious injury, or a threat to the physical integrity of self or others
2. the person's response involved intense fear, helplessness, or horror. Note: In children, this may be expressed instead by disorganized or agitated behavior

B. The traumatic event is persistently reexperienced in one (or more) of the following ways:

1. recurrent and intrusive distressing recollections of the event, including images, thoughts, or perceptions. Note: In young children, repetitive play may occur in which themes or aspects of the trauma are expressed.
2. recurrent distressing dreams of the event. Note: In children, there may be frightening dreams without recognizable content.
3. acting or feeling as if the traumatic event were recurring (includes a sense of reliving the experience, illusions, hallucinations, and dissociative flashback episodes, including those that occur on awakening or when intoxicated). Note: In young children, trauma-specific reenactment may occur.
4. intense psychological distress at exposure to internal or external cues that symbolize or resemble an aspect of the traumatic event
5. physiological reactivity on exposure to internal or external cues that symbolize or resemble an aspect of the traumatic event

DSM-IV-TR Criteria for Posttraumatic Stress Disorder Criteria C, D, E, and F

C. Persistent avoidance of stimuli associated with the trauma and numbing of general responsiveness (not present before the trauma), as indicated by three (or more) of the following:

1. efforts to avoid thoughts, feelings, or conversations associated with the trauma
2. efforts to avoid activities, places, or people that arouse recollections of the trauma
3. inability to recall an important aspect of the trauma
4. markedly diminished interest or participation in significant activities
5. feeling of detachment or estrangement from others
6. restricted range of affect (e.g., unable to have loving feelings)
7. sense of a foreshortened future (e.g., does not expect to have a career, marriage, children, or a normal life span)

D. Persistent symptoms of increased arousal (not present before the trauma), as indicated by two (or more) of the following:

1. difficulty falling or staying asleep
2. irritability or outbursts of anger
3. difficulty concentrating
4. hypervigilance
5. exaggerated startle response

E. Duration of the disturbance (symptoms in Criteria B, C, and D) is more than 1 month.

F. The disturbance causes clinically significant distress or impairment in social, occupational, or other important areas of functioning.

Specify if:

Acute: if duration of symptoms is less than 3 months
Chronic: if duration of symptoms is 3 months or more

Specify if:

With Delayed Onset: if onset of symptoms is at least 6 months after the stressor

DSM-IV-TR Criteria for Obsessive-Compulsive Disorder Criteria A and B

A. Either obsessions or compulsions:

Obsessions as defined by (1), (2), (3), and (4):

1. recurrent and persistent thoughts, impulses, or images that are experienced, at some time during the disturbance, as intrusive and inappropriate and that cause marked anxiety or distress
2. the thoughts, impulses, or images are not simply excessive worries about real-life problems
3. the person attempts to ignore or suppress such thoughts, impulses, or images, or to neutralize them with some other thought or action
4. the person recognizes that the obsessional thoughts, impulses, or images are a product of his or her own mind (not imposed from without as in thought insertion)

Compulsions as defined by (1) and (2):

1. repetitive behaviors (e.g., hand washing, ordering, checking) or mental acts (e.g., praying, counting, repeating words silently) that the person feels driven to perform in response to an obsession, or according to rules that must be applied rigidly
2. the behaviors or mental acts are aimed at preventing or reducing distress or preventing some dreaded event or situation; however, these behaviors or mental acts either are not connected in a realistic way with what they are designed to neutralize or prevent or are clearly excessive

B. At some point during the course of the disorder, the person has recognized that the obsessions or compulsions are excessive or unreasonable. Note: This does not apply to children.

DSM-IV-TR Criteria for Obsessive-Compulsive Disorder Criteria C, D, and E

C. The obsessions or compulsions cause marked distress, are time consuming (take more than 1 hour a day), or significantly interfere with the person's normal routine, occupational (or academic) functioning, or usual social activities or relationships.

D. If another Axis I disorder is present, the content of the obsessions or compulsions is not restricted to it (e.g., preoccupation with food in the presence of an Eating Disorder; hair pulling in the presence of Trichotillomania; concern with appearance in the presence of Body Dysmorphic Disorder; preoccupation with drugs in the presence of a Substance Use Disorder; preoccupation with having a serious illness in the presence of Hypochondriasis; preoccupation with sexual urges or fantasies in the presence of a Paraphilia; or guilty ruminations in the presence of Major Depressive Disorder).

E. The disturbance is not due to the direct physiological effects of a substance (e.g., a drug of abuse, a medication) or a general medical condition.

Specify if:

With Poor Insight: if, for most of the time during the current episode the person does not recognize that the obsessions and compulsions are excessive or unreasonable

CHAPTER SIX

SOMATOFORM AND DISSOCIATIVE DISORDERS

LEARNING OBJECTIVES

1. Identify the defining features of somatoform disorders and distinguish the major features of hypochondriasis from illness phobia and somatization disorder.
2. Describe the major manifestations of conversion disorder as well as the sensory, motor, and visceral symptoms that characterize this disorder.
3. Understand malingering and factitious disorders and their relation to the diagnosis of somatoform (e.g., conversion disorder) and dissociative disorders (e.g., dissociative identity disorder).
4. Be able to distinguish between depersonalization and derealization.
5. Be able to describe and distinguish between the five types of dissociative disorders: depersonalization disorder, dissociative amnesia, dissociative fugue, dissociative trance disorder, and dissociative identity disorder (e.g., alters, host, and a switch).
6. Discuss important etiological and treatment factors, including important known cultural nuances for each of the dissociative disorders.
7. Discuss false memory syndrome in the context of trauma associated with dissociative disorders.

OUTLINE

I. Somatoform Disorders

A. Persons who are overly preoccupied with their health or body appearance are said to have **somatoform disorders** (soma meaning body). What these disorders share in common is that there is usually no identifiable medical condition causing the physical complaints.

1. The DSM-IV-TR lists five basic somatoform disorders: hypochondriasis, somatization disorder, conversion disorder, pain disorder, and body dysmorphic disorder.
2. In each, individuals are pathologically concerned with the appearance or functioning of their bodies.

B. **Hypochondriasis** has ancient Greek roots, referring to the region below the ribs (i.e., hypochondria) and related organs that were believed to affect mental state. In modern times, the term hypochondriasis refers to physical complaints without a clear cause, and particularly severe anxiety focused on the *possibility* of having a serious disease. Medical reassurance does not seem to help.

1. The textbook describes the case of Gail to illustrate hypochondriasis.
2. The essential problem in hypochondriasis is anxiety. The expression of anxiety differs from other anxiety disorders as follows: In hypochondriasis a person is preoccupied with bodily symptoms and misinterprets them as signs

of illness or disease. Such persons almost always present first to their physician.

   a. Hypochondriasis shares many features with anxiety and mood disorders, and rates of comorbidity with such disorders are high.
   b. Another important feature of hypochondriasis is that **reassurance** from numerous doctors that the person is healthy has, at best, only a short-term positive effect. Often such persons will return to the same or other doctors on the assumption that the doctor missed something initially in ruling out medical reasons for the symptoms. This **disease conviction** has become a core diagnostic feature of hypochondriasis.
   c. Persons with hypochondriasis fear the possibility of already *having* a disease, whereas persons with **illness phobia** are fearful of *developing* a disease. A further point of distinction is that those suffering from hypochondriasis are more likely to misinterpret physical symptoms, display higher rates of checking behaviors, have higher levels of trait anxiety, and have a later age of onset than those with illness phobia.
   d. Persons with panic disorder fear the immediate symptom-related catastrophes that may occur during the few minutes following a panic attack, whereas persons with hypochondriasis focus on a long-term process of illness and disease. Persons with panic disorder are also more likely reassured that their symptoms do not have a medical cause compared to those with hypochondriasis. Finally, hypochondriacal concerns are much broader than those seen with panic disorder.

3. Little is known about the **prevalence of hypochondriasis** in the general population. Approximately 3% of medical patients may meet criteria for hypochondriasis and the sex ratio is 50:50. Hypochondriasis may emerge at any time, with peak periods in adolescence, middle age (40s and 50s), and after age 60. Hypochondriasis has a chronic course.
   a. **Koro** is a culture-specific variant of hypochondriasis found mostly in Chinese males, and reflects the belief, accompanied by severe anxiety and sometimes panic, that the genitals are retracting into the abdomen.
   b. In India, males often show anxious concern about losing semen; a disorder called **dhat**.
4. Hypochondriasis is thought to be caused by **distorted cognitive** or **perceptual and emotional factors**. For example, persons with hypochondriasis tend to interpret ambiguous stimuli such as minor pain as threatening. These cognitive distortions and increased self-focusing tend to create anxiety and subsequently more physical symptoms. Persons with hypochondriasis also have a restricted concept of health as being totally symptom free.
   a. Other etiological factors may include genetics vulnerabilities, overreaction to stress, a tendency to view negative life events as unpredictable and uncontrollable, and modeling of adults with hypochondriasis.
   b. In addition, persons with hypochondriasis may develop the disorder in the context of a stressful life event, experience a disproportionate

incidence of familial disease during childhood, and/or receive substantial attention for illness-related behaviors.

5. Little is known about **treating hypochondriasis**. Recent studies suggest that cognitive-behavioral treatments, incorporating identifying and challenging illness-related misinterpretations of physical symptoms, showing patients how to voluntarily produce the symptoms, coaching patients to rely less on reassurance, and stress management tend to be helpful.
    a. Little evidence exists to support traditional psychodynamic treatment for hypochondriasis. More recent approaches attempt to offer more substantial and sensitive reassurance than is typical in a physician's office and with some encouraging results.

C. **Somatization disorder** (also known as **Briquet's syndrome** until 1980), involves an extended history of physical complaints before age 30 and substantial impairment in social or occupational functioning.

1. The textbook presents the case of Linda to illustrate somatization disorder.
2. Persons with somatization disorder are concerned about the symptoms themselves, whereas persons with hypochondriasis are concerned with what the symptoms might mean.
    a. Moreover, they show little urgency to respond to, or take action about, their symptoms, despite feeling continually weak, and ill.
    b. In somatization disorder, the symptoms become a major part of the person's identity.
3. The DSM-IV-TR requires that the person report 8 symptoms to meet diagnostic criteria, whereas the diagnosis **undifferentiated somatoform disorder** is reserved for persons who report fewer than 8 symptoms.
    a. Somatization disorder is rare, and **prevalence rates** range from 4.4% (in a large city) to 20% of a large sample of primary care patients.
    b. The typical age of onset is adolescence, and most persons with somatization disorder are unmarried women of a lower socioeconomic status.
    c. However, males may display more somatization disorder than females in different cultures.
    d. Somatization disorder typically runs a chronic course.
4. Somatization disorder shares features with hypochondriasis, including a history of family illness or injury during childhood. Mixed results exist regarding genetic contributions, although somatization disorder is strongly linked in family studies to **antisocial personality disorder** (ASPD).
    a. Some evidence suggests that somatization disorder and ASPD (as well as substance abuse and attention deficit hyperactivity disorder) share a **neurobiologically-based disinhibition syndrome**. In essence, persons with these disorders may possess a weak **behavioral inhibition system (BIS)** that does not control the **behavioral activation system (BAS)**.
    b. The **BAS** is a brain system that underlies impulsivity, thrill-seeking behavior, and excitability, whereas the **BIS** is involved in sensitivity to

threat or danger and avoidance of situations or cues suggesting that threat or danger is imminent. Many behaviors and traits associated with somatization disorder also seem to reflect short-term gain (i.e., active BAS) and insensitivity for long-term problems (i.e., weak BIS).

The major difference between somatization disorder and ASPD, however, may involve **level of dependency**. Whereas males tend to display aggression and ASPD, females tend to display dependency and little aggression. Therefore, gender socialization may direct a specific biological vulnerability.

5. **Treatment** is exceedingly difficult, and no treatment exists with demonstrated effectiveness. Treatment of somatization disorder typically involves attempts to reduce the person's tendency to visit numerous medical specialists according to the "symptom of the week."
    a. Use of a **gatekeeper physician**, one assigned to screen all physical complaints and decide on whether further evaluation is warranted, can be helpful.
    b. Additional attention is directed at reducing the supportive consequences of relating to significant others on the basis of physical symptoms.

D. **Conversion disorders** refer to physical malfunctioning without any physical or organic pathology to account for the malfunction, especially in sensory-motor areas. Examples include paralysis, aphonia (i.e., difficulty speaking), mutism, analgesia, seizures, blindness, loss of sense of touch, globus hystericus (i.e., sensation of lump in throat), and astasia-abasia (i.e., weakness in legs and loss of balance). Most conversion symptoms suggest some kind of neurological disease, but can mimic the full range of physical functioning. Conversion disorder is illustrated in the textbook with the case of Eloise.

1. Freud popularized the term "conversion," believing that anxiety from unconscious conflicts somehow converted into physical symptoms to find expression (i.e., anxiety is displaced onto a more acceptable object, in this case physical problems).
2. Several differences exist among those with conversion disorder, actual physical disorder, **malingering** (i.e., deliberately faking symptoms), **factitious disorder** (i.e., symptoms are feigned and under voluntary control, but without any obvious reason for doing so aside from to assume the sick role and gain attention) and **factitious disorder by proxy** (i.e., caregiver making others sick; sometimes referred to as munchausen syndrome by proxy).
    a. First, as with somatization disorder, conversion disorder is often (but not always) marked by **la belle indifference**, or a general apathy toward one's symptoms.
    b. Second, conversion symptoms are usually precipitated by some stressful event.
    c. Third, those with conversion disorder often function normally but display little insight into this ability. Still, an awareness of sensory and motor information is disturbed.

    d. In general, those with conversion disorder are dissociated from sensory-motor awareness, whereas those who malinger or have a factitious disorder attempt to fake this effect (e.g., by faking blindness) and often look worse than blind persons who perform at chance levels on visual discrimination tasks.
3. **Unconscious mental processes** are salient features of conversion disorders, as illustrated by the classic case of Anna O. It is known that persons with small, localized damage to certain parts of their brains can identify objects in their field of vision, but without awareness that they could, in fact, see. The textbook presents the case of Celia to illustrate this concept.
4. Conversion disorders are rare, and **prevalence** estimates in neurological settings range from 1 to 30%, whereas in epilepsy setting the range is between 10 and 20% of cases.
    a. Conversion disorders are seen primarily in women and typically develop during adolescence or shortly thereafter.
    b. Such disorders are also seen more often in less educated, lower socioeconomic status groups where knowledge about disease and medical illness is not well developed.
    c. Conversion reactions are not uncommon in soldiers exposed to combat. Symptoms often disappear, but return later in the same or similar form when a new stressor occurs.
    d. Conversion symptoms are common in some cultural and rural fundamental religious groups. However, the symptoms would not meet criteria for a disorder unless they persist and interfere with life functioning.
5. The **Freudian psychodynamic** view postulates four basic processes in the development of conversion disorder:
    a. Experience of a traumatic event, or unacceptable unconscious conflict.
    b. The person represses the unacceptable conflict and resulting anxiety, thereby making it unconscious.
    c. Anxiety continues to fester and increase and threatens to emerge into consciousness. The person converts the conflict into physical symptoms, and thereby relieves the pressure of having to deal directly with the conflict. The reduction in anxiety is the **primary gain** or reinforcing event that maintains the conversion symptom. Primary gain accounts for the la belle indifference as the conversion resolution of the conflict would not be upsetting to the patient.
    d. Individual receives greatly increased attention and sympathy from loved ones. Freud considered attention/avoidance to represent **secondary gain**.
    e. Little data exists to support Freud's account; though the role of trauma does have support. A modification of Freud's approach stipulates that, following the traumatic event, patients develop symptoms purposefully but detach this motivation from consciousness. The behaviors are subsequently maintained by negative reinforcement.

6. **Treatment** of conversion disorder is similar to treatment for somatization disorder. A core strategy is to identify and attend to the trauma or stressful life event and to remove sources of secondary gain such as working to reduce reinforcing or supportive consequences of the conversion symptoms.

E. **Pain disorder** refers to a disorder where there may have been initial clear reasons for pain, but where psychological factors play a large role in the persistence of pain. It is difficult to judge cases where the causes were primarily physical vs. psychological. An important feature of pain disorder is that the pain is real and it hurts. The textbook presents the cases of a medical student and a woman with cancer to illustrate pain disorder.

F. **Body dysmorphic disorder (BDD)** (or imagined ugliness) involves a preoccupation with some *imagined* defect in appearance despite reasonably normal appearance. That is, the focus is on physical appearance.

1. The textbook illustrates BDD with the case of Jim.
2. Reaction to perceived distortions in facial features is common. These persons are fixated on mirrors, engage in suicidal behavior, display ideas of reference (i.e., thinking that events in the world are somehow related to them and their imagined defect) and avoidance, and experience severe disruption in daily functioning. The condition was previous known as dysmorphophobia (i.e., fear of ugliness).
    a. The predominant focus of attention in adolescence is skin and hair. The disorder is largely influenced by cultural standards of beauty. Examples include skin condition, facial width, slope of nose, and lip, neck, and foot size.
    b. Many persons with BDD become fixated on mirrors and frequently check their appearance. Others show a phobic fear and avoidance of mirrors. Suicidal ideation, attempts, and suicide completion are frequent consequences of BDD.
3. Best estimates of the **prevalence of BDD** are that is it more common that previously thought and that it tends to run a lifelong, chronic course if left untreated.
    a. BDD is seen equally in males and females, few marry, and age of onset ranges from early adolescence through the 20s, peaking at age 18 or 19.
    b. BDD is not seen frequently in mental health settings as BDD sufferers frequently seek out plastic surgeons.
4. **Little is known about the causes or treatment of BDD**, including whether BDD runs in families, biological and predisposing vulnerabilities. Obsessive-compulsive disorder tends to co-occur with BDD and both disorders share similar features (e.g., intrusive thoughts, checking).
    a. There are two and only two treatments for BDD with any evidence of effectiveness:
    b. **SSRIs**, such as clomipramine (Anafranil) and fluvoxamine (Luvox) provide relief for some people; both drugs also work for OCD.

c. **Cognitive-behavior therapy**, specifically exposure and response prevention, has been successful with BDD and OCD.

5. BDD is big business for **plastic surgeons.** As many as 25% of persons requesting plastic surgery meet criteria for BDD. Persons with BDD do not benefit from plastic surgery, and preoccupation with imagined ugliness may actually increase following plastic surgery.

II. Dissociative Disorders

A. **Dissociative disorders** are characterized by alterations or detachments in consciousness or identity involving either dissociation or depersonalization. Dissociative disorders include depersonalization disorder, dissociative amnesia, dissociative fugue, dissociative trance disorder, and dissociative identity disorder. Each involves extreme manifestations of normal variants of depersonalization and derealization experiences.

1. **Depersonalization** involves distortion in perception such that a sense of reality is lost. Symptoms of unreality are characteristic of dissociative disorders because depersonalization is a psychological mechanism whereby one dissociates from reality.
2. **Derealization** involves losing a sense of the external world (e.g., things may seem to change shape or size; people may appear dead or mechanical).
3. Feelings of depersonalization and derealization are also part of other disorders, including panic and acute stress disorder.

B. **Depersonalization disorder** is a very rare condition involving severe and frightening feelings of unreality and detachment such that they dominate an individual's life and interfere with normal functioning. The textbook illustrates depersonalization disorder with the case of Bonnie.

1. Primary problem involves depersonalization and derealization.
2. Limited data suggest that 50% of persons suffering from depersonalization disorder also have another mood or anxiety disorder; mean onset is approximately 16 years of age, and the disorder tends to be chronic.
3. Depersonalization is related to a **distinct cognitive profile**, reflecting cognitive deficits in attention, short-term memory, and spatial reasoning. Such persons are easily distracted. Such deficits correspond with reports of **tunnel vision** (i.e., perceptual distortions) and **mind emptiness** (i.e., difficulty absorbing new information).

C. **Dissociative amnesia** represents several forms of psychogenic memory loss and is most often found in females. The textbook illustrates dissociative amnesia with the case of "The Woman Who Lost Her Memory."

1. Those with **generalized amnesia** are unable to recall anything, including their identity. Generalized amnesia may be lifelong or may extend from a period in the more recent past.
2. More common is **localized or selective amnesia**, or a failure to recall specific (usually traumatic) events during a specific period of time. In most cases of

amnesia, the forgetting is very selective for traumatic events or memories rather than generalized.

D. **Dissociative fugue** is related to dissociative amnesia. Persons with dissociative fugue just take off, and later find themselves in a new place, unable to remember why or how they got there, including an inability to recall their past. Often a new identity is assumed. Dissociative amnesia and fugue usually begin in adulthood, with rapid onset and dissipation, and most are female.

1. Dissociative fugue is illustrated in the textbook with the case of the misbehaving sheriff.
2. A related non-Western variation of dissociative fugue is called **amok** (as in running amok). This disorder is most often seen in males and involves a trancelike state where the person often brutally assaults or sometimes kills persons or animals. Such persons usually do not remember the episode.

E. **Dissociative trance disorder** represents a condition that differs in important ways across cultures. In this condition, the symptoms resemble those of other dissociative disorders, with the exception that dissociative symptoms and sudden changes in personality are attributed to possession of a spirit known to a particular culture. This disorder is more common in women and is often associated with some life stressor. Dissociative traces commonly occur in India, Nigeria, Thailand, and other Asian and African countries. This condition is considered abnormal only if the trance is undesirable and pathological by members of the particular culture.

F. **Dissociative identity disorder (DID)** involves the adoption of new identities (as many as 100), all simultaneously coexisting. In some cases, these identities are complete, each with its own unique set of behaviors, voice, and posture. But in many cases, only a few characteristics are distinct, because identities are partially independent. The textbook illustrates DID with the case of "Jonah: Bewildering Blackouts."

1. Clinical Description
    a. **Alter** refers to the different identities or personalities in DID. Many patients have at least 1 impulsive alter, and cross-gendered alters are not uncommon.
    b. DSM-IV-TR criteria include amnesia, as in dissociative amnesia and dissociative fugue. However, here the defining feature is that certain aspects of the person's identity are dissociated.
2. Characteristics
    a. A **host** is typically the identity that seeks treatment and the identity that tries to keep fragments of identity together; though the host often ends up becoming overwhelmed in the process. The host identity often develops later than the other identities.
    b. **Switch** refers to the transition from one personality to another. Often a switch is instantaneous and may include physical transformations (e.g., posture, facial patterns).

3. Can DID be faked?
    a. First, evidence indicates that persons with DID are suggestible, creating the possibility that personalities are developed from therapists' leading questions. The example of Kenneth Bianchi is presented. The symptoms of DID could be accounted for by therapists who inadvertently suggest the existence of alters to suggestible individuals – a model known as a **sociocognitive model**.
    b. A recent survey of American psychiatrists showed little consensus on the scientific validity of DID.
    c. Objective tests suggest that many people with fragmented identities are not consciously or voluntarily faking (e.g., optical changes, measures of visual acuity, eye muscle balance).
    d. Persons with DID, unlike malingerers, are more likely to hide their symptoms.
4. Average number of identities in DID patients is close to 15.
    a. The ratio of females to males with DID is high (9:1).
    b. Onset of DID is almost always in childhood, often as young as 4 years of age. DID tends to run a chronic lifetime course if left untreated.
    c. Good prevalence data are lacking, but estimates range from 3 to 6% in the United States. DID is associated with high rates of comorbidity.
5. Almost all patients presenting with DID have histories of horrible, unspeakable, child abuse, usually **sadistic sexual or physical abuse**. It is believed that DID is rooted in a natural tendency to escape or dissociate from the unremitting negative affect associated with severe abuse. A lack of social support during the abuse is also important.
    a. There is a growing opinion that DID is a very extreme subtype of PTSD, with an emphasis on the process of dissociation in DID over anxiety as in PTSD.
    b. DID is unlikely to develop after age 9.
6. Persons who eventually develop DID may have a tendency to be **highly suggestible** or possess the ability to have a creative fantasy life. For example, 50% of those with DID remember imaginary playmates in childhood. It is therefore possible that those who are suggestible or hypnotizable are also those who can use dissociation as a defense against traumatic events **(i.e., autohypnotic model)**.
7. There is a biological vulnerability to DID, but it is difficult to pinpoint. For example, about half of patients with **temporal lobe epilepsy** display some type of dissociative symptoms (e.g., development of a new identity fragment). In addition, dissociative symptoms are not associated with trauma in seizure patients, as they are with DID patients without seizure disorders.
8. Evidence supporting the existence of **distorted or illusory memories** comes from experiments by Elizabeth Loftus and her colleagues. The evidence across numerous studies suggests that memories can be planted by strong suggestions by authority figures.

G. Persons with dissociative amnesia and fugue state usually get better on their own without treatment and remember what they have forgotten. For DID, however, the focus is on reintegration of identities and much of the treatment follows similar treatments for PTSD.

1. The fundamental treatment goal with DID is to identify cues or triggers that provoke memories of trauma and/or dissociation and to neutralize them.
2. The patient must also confront and relive the early trauma and gain control over memories of the horrible events.
3. There is no evidence that hypnosis is a necessary part of treatment.

OVERALL SUMMARY

This chapter outlines the primary features of somatoform and dissociative disorders. With respect to the former, the symptoms, prevalence, etiology, and treatment of hypochondriasis, somatization disorder, conversion disorder, and body dysmorphic disorder are discussed. For dissociative disorders, depersonalization, amnesia, and fugue are discussed. The chapter also describes the relation between malingering and factitious disorders in the context of conversion reactions and dissociative identity disorder. In addition, the major characteristics of dissociative trance and dissociative identity disorder are described, including available treatment approaches.

KEY TERMS

Alters (p. 191)
Body dysmorphic disorder (p. 182)
Conversion disorder (p. 177)
Depersonalization disorder (p. 188)
Derealization (p. 187)
Dissociative amnesia (p. 188)
Dissociative disorders (p. 187)
Dissociative fugue (p. 189)
Dissociative identity disorder (p. 191)
Dissociative trance disorder (p. 190)
Factitious disorders (p. 178)
Generalized amnesia (p. 188)
Hypochondriasis (p. 169)
Localized or selective amnesia (p. 189)
Malingering (p. 177)
Pain disorder (p. 182)
Somatization disorder (p. 173)
Somatoform disorders (p. 169)

INFOTRAC KEY TERM EXERCISES

Each exercise is linked to key terms from the Wadsworth InfoTrac on-line searchable database. Key terms must be entered exactly as written.

Exercise 1: **How do Behavior Analysts Explain Dissociative Identity Disorder?**
Article: A99514094
Citation: (Dissociative identity disorder: The relevance of behavior analyis). Brady J. Phelps.
The Psychological Record, Spring 2000 v50 i2 p235

Behavior analytic accounts of Dissociative Identity Disorder, formerly known as Multiple Personality Disorder, are rarely presented in detail. This lack of depth may be due to misunderstanding the relevance of the behavior analytic position on personality, abnormality, and related issues. Review this InfoTrac article and answer the following questions: (a) how is personality explained in behavioral terms?, (b) what is dissociative identity disorder, (c) how common is this problem?, and (d) how does behavioral theory explain this disorder and what treatment implications stem from this account? Limit your answer to 3-5 typed double-spaced pages.

Exercise 2: **Somatoform Disorders in Children and Adolescents**
Key Term: *Somatoform Disorders in Children*

Much of the literature regarding somatoform disorders is focused on adults; however, there are indications that such problems often begin in childhood and adolescence and have a strong familial component. Review the InfoTrac article(s) on somatoform disorders in children and adolescence. Then, pretend that your task is to re-write portions of the textbook on somatoform disorders. Select a section describing one of the somatoform disorders from the text and revise the material in light of what you have learned about a somatoform disorder in children. Based on your reading, what information would you include regarding children and adolescents and why? Limit your answer to 3-5 typed double-spaced pages.

Exercise 3 (Future Trend): Hypnotic States and Dissociative Disorders

Persons suffering from dissociative disorders are often highly suggestible and the psychological phenomena resembles what looks very much like a hypnotic state. The term hypnosis is familiar to many, and is often associated with psychotherapy. Yet, the nature of hypnosis is not well understood, including its relation to dissociative disorders. Students will typically find discussion of hypnosis interesting. It remains a highly controversial intervention technique, particularly in the context of dissociative disorders. You can discuss hypnotic states, procedures used to induce them, and their efficacy and effectiveness. This is also an opportunity to relate hypnotic procedures with false memory syndrome. The links below should serve as good starting points.

http://www.apa.org/divisions/div30/hypnosis.html
http://serendip.brynmawr.edu/bb/neuro/neuro00/web3/Arnaudo.html
http://ist-socrates.berkeley.edu/~kihlstrm/hypnosis_L&M2003.htm
http://www.selfgrowth.com/articles/Shelp6.html
http://www.ruf.rice.edu/~sch/beliefs/b-mpd.htm

CLASSROOM ACTIVITIES, DEMONSTRATIONS, AND LECTURE TOPICS

1. **Activity: When Have I Assumed the Sick Role?** To expose students to characteristics endorsed by people diagnosed with a somatoform disorder, including features of malingering or factitious disorders, you could ask students if they have ever used or faked physical symptoms to get out of having to perform important life activities (e.g., exams, classes, work, social functions), including use of such tactics to gain attention and sympathy from others.

2. **Activity: Understanding Hypochondriasis.** You could administer the Hypochondriasis scale of the MMPI-2 to your students. After scoring the scale, you could discuss results and how the test items relate to the DSM-IV-TR diagnosis. To depict the process of a person with hypochondriasis, ask your students to keep a log of their bodily sensations for a few days. Ask your students to pay very close attention to any bodily sensation they experience. Examples may include stomach rumblings, headaches, muscle soreness, frequent urination, stiffness, tingling sensations, skin color changes, perspiration, and fatigue among others. Have your students bring in their record and ask them to consider how a person with hypochondriasis might interpret these normal sensations. What physical ailment could they represent? Also, discuss with them why anxiety is so prevalent among people with this disorder.

3. **Activity: "Normal" Dissociations.** Before exploring the dissociative disorders, ask your students to identify periods of dissociation that are normal. For example, most students have had the experience of wanting to drive to a friend's house, but ending up at their school or office because they are so used to driving that route. Others have had experiences of driving on the highway only to find that they have no recollection of the last 10 or so miles they have driven, including obvious landmarks they had passed along the way. Alternatively, many have had the experience of dialing a phone number intending to talk to one particular friend, only to have dialed the number of someone else without being consciously aware of doing so. These examples illustrate that one can fail to be conscious of what one is doing, and yet safely guide oneself through a task. Another example occurs when studying. Again, almost every student has had the experience of reading pages of material (perhaps in their Abnormal text!), only to snap out of their "trance" and realize that, although their eyes were moving over the words, they were thinking about very different things besides their textbook material. That is, they get to the bottom of a page and have no idea how they got there. Finally, many students may have experienced some form of trauma in which they felt "cut-off" from feelings or numb from shock. Highlighting these experiences helps illustrate that dissociative disorders are not as "bizarre" as they first appear. Emphasizing the continuum of behavior is important here to enhance student empathy for people with this class of disorders. We are all capable of forms of dissociation, and people with severe dissociative disorders may be simply using a natural process to protect themselves from the ongoing onslaught of trauma.

4. **Activity: Invited Hypnotist or Pain Specialist.** A useful class activity can be to invite a guest lecturer with expertise in hypnotism or the treatment of pain-related disorders to come and speak to your class.

5. **Video Activity: Abnormal Psychology, Inside/Out, Vol. 2.** This video segment presents a case of Mike, who suffered a brain injury after racing his car and cannot learn or remember new information. After describing dissociative amnesia, play this video segment and ask the class to determine whether Mike would meet diagnostic criteria for a dissociative amnesia disorder. Use this video clip to illustrate important facets of amnesia and the critical features that would not warrant a diagnosis of dissociative amnesia in this case.

SUPPLEMENTARY READING MATERIAL FOR CHAPTER SIX

(i = These sources can be found on "*Infotrac, the online library*" provided by Wadsworth and Brooks/Cole Publishing.)

Bliss, E. L. (1980). Multiple personalities?: A report of 14 cases with implications for schizophrenia and hysteria. Archives of General Psychiatry, 37, 1388-1397.

i Chapman, J., & Lopresti, R. (2000). Lilienfeld, Scott O., et al. "Dissociative identity disorder and the sociocognitive model: Recalling the lessons of the past." Skeptical Inquirer, 24, i1 58.

Chase, T. (1990). When rabbit howls. New York: Jove.

i Fritz, G. K., Fritsch, S., & Hagino, O. (1997). Somatoform disorders in children and adolescents: A review of the past 10 years. Journal of the American Academy of Child and Adolescent Psychiatry, 36, 1329(10).

Kellner, R. (1991). Psychosomatic syndromes and somatic symptoms. Washington, DC: American Psychiatric Press.

Kellner, R. (1986). Somatization and hypochondriasis. New York: Praeger.

Kluft, R. P. (1991). Multiple personality disorder. In A. Tasman & S. M. Goldfinger (Eds.), American psychiatric press review of psychiatry, vol. 10. Washington, DC: American Psychiatric Press.

Loewenstein, R. J. (1991). Psychogenic amnesia and psychogenic fugue: A comprehensive review. In A. Tasman & S.M. Goldfinger (Eds.), American psychiatric press review of psychiatry, vol. 10. Washington, DC: American Psychiatric Press.

Lynn, S. J., & Rhue, J. W. (1994). Dissociation: Clinical and theoretical perspectives. New York: Guilford.

Miller, M., & Bowers, K. S. (1993). Hypnotic analgesia: Dissociated experience or dissociated control? Journal of Abnormal Psychology, 102, 29-38.

Phelps, B. J. (2000). Dissociative identity disorder: The relevance of behavior analysis. The Psychological Record, 50, i2, 235.

Spanos, N. P. (1997). Multiple identities and false memories: A sociological perspective. Washington, DC: American Psychological Association.

Thigpen, C. H., & Cleckley, H. M. (1957). The three faces of Eve. New York: McGraw-Hill.

Waites, E. A. (1993). Trauma and survival: Post-traumatic and dissociative disorders in women. New York: Norton.

Weintraub, M. I. (1983). Hysterical conversion reactions: A clinical guide to diagnosis and treatment. New York: SP Medical and Scientific Books.

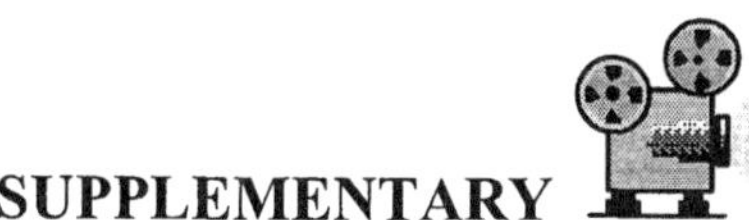

SUPPLEMENTARY VIDEO RESOURCES FOR CHAPTER SIX

Abnormal psychology, inside/out, vol. 2. *(available through your International Thomson Learning representative).* The video segment presents a case of Mike, who suffered a brain injury after racing his car and cannot learn or remember new information. However, he has retained over-learned memories, such as how to build an engine. He carries a notebook with information with him at all times with activities he must do every half hour. He has developed a temper problem, depression and has lost his job, wife and home as a result of the trauma. Finally, Mike describes a repetition technique he uses to help remember short term information.

A second segment provides an overview of the characteristics of dissociative identity disorder (DID), where a female client describes her alters, and what it is like to suffer from DID. This volume of inside/out also includes a segment on the relation of early history of child abuse and DID. (5 min)

Abnormal psychology, inside/out, vol. 3. *(available through your International Thomson Learning representative).* Katherine A. Phillips of Brown University interviews one of her body dysmorphic clients to show the nature of the disorder, its symptoms, and the devastating impact it had on his life--his marriage, his work and his family relationships.

Agnes of God. (Hollywood Film; Mystery). Jane Fonda plays a court-appointed psychiatrist who must make sense out of pregnancy and apparent infanticide in a local convent. The film illustrates stigmata as an example of a conversion reaction.

Cyrano de Bergerac. (Hollywood Film; Romance). This film depicts Cyrano; a man obsessed with the size of his nose and who is convinced that he is forever unlovable because of this presumed defect.

Freud. (Hollywood Film; Biography). This film illustrates several clinical manifestations of somatoform disorders (e.g., paralysis, false blindness, and false pregnancy).

Hanna and her sisters. (Hollywood Film; Comedy/Drama). Woody Allen stars as a hopeless hypochondriac who spends his days worry about brain tumors, cancer, and cardiovascular disease.

The devils. (Hollywood Film; Drama/Historical). This film, adapted from Aldous Huxley's book, The Devils of Loundun, traces the lives of 17th century French nuns who experienced highly erotic dissociative states attributed to possession by the devil.

Multiple personalities. (Insight Media: 2162 Broadway, New York, NY 10024/ (800)-233-9910). Multiple Personality Disorder (i.e., Dissociative Identity Disorder) remains one of the most misunderstood mental disorders today. Although it is usually triggered by abuse or trauma, there are many cases with no apparent cause behind the onset of the affliction. This program enters the minds of several people who have battled Multiple Personality Disorder, offering an intimate look at what life is like for those who live with strangers in their own minds. It takes an in-depth look at the Sybil case. (50 min)

Multiple personalities. (Insight Media: 2162 Broadway, New York, NY 10024/ (800)-233-9910). This program explores the causes and characteristics of multiple personality disorder. Presenting three case studies, it shows therapists working with their clients and explains that multiple personalities are often created to deal with difficult experiences in childhood. (30 min)

Neurotic, stress-related, and somatoform disorders. (Insight Media: 2162 Broadway, New York, NY 10024/ (800)-233-9910). This program examines neurotic, stress-related, and somatoform disorders, discussing differential diagnoses and showing interviews with patients who exhibit characteristic symptoms. It explores such disorders as obsessive-compulsive disorder, phobic anxiety, anxiety, stress reactions and adjustment, and dissociative disorders. It also looks at such sub-disorders as Korsakov's syndrome, agoraphobia and social phobia, panic disorder, and post-traumatic stress syndrome. (45 min)

Primal fear. (Hollywood Film; Drama). The film depicts a man who commits heinous crimes, purportedly as a result of a dissociative disorder. The film raises questions about the problem of malingering and differential diagnosis.

The many faces of Marsha. (Insight Media: 2162 Broadway, New York, NY 10024/ (800)-233-9910). This 48 Hours video illuminates the mysteries of multiple personality disorder through the case of one woman trapped in a maze of over 200 personalities. It shows how the personalities interact with each other and documents how Marsha's therapists tried to cure her illness. (48 min)

The three faces of eve. (Hollywood Film; Drama). The film portrays a woman with three personalities (i.e., Eve White, Eve Black, and Jane).

Twelve o'clock high. (Hollywood Film; War). This film depicts a general who develops conversion disorder (i.e., paralysis) in response to his role in the death of several of his subordinates. This film is based on a true story.

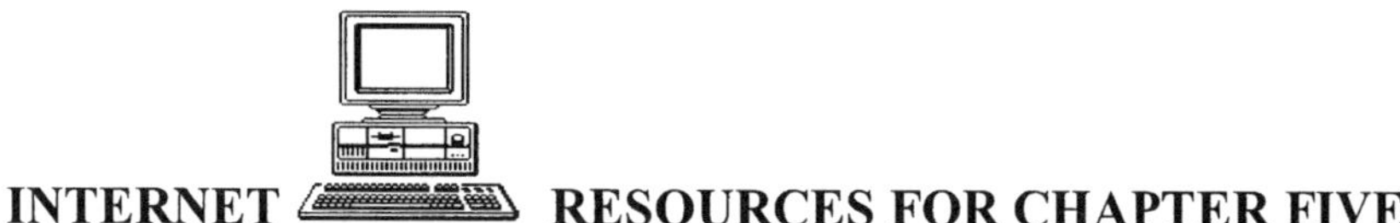

INTERNET RESOURCES FOR CHAPTER FIVE

American Society for Clinical Hypnosis
http://www.hypnosis-research.org/hypnosis/
A good resource for research relevant to altered states of consciousness.

Child Abuse: Statistics, Research, and Resources
http://www.jimhopper.com/abstats/
A good resource for current research and informational links related to child abuse.

Conversion and Somatization Disorders
http://www.mc.vanderbilt.edu/peds/pidl/adolesc/convreac.html
This web page has material on somatoform disorders, including statistics on the prevalence of theses disorders, and references for further information.

International Society for the Study of Dissociation
http://www.issd.org/
Offers information about diagnosis and treatment of dissociative disorders.

Mental Health Net Dissociative Disorders
http://www.cmhc.com
Offers information and connections to other web sites related to dissociative disorders.

Munchausen Syndrome and Factitious Disorders
http://ourworld.compuserve.com/homepages/Marc_Feldman_2/
An interesting starting point for the exploration of Munchausen syndrome and factitious disorders.

Recovered Memories of Sexual Abuse
http://www.jimhopper.com/memory/
A useful scholarly source of information and links related to recovered memories of sexual abuse.

WARNING SIGNS FOR HYPOCHONDRIASIS

- Frequent visits to the doctor
- Fixation on a disease that no doctor has diagnosed
- Rejection of a doctor's reassurance that there is nothing seriously wrong with you
- Continuous doctor-shopping
- Checking your body many times a day/week for peculiarities
- Preoccupation with an illness that you see on television or in the newspaper
- Excessive concern about fear or pain
- Frequent thoughts of death

WARNING SIGNS FOR MUNCHAUSEN BY PROXY SYNDROME

Experts say any of these warning signs may point to the possibility that Munchausen by Proxy syndrome may be a factor in a child's apparent illness:

- Illness that persists in spite of traditionally effective treatments
- The child has been to many doctors without a clear diagnosis
- The parent (usually the mother) seems eager for the child to undergo additional tests, treatments or surgeries
- The parent is very reluctant to have the child out of her sight
- Another child in the same family has had an unexplained illness
- Parent has a background in health care
- Symptoms appear only when the parent is present

WARNING SIGNS FOR BODY DYSMORPHIC DISORDER

- Constant and excessive use or avoidance of mirrors
- Spending lots of time (i.e. 1+ hours) grooming every day
- Attempts to hide parts of body that one does not like
- Experience of distress over performing grooming rituals that one feels compelled to do
- Constant seeking of reassurance about looks, and subsequent discounting of the feedback
- Anxiety or depression about one's appearance

WARNING SIGNS FOR DISSOCIATIVE IDENTITY DISORDER

The following symptoms may indicate dissociative identity disorder:

- Two or more distinct personalities exist within one person
- Each personality has its own way of thinking about things and relating to others
- At least two of the identities take control of the person's behavior
- The person is unable to recall important personal information

Transparency 6-1

DSM-IV-TR Criteria for Hypochondriasis

A. Preoccupation with fears of having, or the idea that one has, a serious disease based on the person's misinterpretation of bodily symptoms.

B. The preoccupation persists despite appropriate medical evaluation and reassurance.

C. The belief in Criterion A is not of delusional intensity (as in Delusional Disorder, Somatic Type) and is not restricted to a circumscribed concern about appearance (as in Body Dysmorphic Disorder).

D. The preoccupation causes clinically significant distress or impairment in socia occupational, or other important areas of functioning.

E. The duration of the disturbance is at least 6 months.

F. The preoccupation is not better accounted for by Generalized Anxiety Disorde Obsessive-Compulsive Disorder, Panic Disorder, a Major Depressive Episode, Separation Anxiety, or another Somatoform Disorder.

Specify if:

> **With Poor Insight**: if, for most of the time during the current episode, the person does not recognize that the concern about having a serious illness is excessive or unreasonable.

DSM-IV-TR Criteria for Somatization Disorder

A. A history of many physical complaints beginning before age 30 years that occur over a period of several years and result in treatment being sought or significant impairment in social, occupational, or other important areas of functioning.

B. Each of the following criteria must have been met, with individual symptoms occurring at any time during the course of the disturbance:

1. four pain symptoms: a history of pain related to at least four different sites or functions (e.g., head, abdomen, back, joints, extremities, chest, rectum, during menstruation, during sexual intercourse, or during urination)
2. two gastrointestinal symptoms: a history of at least two gastrointestinal symptoms other than pain (e.g., nausea, bloating, vomiting other than during pregnancy, diarrhea, or intolerance of several different foods)
3. one sexual symptom: a history of at least one sexual or reproductive symptom other than pain (e.g., sexual indifference, erectile or ejaculatory dysfunction, irregular menses, excessive menstrual bleeding, vomiting throughout pregnancy)
4. one pseudoneurological symptom: a history of at least one symptom or deficit suggesting a neurological condition not limited to pain (conversion symptoms such as impaired coordination or balance, paralysis or localized weakness, difficulty swallowing or lump in throat, aphonia, urinary retention, hallucinations, loss of touch or pain sensation, double vision, blindness, deafness, seizures; dissociative symptoms such as amnesia; or loss of consciousness other than fainting)

C. Either (1) or (2):

1. after appropriate investigation, each of the symptoms in Criterion B cannot be fully explained by a known general medical condition or the direct effects of a substance (e.g., a drug of abuse, a medication)
2. when there is a related general medical condition, the physical complaints or resulting social or occupational impairment are in excess of what would be expected from the history, physical examination, or laboratory findings

D. The symptoms are not intentionally feigned or produced (as in Factitious Disorder or Malingering).

DSM-IV-TR Criteria for Conversion Disorder

A. One or more symptoms or deficits affecting voluntary motor or sensory function that suggest a neurological or other general medical condition.

B. Psychological factors are judged to be associated with the symptom or deficit because the initiation or exacerbation of the symptom or deficit is preceded by conflicts or other stressors.

C. The symptom or deficit is not intentionally produced or feigned (as in Factitious Disorder or Malingering).

D. The symptom or deficit cannot, after appropriate investigation, be fully explained by a general medical condition, or by the direct effects of a substance, or as a culturally sanctioned behavior or experience.

E. The symptom or deficit causes clinically significant distress or impairment in social, occupational, or other important areas of functioning or warrants medical evaluation.

F. The symptom or deficit is not limited to pain or sexual dysfunction, does not occur exclusively during the course of Somatization Disorder, and is not better accounted for by another mental disorder.

Specify type of symptom or deficit:

With Motor Symptom or Deficit
With Sensory Symptom or Deficit
With Seizures or Convulsions
With Mixed Presentation

DSM-IV-TR Criteria for Pain Disorder

A. Pain in one or more anatomical sites is the predominant focus of the clinical presentation and is of sufficient severity to warrant clinical attention.

B. The pain causes clinically significant distress or impairment in social, occupational, or other important areas of functioning.

C. Psychological factors are judged to have an important role in the onset, severity, exacerbation, or maintenance of the pain.

D. The symptom or deficit is not intentionally produced or feigned (as in Factitious Disorder or Malingering).

E. The pain is not better accounted for by a Mood, Anxiety, or Psychotic Disorder and does not meet criteria for Dyspareunia.

Code as follows:

> **Pain Disorder Associated With Psychological Factors**: psychological factors are judged to have the major role in the onset, severity, exacerbation, or maintenance of the pain. (If a general medical condition is present, it does not have a major role in the onset, severity, exacerbation, or maintenance of the pain.) This type of Pain Disorder is not diagnosed if criteria are also met for Somatization Disorder.

DSM-IV-TR Criteria for Pain Disorder Additional Specifiers

Specify if:

Acute: duration of less than 6 months
Chronic: duration of 6 months or longer
Pain Disorder Associated With Both Psychological Factors and a General Medical Condition: both psychological factors and a general medical condition are judged to have important roles in the onset, severity, exacerbation, or maintenance of the pain. The associated general medical condition or anatomical site of the pain (see below) is coded on Axis III.

Specify if:

Acute: duration of less than 6 months
Chronic: duration of 6 months or longer

Note: The following is not considered to be a mental disorder and is included here to facilitate differential diagnosis.

Pain Disorder Associated With a General Medical Condition: a general medical condition has a major role in the onset, severity, exacerbation, or maintenance of the pain. (If psychological factors are present, they are not judged to have a major role in the onset, severity, exacerbation, or maintenance of the pain.) The diagnostic code for the pain is selected based on the associated general medical condition if one has been established or on the anatomical location of the pain if the underlying general medical condition is not yet clearly established--for example, low back (724.2), sciatic (724.3), pelvic (625.9), headache (784.0), facia (784.0), chest (786.50), joint (719.4), bone (733.90), abdominal (789.0), breast (611.71), renal (788.0), ear (388.70), eye (379.91), throat (784.1), tooth (525.9), and urinary (788.0).

DSM-IV-TR Criteria for Body Dysmorphic Disorder

A. Preoccupation with an imagined defect in appearance. If a slight physical anomaly is present, the person's concern is markedly excessive.

B. The preoccupation causes clinically significant distress or impairment in social, occupational, or other important areas of functioning.

C. The preoccupation is not better accounted for by another mental disorder (e.g., dissatisfaction with body shape and size in Anorexia Nervosa).

Transparency 6-7

DSM-IV-TR Criteria for Depersonalization Disorder

A. Persistent or recurrent experiences of feeling detached from, and as if one is an outside observer of, one's mental processes or body (e.g., feeling like one is in a dream).

B. During the depersonalization experience, reality testing remains intact.

C. The depersonalization causes clinically significant distress or impairment in social, occupational, or other important areas of functioning.

D. The depersonalization experience does not occur exclusively during the course of another mental disorder, such as Schizophrenia, Panic Disorder, Acute Stress Disorder, or another Dissociative Disorder, and is not due to the direct physiological effects of a substance (e.g., a drug of abuse, a medication) or a general medical condition (e.g., temporal lobe epilepsy).

DSM-IV-TR Criteria for Dissociative Amnesia

A. The predominant disturbance is one or more episodes of inability to recall important personal information, usually of a traumatic or stressful nature, that is too extensive to be explained by ordinary forgetfulness.

B. The disturbance does not occur exclusively during the course of Dissociative Identity Disorder, Dissociative Fugue, Posttraumatic Stress Disorder, Acute Stress Disorder, or Somatization Disorder and is not due to the direct physiological effects of a substance (e.g., a drug of abuse, a medication) or a neurological or other general medical condition (e.g., Amnestic Disorder Due to Head Trauma).

C. The symptoms cause clinically significant distress or impairment in social, occupational, or other important areas of functioning.

DSM-IV-TR Criteria for Dissociative Fugue

A. The predominant disturbance is sudden, unexpected travel away from home or one's customary place of work, with inability to recall one's past.

B. Confusion about personal identity or assumption of a new identity (partial or complete).

C. The disturbance does not occur exclusively during the course of Dissociative Identity Disorder and is not due to the direct physiological effects of a substance (e.g., a drug of abuse, a medication) or a general medical condition (e.g., temporal lobe epilepsy).

D. The symptoms cause clinically significant distress or impairment in social, occupational, or other important areas of functioning.

DSM-IV-TR Research Criteria for Dissociative Trance Disorder

A. Either (1) or (2):

1. Trance, i.e., temporary marked alteration in the state of consciousness or loss of customary sense of personal identity without replacement by an alternate identity, associated with at least one of the following:
    a. narrowing of awareness of immediate surroundings, or unusually narrow and selective focusing on environmental stimuli
    b. Stereotyped behaviors or movements that are experienced as being beyond one's control

2. Possession trance, a single or episodic alteration in the state of consciousness characterized by the replacement of customary sense of personal identity by a new identity. This is attributed to the influence of a spirit, power, deity, or other person, as evidenced by one (or more) of the following:
    a. stereotyped and culturally determined behaviors or movements that are experienced as being controlled by the possessing agent
    b. full or partial amnesia for the event

B. The trance or possession trance state is not accepted as a normal part of a collective cultural or religious practice.

C. The trance or possession trance state causes clinically significant distress or impairment in social, occupational, or other important areas of functioning.

D. The trance or possession trance state does not occur exclusively during the course of a Psychotic Disorder (including Mood Disorder With Psychotic Features and Brief Psychotic Disorder) or Dissociative Identity Disorder and is not due to the direct physiological effects of a substance or a general medical condition.

DSM-IV-TR Criteria for Dissociative Identity Disorder

A. The presence of two or more distinct identities or personality states (each with its own relatively enduring pattern of perceiving, relating to, and thinking about the environment and self).

B. At least two of these identities or personality states recurrently take control of the person's behavior.

C. Inability to recall important personal information that is too extensive to be explained by ordinary forgetfulness.

D. The disturbance is not due to the direct physiological effects of a substance (e.g., blackouts or chaotic behavior during Alcohol Intoxication) or a general medical condition (e.g., complex partial seizures). Note: In children, the symptoms are not attributable to imaginary playmates or other fantasy play.

DSM-IV-TR Criteria for Factitious Disorders

A. Intentional production or feigning of physical or psychological signs or symptoms.

B. The motivation for the behavior is to assume the sick role.

C. External incentives for the behavior (such as economic gain, avoiding legal responsibility, or improving physical well-being, as in Malingering) are absent.

Specify type:

With Predominantly Psychological Signs and Symptoms: if psychological signs and symptoms predominate in the clinical presentation

With Predominantly Physical Signs and Symptoms: if physical signs and symptoms predominate in the clinical presentation

With Combined Psychological and Physical Signs and Symptoms: if both psychological and physical signs and symptoms are present but neither predominates in the clinical presentation

Transparency 6-13

DSM-IV-TR Research Criteria for Factitious Disorder by Proxy

A. Intentional production or feigning of physical or psychological signs or symptoms in another person who is under the individual's care.

B. The motivation for the perpetrator's behavior is to assume the sick role by proxy.

C. External incentives for the behavior (such as economic gain) are absent.

D. The behavior is not better accounted for by another mental disorder.

CHAPTER SEVEN

MOOD DISORDERS AND SUICIDE

LEARNING OBJECTIVES

1. Differentiate a depressive episode from a manic and hypomanic episode.
2. Describe the clinical symptoms of major depression.
3. Describe the clinical symptoms of bipolar disorder, including mania.
4. Differentiate major depression from dysthymic disorder.
5. Differentiate bipolar disorder from cyclothymic disorder.
6. Understand the different symptom and longitudinal course specifiers for mood disorders, including their relation with prognosis and treatment.
7. Describe the differences in prevalence of mood disorders across the life span.
8. Describe the biological, psychological, and sociocultural contributions to the development of unipolar and bipolar mood disorders, including what is known about such disorders in children.
9. Describe medical and psychological treatments that have been successful in treating mood disorders.
10. Describe the relationship between suicide and mood disorders.
11. Elucidate known risk factors for suicide and approaches to suicide prevention and treatment.

OUTLINE

I. Understanding and Defining Mood Disorders
    A. An overview of depression and mania
        1. The disorders described in this chapter used to be called "depressive disorders," affective disorders," or even "depressive neuroses." Beginning with the DSM-III, these problems were grouped under the heading **mood disorders** because they all represent gross deviations in mood.
        2. The experience of depression and mania contribute, either alone or in combination, to all mood disorders.
        3. **Major depressive episode** is most commonly diagnosed and most severe form of depression (see DSM-IV-TR diagnostic criteria for Major Depression). The textbook illustrates clinical depression with the case of Katie. DSM-IV-TR criteria for major depressive episode includes:
            a. Extremely depressed mood state lasting at least 2 weeks.
            b. Cognitive symptoms (e.g., feeling worthless, indecisiveness).
            c. Disturbed physical functions (e.g., altered sleep patterns, changes in appetite/weight, loss of energy), often referred to as **somatic or vegetative symptoms**. Such symptoms are central to this disorder.
            d. **Anhedonia**, or the loss of interest or pleasure in usual activities.
            e. Average duration of an untreated major depressive episode is 9 months.

4. **Mania** refers to abnormally exaggerated elation, joy, or euphoria. Such episodes are accompanied by extraordinary activity (i.e., hyperactivity), require decreased need for sleep, and may include grandiose plans (i.e., believing that one can accomplish anything). Speech is typically rapid and may become incoherent, and may involve a flight of ideas (i.e., attempt to express many ideas at once). A **hypomanic** (hypo means below) episode is a less severe version of a manic episode that does not cause marked impairment in social or occupational functioning. DSM-IV-TR criteria for a manic episode includes:
    a. A duration of 1 week; less if the episode is severe enough to require hospitalization.
    b. Irritability often accompanies the manic episode toward the end of its duration.
    c. Anxiousness and depression are often part of a manic episode.
    d. Average duration of an untreated manic episode is 3-6 months.

B. The structure of mood disorders

1. **Unipolar disorder** refers to the experience of either depression or mania, and most individuals with this condition suffer from unipolar depression. **Bipolar disorder** refers to alternations between depression and mania. Feeling depression and manic at the same time is referred to as a **dysphoric manic or mixed episode**.
2. An important feature of major depressive episodes is that they are **time limited**, lasting 2 weeks to 9 months if left untreated.
3. Almost all major depressive episodes remit without treatment. Manic episodes remit without treatment after six months. Thus, it is important to determine the **course or temporal patterning** of the depressive and manic episodes. Different patterns appear in the DSM-IV-TR under the heading course modifiers for mood disorders.
    a. **Course modifiers** characterize the past mood state and are helpful to predict the future course of the disorder. Understanding the course is related to predicting future occurrences of mood changes and in helping to prevent them.

C. Depressive disorders

1. **Major depressive disorder, single episode** is defined, in part, by the absence of manic or hypomanic episodes before or during the episode. The occurrence of 1 isolated depressive episode in a lifetime is rare, and unipolar depression is almost always a chronic condition that waxes and wanes over time, but seldom disappears.
2. **Major depressive disorder, recurrent** requires that two or more major depressive episodes occur and are separated by a period of at least 2 months during which the individual is not depressed. Recurrent major depression is associated with a family history of depression. As many as 85% of single-episode cases later have a second episode of major depression.

a. The median lifetime number of major depressive episodes is four, and the median duration is 4 to 5 months.
b. Mean age of onset for major depression is 25 years for persons not in treatment, and 29 years for persons who are in treatment. The length of major depressive episodes is variable, with some lasting as little as 2 weeks to as long as several years in more severe cases.
c. The average age of onset of major depression appears to be decreasing.

3. **Dysthymic disorder** shares many of the symptoms of major depressive, but unlike major depression, the symptoms in dysthymia tend to be milder and remain relatively unchanged over long periods of time, as much as 20 or 30 years. Dysthymic disorder is defined by persistently depressed mood that continues for at least 2 years. During this time, the person cannot be symptom free for more than 2 months at a time. Many eventually experience a major depressive episode at some point.
    a. The mean age of onset for dysthymia is typically in the early 20s (i.e., **late onset**). The onset of dysthymia before age 21 (i.e., **early onset**) is associated with (a) greater chronicity, (b) relatively poor prognosis (i.e., response to treatment), and (c) stronger likelihood of the disorder running in the family.
    b. The median duration of dysthymic disorder is approximately 5 years in adults and 4 years in children.
    c. Patients suffering from dysthymia have a higher likelihood of attempting suicide than those suffering from major depressive disorder.
4. **Double depression** refers to both major depressive episodes and dysthymic disorder.
    a. Dysthymic disorder often develops first, and this condition is associated with severe psychopathology and problematic future course. Indeed, many do not recover after two years, and relapse rates are very high.
    b. Double depression is common, with as many as 79% of persons with dysthymia reporting a major depressive episode at some point in their lives.
5. The frequency of severe depression following the **death of a loved one** is quite high. Most mental health professionals do not consider depression associated with death or loss a disorder unless very severe symptoms appear (e.g., psychotic features, suicidal ideation, or the less-alarming symptoms last longer than 2 months). **Grief** is usually resolved within several months post loss, but may be exacerbated at significant anniversaries, such as the birthday of the loved one or during holidays.
    a. If grief lasts longer than 1 year or so the chance of recovering from severe grief is greatly reduced and mental health professionals may become concerned.
    b. A history of major depressive episodes may predict the development of a **pathological grief reaction** or **impacted grief reaction**, which include symptoms of intrusive memories and strong yearnings for the

loved one, and avoiding people and places associated with the loved one.

D. Bipolar disorders

1. The core identifying feature of bipolar disorders is the tendency of manic episodes to alternate with major depressive episodes. Beyond that, bipolar disorders parallel depressive disorders (e.g., a manic episode can occur once or repeatedly. The textbook presents the case of Jane to illustrate Bipolar II disorder.
2. **Bipolar I disorder** is the alternation of full manic episodes and depressive episodes. The textbook presents the case of Billy to illustrate a full manic episode.
    a. Average age on onset is 18 years, but can begin in childhood.
    b. Tends to be chronic.
    c. Suicide is a common consequence.
3. In **bipolar II disorder**, major depressive episodes alternate with hypomanic episodes.
    a. Average age on onset is 22 years, but can begin in childhood.
    b. Only 10 to 13% of cases progress to full bipolar I disorder.
    c. Tends to be chronic.

4. **Cyclothymic disorder** is a more chronic version of bipolar disorder where manic and major depressive episodes are less severe. Such persons tend to remain in either a manic or depressive mood state for several years with very few periods of neutral (or euthymic) mood. For the diagnosis, the pattern must last for at least 2 years (1 year for children and adolescents). Such persons are also at increased risk for developing Bipolar I or II disorder.
    a. Average age on onset is about 12 or 14 years.
    b. Cyclothymia tends to be chronic and lifelong.
    c. Most are female.

E. Additional defining criteria for mood disorders

1. Symptom specifiers are often helpful in determining the most effective treatment and are of two broad types: those that describe the most recent episode of the disorder, and those that describe its course of temporal pattern.
2. Specifiers for recent episodes include the following:
    a. **Atypical features specifier** modifies depressive episodes and dysthymia but not manic episodes. Individuals with this specifier oversleep, overeat, gain weight, and show much anxiety. These persons are able to experience some pleasure in their lives. Depression with atypical features is associated with an earlier age of onset and a greater percentage of women.
    b. **Melancholic features specifier** applies only if the full criteria for a major depressive episode have been met; it does not apply to dysthymia. This group includes more severe somatic symptoms (e.g., early morning awakenings, weight loss, loss of sex drive, excessive

guilt, and anhedonia). Signifies a more severe type of depressive episode.

c. **Chronic features specifier** can be applied only if the full criteria for major depressive episode have been met continuously for at least the past 2 years. Does not apply to dysthymic disorder.
d. **Catatonic features specifier** applies to major depressive episodes and manic episodes, though it is very rare. This is a very serious condition involving the total absence of movement (i.e., a stuporous state) or **catalepsy** (i.e., muscles are waxy and semi-rigid).
e. **Psychotic features specifiers** applies to cases where psychotic symptoms (i.e., hallucinations, delusions) are experienced during the major depressive or manic episode. Hallucinations and delusions may be **mood congruent** (i.e., symptom content are directly related to depressed mood) or **mood incongruent**. Examples of these symptoms include auditory hallucinations and somatic or grandeur delusions. Psychotic depressive episodes are rare but associated with poor response to treatment.
f. **Postpartum onset specifier** applies to both major depressive and manic episodes and is used to characterize severe manic or depressive episodes of a psychotic nature that first occur during the postpartum period (i.e., 4-week period immediately following childbirth). 13% of women giving birth meet criteria for a major depressive episode. This specifier is not applied to mild depressive episodes following childbirth.

3. Specifiers describing the course of mood disorders include the following:
    a. **Longitudinal course specifiers** are used to address whether a person has had a past episode of depression or mania and whether the person recovered fully from past episodes. For example, one should determine whether dysthymia preceded a major depressive episode or whether cyclothymic disorder preceded bipolar disorder. Both scenarios tend to decrease chances of recovery and increase length of treatment.
    b. **Rapid cycling pattern** applies only to bipolar I and II disorders. Rapid cycling pattern is used when a person has at least 4 manic or depressive episodes within a period of 1 year. Rapid cycling is a more severe form of bipolar disorder that does not respond well to treatment, and appears to be associated with higher rates of suicide. Alternative drug treatments (e.g., anticonvulsants, mood stabilizers) are typically utilized with individuals meeting criteria for this specifier.
    c. **Seasonal pattern** applies to bipolar disorders and recurrent major depression and is used to indicate whether episodes occur during certain seasons, usually wintertime. Those with winter depressions display excessive sleep and weight gain. Seasonal affective disorder may be related to circadian and seasonal changes in the increased production of melatonin (i.e., a hormone secreted by the pineal gland). Phototherapy is a recommended effective treatment for this condition.

II. Prevalence of Mood Disorders

A. About 16% of the population experience some type of mood disorder during their lifetime, and 6.5% in the last 10 months. Females are twice as likely to have a mood disorder compared to males. The imbalance between males and females is accounted for solely by major depressive disorder and dysthymia. Bipolar disorders are distributed equally between males and females. The prevalence of major depressive disorder and dysthymia is also significantly lower among African Americans than European Americans and Hispanics, although once again, this difference is not seen for bipolar disorders.

B. Mood disorders are fundamentally similar in children and adults. Thus, there are no childhood mood disorders in the DSM-IV-TR. How depression presents does change with age. Estimates of the prevalence of mood disorders in **children and adolescents** vary widely. The consensus is that depressive disorder occurs less often in children than adults but that this difference closes somewhat during adolescence, where depression becomes more frequent compared to adults. Children less than 9 years of age show more irritability and emotional swings rather than classic manic states, and are often mistaken as hyperactive. Bipolar disorder is rare in childhood, but rises substantially in adolescence and so does suicide.

C. As many as 18% to 20% of **elderly** nursing home residents may experience major depressive episodes, which are likely to be chronic. Late-onset depression is associated with marked sleep problems, hypochondriasis, and agitation. It is difficult to diagnose depression in the elderly due to medical illnesses and symptoms of dementia. Generally, the prevalence of major depressive disorder is the same or slightly lower in the elderly as in the general population. Anxiety disorders often accompany depression in the elderly. The gender imbalance in depression disappears after age 65.

D. **Across cultures**, feelings of weakness or tiredness tend to characterize depression. However, more difficulty is found when comparing subjective feelings that accompany depressive disorders. Societies that are more individualistic tend to produce depressive statements with the "I" pronoun, whereas societies that are more integrated focus on "our" statements. Still, the prevalence of depression seems to be similar across subcultures, although more so in economically depressed areas.

E. Speculation has been made as to whether mood disorders and **creativity** are related, possibly genetically. The correlation between famous writers and bipolar disorder is one example.

III. The Overlap of Anxiety and Depression

A. Substantial overlap exists between the emotional states of anxiety and depression. Evidence for this is based on neurobiological findings that familial anxiety is related to familial depression. In addition, drug therapies for both conditions are similar.

B. *Most persons with depression do display anxiety symptoms, but not all anxious patients are depressed.* Symptoms common to anxiety and depressive disorders are referred to as **negative affect.** This may contribute to the creation of a mixed anxiety/depression diagnosis. Core symptoms of depression not found in anxiety states include **anhedonia** (inability to experience pleasure), psychomotor retardation, and negative cognitive content.

IV. Causes of Mood Disorders

A. Biological dimensions

1. **Family studies** indicate that the rate of mood disorders in relatives of probands (i.e., the person known to have the disorder) with mood disorders is generally two to three times greater than the rate in relatives of normal probands. The most frequent mood disorder in relatives of persons suffering from mood disorders is unipolar depression.
2. **Twin studies** reveal that if one identical twin presents with a mood disorder, the other twin is 3 times more likely than a fraternal twin to have a mood disorder, particularly for bipolar disorder. Severe mood disorders may have a stronger genetic contribution than less severe disorders. There also appears to be sex differences in genetic vulnerability to depression, with heritability rates being higher for females compared to males. The environment appears to play a larger role in causing depression in males than females. Twinstudies also support the contention that unipolar and bipolar disorder are inherited separately.
3. Data from family and twin studies also suggest that the biological vulnerability for mood disorders may reflect a more general vulnerability for anxiety disorders as well.
4. Research indicates low levels of **serotonin** in the etiology of mood disorders but only in relation to other neurotransmitters, including norepinephrine and dopamine. One of the functions of serotonin is to regulate systems involving norepinephrine and dopamine. The **permissive hypothesis** stipulates that when serotonin levels are low, other neurotransmitters are permitted to range more widely, become dysregulated, and contribute to mood irregularities.
5. Another theory of depression has implicated the endocrine system, particularly elevated levels of **cortisol**. This has led to the controversial **dexamethasone suppression test (DST).** Dexamethasone is a glucocorticoid that suppresses cortisol secretion. As many as 50% of those with depression, when given dexamethasone, show less suppression of cortisol. However, persons with anxiety disorders also demonstrate nonsuppression. New research findings indicate that elevated levels of stress hormones in the long term may interfere with the production of new neurons (i.e., neurogenesis), especially in the hippocampus, which may result in disrupt memory processes.
6. **Sleep disturbances** are a hallmark of most mood disorders. Depressed persons move into the period of **rapid eye movement sleep (REM)** more quickly than nondepressed persons and also show diminished slow wave sleep

(i.e., the deepest and most restful part of sleep). This REM effect is reduced for persons who have depression related to recent life stress. REM activity is intense in depressed persons. Depriving depressed persons of sleep improves their depression. Persons with bipolar disorder and their children show increased sensitivity to light (i.e., greater suppression of melatonin when exposed to light at night). A relationship between seasonal affective disorder, sleep disturbance, and disturbance in biological rhythms has thus been proposed.

B. Brain wave activity

1. Different **alpha electroencephalogram (EEG)** values have been reported in the two hemispheres of brains of depressed persons. Depressed persons show greater right-side anterior activation of the cerebral hemispheres (i.e., left-side activation) than nondepressed persons. This type of brain function may be an indicator of a biological vulnerability for depression.

C. Psychological dimensions

1. Stressful and traumatic events influence mood disorders, although the context, meaning, and memory of an event must be considered. In general, a marked relationship has been found between severe life events, onset of depression, poorer response to treatment, and longer time before remission. New research suggests that one third of the association between stressful life events and depression is due to a vulnerability whereby depressed persons place themselves in high risk stressful situations (i.e., **reciprocal gene-environment model**). In addition, stressful life events and circadian rhythm disturbances may trigger manic episodes. However, only a minority of people experiencing a negative life event develop a mood disorder; therefore, interaction with a biological vulnerability is likely. The textbook illustrates the relation between life stress and depression by returning to a discussion of the case of Katie.
2. According to the **learned helplessness theory of depression**, people develop depression and anxiety when they assume they have no control over life stress. A depressive attributional style has the following three characteristics.
   a. First, the *attribution is internal* in that one believes negative events are one's fault.
   b. Second, the *attribution is stable* in that one believes that future negative events will be one's fault.
   c. Third, the *attribution is global* in that the person believes negative events will influence many life activities.
   d. Evidence is mixed as to whether learned helplessness is a cause or side effect of depression. Attributions are important as a vulnerability that contributes to a sense of **hopelessness**; a feature that distinguishes depressed from anxious individuals.
3. Aaron T. Beck proposed that depression results from a tendency to interpret life events in a negative way. Persons with depression often engage in several **cognitive errors** and think the worst of everything. The following examples of cognitive errors are illustrated in the textbook:

a. **Arbitrary inference** refers to the tendency of depressed persons to emphasize the negative rather than positive aspects of a situation.
b. **Overgeneralization** refers to the tendency to take one negative consequence of some event and generalize to all related aspects of the situation.

4. According to Beck, persons with depression make such cognitive errors all the time, as represented in thinking negatively about themselves, their immediate world, and their future (called the **depressive cognitive triad**). These beliefs may comprise a **negative schema**, or an automatic and enduring cognitive bias about aspects of life. Substantial empirical evidence supports this theory, although it has been difficult to establish the existence of negative schemas prior to major depressive episodes.

D. Social and cultural dimensions

1. **Marital dissatisfaction** and depression are strongly related, and marital disruption often precedes depression. This seems particularly true for men. In addition, high marital conflict and/or low marital support are important in the etiology and recurrence of depression. Conversely, continuing depression may lead to the deterioration of a marital relationship.
2. **Gender imbalances** occur across the mood disorders (with the exception of bipolar disorder) and this is a world-wide phenomenon. Several theories have arisen to explain why females display more anxiety and depressive disorders than males. Part of this may be due to perceptions of uncontrollability. Such perceptions are strongly influenced by socialization, where females are expected to be passive and sensitive to others. In addition, females may place more emphasis on intimate relationships and be more disturbed by problems in this area than males. Females may also be self-deprecating in times of stress. Finally, females are subjected to more discrimination, poverty, sexual harassment, and abuse than males.
3. The number and frequency of social relationships and contact may be related to depression. A lack of social support appears to predict the later onset of depressive symptoms, and high expressed emotion or dysfunctional families may predict relapse. Conversely, substantial social support is related to rapid recovery from depression.

E. An integrative theory of the etiology of mood disorders

1. Depression and anxiety may share common biological/genetic vulnerabilities, such as an overactive neurobiological response to stressful life events.
2. The onset of stressful life events may then activate stress hormones that affect certain neurotransmitter systems, including turning on certain genes. Extended stress may also affect circadian rhythms and activate a dormant psychological vulnerability characterized by negative thinking and a sense of helplessness and hopelessness.
3. In addition, psychological vulnerabilities such as feelings of uncontrollability may be triggered. All of this is dependent, however, on mediating environmental factors such as interpersonal relationships.

V. Treatment of Mood Disorders

A. Three types of antidepressant medications are used to treat depressive disorders:

1. **Tricyclic antidepressants** are widely used treatments for depression, and include imipramine (Tofranil) and amitriptyline (Elavil). It is not yet clear how these drugs work, but initially at least they block the reuptake of norepinephrine and other neurotransmitters (i.e., down-regulation). This process may take anywhere between 2 to 8 weeks, and patients often feel worse and develop side effects before feeling better. Side effects include blurred vision, dry mouth, constipation, difficulty urinating, drowsiness, weight gain, and sexual dysfunction. Because of the side effects, about 40% of patients stop taking the drugs. Tricyclics alleviate depression in 50% of cases to as high as 65% to 70% of cases. Tricyclics may be lethal in excessive doses.
2. **Monoamine oxidase (MAO) inhibitors** work by blocking an enzyme monoamine oxidase that breaks down serotonin and norepinephrine. MAO inhibitors are slightly more effective than tricyclics and have fewer side effects. However, ingestion of tyramine foods (e.g., cheese, red wine, beer) or cold medications with the drug can lead to severe hypertensive episodes and occasionally death. New MAO inhibitors (not yet widely available) are more selective, short acting, and do not interact negatively with tyramine. MAO inhibitors are usually prescribed only when tricyclics prove to be ineffective.
3. **Selective serotonergic reuptake inhibitors** (SSRIs) specifically block the pre-synaptic reuptake of serotonin, thus increasing levels of serotonin at the receptor site. Fluoxetine (Prozac) is the most popular SSRI. Risks of suicide or acts of violence are no greater with Prozac than with any other antidepressant medication. Common side effects of Prozac are physical agitation, sexual dysfunction or low desire, insomnia, and gastrointestinal upset.
4. St. John's Wort (hypericum) is receiving increasing attention as an herbal solution for depression. Preliminary studies suggest that St. John's Wort works better than placebo in alleviating depression and works as well as low doses of other antidepressant medications. St. John's Wort also appears to alter serotonin function and has few side effects.
5. Current studies indicate that these drug treatments are effective with adults, but not necessarily with children, and may cause substantial negative side effects in children. Similar concerns are evident for the elderly population. Overall, recovery from depression may not be as important in treatment as preventing the next episode of depression from occurring. Drug treatment is therefore extended well past the end of a patient's current depressive episode. Approximately 40% to 50% of depressed persons do not respond to these medications, and females of childbearing age must avoid conceiving while taking antidepressants.
6. **Lithium** is a common salt found in the natural environment, including drinking water. Lithium is the primary drug of choice in the treatment of bipolar disorder. Side effects may be severe, and dosage must be carefully regulated to prevent toxicity (poisoning) and lowered thyroid functioning.

Substantial weight gain is also a common side effect. Debate exists as to how lithium works, but possibilities include the reduction of dopamine and norepinephrine or changes in neurohormones. About 30-60% of persons with bipolar disorder respond well to lithium treatment. In other cases of bipolar disorder, antiseizure medication may be effective.

B. **Electroconvulsive therapy (ECT)** is the treatment of choice for very severe depression. The patient is anesthetized and is given muscle-relaxing drugs to prevent bone breakage from convulsions during seizures and is then administered a brief (less than 1 second) electric shock introduced to the brain. The result is brief convulsions lasting for several minutes. Treatments are usually administered once every other day for a total of 6 to 10 treatments. Side effects are few and are limited to short-term memory loss and confusion; both of which usually disappear after a week or two. Approximately 50-70% of those persons not responding to medication benefit from ECT. However, relapse is seen in 60% of cases. The mechanism of action for ECT is unclear. **Transcranial magnetic stimulation (TMS)** is a new procedure that is related to ECT, but involves setting up a strong magnetic field around the brain. No good data exist yet to support the efficacy of TMS.

C. At least three major **psychosocial treatments** are available for depressive disorders.

1. Aaron Beck's **cognitive therapy** involves teaching clients to examine the types of thinking processes they engage in while depressed and recognize cognitive errors when they occur. Clients are informed about how these processes lead to depression and faulty thinking patterns are modified. Clients also monitor and record their thoughts between therapy sessions and are assigned homework to change their behavior. Increased behavioral activity to elicit social reinforcement is also mandated. Treatment usually takes 10 to 12 sessions. The textbook illustrates Beck's cognitive therapy with a dialogue between Beck and a patient named Irene.
2. Lewinson and Rehm developed a form of cognitive-behavior therapy for depression that focused initially on reactivating depressed patients and countering their mood by bringing them in contact with reinforcing events. More recent approaches have also stressed the preventing avoidance of social and environmental cues that produce negative affect or depression. Exercise, increasing positive activities alone can improve self-concept and lift depression.
3. **Interpersonal therapy (IPT)** focuses on resolving problems in existing relationships and/or building skills to develop new relationships. Like cognitive-behavioral approaches, IPT is highly structured and seldom takes longer than 15 to 20 weekly sessions. The therapist and client identify life stressors that precipitate depression, and then address interpersonal role disputes, adjustments to losing a relationship, acquisition of new relationships, and social skills deficits.

4. Recent studies comparing the results of cognitive therapy and IPT to those of tricyclic antidepressants and other control conditions for major depressive disorder and dysthymia have shown that psychosocial approaches and medication are equally effective, and that all treatments are better than placebo and brief psychodynamic therapy.

D. Current data suggest that **combining medication and psychosocial treatments** do not confer any immediate advantage over separate medication or psychosocial treatment. Medication alone typically works more quickly than psychosocial treatment. However, over 50% of patients on antidepressant medication relapse if their medication is stopped within 4 months after their last depressive episode. Psychosocial interventions (i.e., cognitive therapy and IPT) seem helpful in preventing relapse. Findings provide strong support for continuing drug treatment in severe patients who are at high risk for relapse and who have had an initial positive response to antidepressant medication.

E. Though **medication is the preferred treatment for bipolar disorder**, most clinicians emphasize the need for psychosocial interventions to manage interpersonal and practical problems, particularly noncompliance with medication regimen and family stress that has been show to be related to increased risk of relapse.

VI. Suicide

A. Suicide is the eighth leading cause of death in the United States, although many unreported suicides occur. **Suicidal ideation** refers to serious contemplation about committing suicide, whereas **suicidal attempt** refers to surviving an attempted suicide. Suicide is overwhelmingly a white phenomenon and African Americans and Hispanics seldom commit suicide. Suicide rates are also quite high in Native Americans. The rate of suicide is increasing, especially among adolescents and the elderly. Males are 4-5 times more likely to commit suicide than females, although females are three times more likely to attempt suicide than men. This is explained by the fact that men choose more lethal methods of suicide than women. However, in China, females commit suicide more often than males, and the reason seems related to the absence of stigma about suicide in Chinese society (i.e., it is viewed as honorable and a reasonable solution to problems).

1. Emile Durkeim, a sociologist, defined a number of suicide types related to the cause of suicide:
    a. **Formalized** or **altruistic suicide** is socially or familially sanctioned (e.g., killing oneself to avoid dishonor to self or family).
    b. **Egoistic suicide,** which may be common in the elderly, is suicide caused by disintegration of social support.
    c. **Anomic suicides** occur following some major disruption in one's life (e.g., sudden loss of a high prestige job). Anomie means lost and confused.
    d. **Fatalistic suicides** refer to suicide related to a loss of control over one's destiny (e.g., mass suicide of Heaven's Gate cult members).

2. Freud believed that suicide was the result of unconscious hostility expressed inwardly to the self.

B. Risk factors for suicide include the following:
1. If a family member commits suicide, there is an increased risk that someone else in the family will also do so.
2. Low levels of serotonin may be associated with suicide and with violent suicide attempts. Low levels of serotonin are associated with impulsivity, instability, and the tendency to overreact to situations.
3. Existence of a psychological disorder is related to suicide, as over 90% of people who kill themselves suffer from a psychological disorder. As many as 60% of suicides occur in persons suffering from a mood disorder. Depression and suicide are still considered independent as suicide can occur without a mood disorder and not all persons with mood disorders try to kill themselves.
4. Alcohol use and abuse are associated with 25% to 50% of suicides.
5. Past suicide attempts is another strong risk factor in predicting subsequent suicide attempts.
6. Most important risk factor for suicide is a severe, stressful event that is experienced as shameful or humiliating.

C. Publicity about suicide appears to increase rates of suicide, and clusters of suicides (i.e., several people copying one person who committed suicide) seems to predominate in teenagers. The reasons for imitation or modeling of suicide are complex, but may be due to the media romanticizing suicide, the media spelling out methods used to commit suicide.

D. Predicting suicide is difficult, but mental health professionals routinely assess for suicide, often directly via intent, a plan, and a means to carry it out. In general, the more detailed the plan, the more one is at risk for committing suicide. A suicide contract may be used to prevent a patient from killing him or herself, and at times, hospitalization is required. Programs to reduce suicide include curriculum-based programs that are designed to educate students about suicide and to provide means for handling stress.

E. Treatments for persons at risk for suicide may employ a problem-solving cognitive-behavioral intervention, coping-based interventions, and stress reduction techniques. Of these, the problem solving approach seems most effective.

OVERALL SUMMARY

This chapter outlines the characteristic features of mood disorders (i.e., depression and mania). Specifically, the epidemiology, etiology, and treatment of major depressive episodes, dysthymia, cyclothymia, and bipolar disorder I and bipolar disorder II are described. Symptom feature modifiers, or those additional factors that have implications for predicting course or response to treatment, are also covered. The chapter is also devoted to the phenomenon of suicide, including prevention and intervention of suicidal ideation and intent. Various clinical examples are presented throughout the chapter.

KEY TERMS

Bipolar I disorder (p. 213)
Bipolar II disorder (p. 213)
Catalepsy (p. 216)
Cognitive therapy (p. 239)
Cyclothymic disorders (p. 214)
Delusions (p. 216)
Depressive cognitive triad (p. 231)
Double depression (p. 208)
Dysphoric manic or mixed episode (p. 207)
Dysthymic disorder (p. 208)
Electroconvulsive therapy (ECT) (p. 239)
Hallucinations (p. 216)
Hypomanic episode (p. 206)
Interpersonal psychotherapy (p. 241)
Learned helplessness theory of depression (p. 230)
Maintenance treatment (p. 243)
Major depressive disorder, single or recurrent episode (p. 208)
Major depressive episode (p. 206)
Mania (p. 206)
Mood disorders (p. 206)
Neurohormones (p. 227)
Pathological or impacted grief reaction (p. 211)
Psychological autopsy (p. 248)
Seasonal affective disorder (p. 217)
Suicidal attempts (p. 247)
Suicidal ideation (p. 247)

INFOTRAC KEY TERM EXERCISES

Each exercise is linked to key terms from the Wadsworth InfoTrac on-line searchable database. Key terms must be entered exactly as written.

Exercise 1: Use of Electroconvulsive Therapy in Children: Is it Safe?, and Does it Work?
Article: A19912690
Citation: (Use of electroconvulsive therapy with children: an overview and case report.) Catherine L. Willoughby; Elizabeth A. Hradek; Nancy R. Richards.
Journal of Child and Adolescent Psychiatric Nursing, July-Sept 1997 v10 n3 p11(7)

Your textbook notes that Electroconvulsive Therapy (ECT) is efficacious as a late line treatment for severe cases of adult depression. Increasing, however, ECT is being used with children and adolescence. This InfoTrac article reviews research using ECT in children and adolescence, and then provides limited data on the use of ECT with 8-year-old girl who suffered from psychotic depression. You are to review this article and address the following questions: (a) what is the state of research evidence supporting ECT in children and adolscence? (e.g., how many studies, does ECT work and for what age group), (b) describe guidelines for use of ECT in children/adolescents, and (c) provide a summary of the case report that follows. Was ECT effective for this young girl? Knowing what you know about ECT, what kinds of concerns would you have about its use with small children and young adolescents? Limit your answer to 3-5 typed double-spaced pages.

Exercise 2: Facts About St. John's Wort in the Treatment of Depression
Key Term: *St. John's Wort; Subdivision: Evaluation*

St. John's Wort is receiving increasing attention as a viable over-the-counter solution for the treatment of depression. St. John's Wort is available without a prescription at most health food stores and pharmacies. Your task here is to evaluate the current evidence regarding the effectiveness of St. John's Wort as a treatment for depression, including the known contraindications and side effects. In so doing, think whether the evidence is there to warrant consumers or physicians turning to St. John's as a solution for depression. Review the InfoTrac article(s) on this topic and provide a review and case for or against the utility of St. John's Wort, backed by appropriate evidence. Limit your answer to 3-5 typed double-spaced pages.

Exercise 3 (Future Trend): Psychologists as Gatekeepers for Physician-Assisted Suicide?

Suicide in the deliberate taking of one's life, and most of us tend to think of suicide as the least functional outcome of a human life. Mental health professionals go to great lengths to prevent suicide and to alleviate the suffering that contributes to it. Physician assisted suicide, by contrast, is a case where medical professionals appear to be facilitating suicide in terminally ill individuals, not acting to preventing it. Though psychologist have not assumed an active role in assisting suicide directly, there is great debate about the role(s) psychologists ought to take in such cases. It could be argued that psychologists, by virtue of their unique training and assessment skills, are best positioned to serve as gatekeepers for physician-assisted suicide. Given trends for prescription authority for psychologists one may even wonder whether psychologists may someday function as some physicians do now in assisting terminally ill patients take their own lives. This topic spans a range of ethical, moral, and legal issues that lend themselves to a debate format, or in class discussion about suicide and the role of psychologists in the prevention and alleviation of suffering. The links below provide some additional information and resources on this topic.

http://www.apa.org/pi/aseol/introduction.html
http://www.apa.org/ppo/issues/asresolu.html
http://www.psychiatrictimes.com/p040101b.html
http://www.nrlc.org/euthanasia/asisuid1.html

Fenn, D. S., & Ganzini, L. (1999). Attitudes of Oregon psychologists toward physician-assisted suicide and the Oregon Death With Dignity Act. Professional Psychology: Research and Practice, 30, 235–244. http://www.apa.org/journals/pro/pro303235.html

CLASSROOM ACTIVITIES, DEMONSTRATIONS, AND LECTURE TOPICS

1. **Activity: Suicide Questionnaire.** Give students HANDOUT 7.1 to enable them to test their knowledge about suicide. After they have completed the handout, discuss the correct answers with them and address concerns voiced by class members. Correct answers:
   a. (F) Although there may be some people who talk about suicide but never follow through, those who talk about suicide are at high risk for suicide. Many who successfully kill themselves have made earlier threats to do so.
   b. (F) Many people are suicidal for a short period of time; some who make it through a suicidal crisis recover completely.
   c. (F) Many people offer clues they are considering suicide before they attempt to kill themselves. About 80% of suicide attempts are preceded by a warning of some kind.
   d. (F) Talking about suicide can be helpful in prevention and does not trigger the act. In fact, you may show the person that you are not frightened and are willing to talk about it with them.
   e. (T) A depressed person who gives away valued possessions may be preparing for suicide.
   f. (F) A sudden recovery from depression is a clue the person is considering suicide and has attained peace of mind as a consequence of their plan.

2. **Activity: Suicide Prevention.** You may want to give your students HANDOUT 7.2 on suicide prevention. Discuss students' reactions to the suggestions and add any recommendations that class members may have regarding helping someone who is suicidal. You may also use the discussion as an opportunity to talk about assisted suicide.

3. **Activity: A Self-Rating Depression Scale.** A self-assessment inventory was developed by Zung (1965) to measure both the feelings and physical factors associated with depression (e.g., changes in eating and sleeping habits, lethargy, etc.). Though the clinical utility and psychometric properties of this measure are questionable, the scale nicely illustrates components of depression and takes only a few minutes to complete.

   Source Information. Zung, W. (1965) A self-rating depression scale. Archives of General Psychiatry, 12, 63-70.

4. **Activity: Bipolar Disorder Screening.** You may want to also give your students HANDOUT 7.3 that depicts items developed by the Depression and Bipolar Support Alliance as a brief screening tool for bipolar disorder. The items give students a sense of some of the problems associated with bipolar disorder.

   Source Information. This screening tool was developed by the Depression and Bipolar Support Alliance and is available on line at http://www.dbsalliance.org/questionnaire/screening_intro.asp.

5. **Video Activity: Abnormal Psychology, Inside/Out, Vol. 1.** After reviewing the nature of depressive disorders, present the video segment depicting Barbara, but do not let on

about her diagnosis. Ask students to see if they can arrive at a diagnosis for Barbara. The correct answer is Unipolar Depression, without Psychosis.

HANDOUT 7.1

WHAT DO YOU KNOW ABOUT SUICIDE?

Respond to each of the following questions by answering true or false:

1. _____ People who talk about suicide rarely follow through and actually attempt or commit suicide.

2. _____ People who are suicidal will remain suicidal their entire lives.

3. _____ Almost all suicides take place with little or no warning.

4. _____ Talking about suicide often precipitates a desire to follow through and do it.

5. _____ Giving away valued possessions is a clue that a person may be considering suicide.

6. Someone who is recovering from severe depression and suddenly develops a positive outlook on life rarely commits suicide.

HANDOUT 7.2

SUICIDE PREVENTION

Although there is no one best way to approach a situation where suicide may be a possibility, the guidelines that follow may be helpful.

1. Treat the person as a normal human being.

2. Don't consider the person too vulnerable or fragile to talk about the possibility of suicide. Raise the subject yourself by asking the person directly. For example, "It sounds like you are feeling depressed. Have you been thinking about harming or hurting yourself or committing suicide?"

3. Show the person you care about them even if you don't know them very well.

4. Help the person talk about and clarify the problem. Those who are depressed may have difficulty pinpointing the problem and may feel frustrated and confused.

5. Listen carefully. People who are considering suicide are in mental and/or physical pain, although you may not be able to guess the type of pain or the source of the problem. Be there to help the person talk about the issue. You don't need to fix the problem.

6. Suicide is often viewed as the final solution to an overwhelming problem. The person who is depressed may have difficulty sorting out alternative solutions to the problem(s) he/she faces.

7. Encourage the person to seek professional assistance. Crisis hotlines are available in many communities. If an immediate danger of suicide exists, do not leave the person alone. If the crisis seems to be improved for thc moment, be sure you have a plan of action regarding professional help before leaving the person. Have the person promise to call you before doing any harm to him/herself. Offer to accompany him/her to see a mental health professional.

8. If a friend refuses help, you may need to contact someone close to him/her such as a family member to share your concerns.

9. Maintain contact with your friend.

HANDOUT 7.3

THE MOOD DISORDER QUESTIONNAIRE

Items in this questionnaire are intended as a screening instrument. Please answer each question as best you can by circling either yes or no.

1. Has there ever been a period of time when you were not your usual self and...

Yes	No	...you felt so good or so hyper that other people thought you were not your normal self or you were so hyper that you got into trouble?
Yes	No	...you were so irritable that you shouted at people or started fights or arguments?
Yes	No	...you felt much more self-confident than usual?
Yes	No	...you got much less sleep than usual and found you didn't really miss it?
Yes	No	...you were much more talkative or spoke much faster than usual?
Yes	No	...thoughts raced through your head or you couldn't slow your mind down?
Yes	No	...you were so easily distracted by things around you that you had trouble concentrating or staying on track?
Yes	No	...you had much more energy than usual?
Yes	No	...you were much more active or did many more things than usual?
Yes	No	...you were much more social or outgoing than usual, for example, you telephoned friends in the middle of the night?
Yes	No	...you were much more interested in sex than usual?
Yes	No	...you did things that were unusual for you or that other people might have thought were excessive, foolish, or risky?
Yes	No	...spending money got you or your family into trouble?

2. If you checked YES to more than one of the above, have several of these ever happened during the same period of time? Yes No

3. How much of a problem did any of these cause you - like being unable to work; having family, money or legal troubles, getting into arguments or fights? Please select one response only.

No Problem Minor Problem Moderate Problem Serious Problem

Source Information. This screening tool was developed by National Depressive and Manic-Depressive Association and is available on line at http://www.ndmda.org/screening.asp.

SUPPLEMENTARY READING MATERIAL FOR CHAPTER SEVEN

(= These sources can be found on "*Infotrac, the online library*" provided by Wadsworth and Brooks/Cole Publishing.)

Beck, A. T. (1987). Cognitive therapy of depression. New York: Guilford.

Bernard, M. E., & DiGuiseppe, R. (Eds.) (1989). Inside rational-emotive therapy. New York: Academic Press.

Burns, D. D. (1989). The feeling good handbook. New York: Plume.

Clark, D. A., & Beck, A. T. (1999). Scientific foundations of cognitive theory and therapy of depression. Philadelphia: Wiley.

Copeland, M. E. (1994). Living without depression and manic depression: A workbook for maintaining mood stability. New York: New Harbinger.

Faedda, G., Tondo, L., & Ross, J. (1993). Seasonal mood disorders: Patterns of seasonal recurrence in mania and depression. Archives of General Psychiatry, 50, 17-23.

Fremouw, W. J., Perczel, W. J., & Ellis, T. E. (1990). Suicide risk: Assessment and response guidelines. New York: Pergamon.

Geller, B., & Luby, J. (1997). Child and adolescent bipolar disorder: A review of the past 10 years. Journal of the American Academy of Child and Adolescent Psychiatry, 36, 1168(9).

Geller, B., Reising, D., Leonard, H., Riddle, M. A., & Walsh, B. T. (1999). Critical review of tricyclic antidepressant use in children and adolescents. Journal of the American Academy of Child and Adolescent Psychiatry, 38, 513(4).

Goodwin, F., & Jamison, K. (1990). Manic-depressive illness. New York: Oxford University.

Gotlib, I. H. (1987). Treatment of depression: An interpersonal systems approach. New York: Pergamon.

Lewinsohn, P. M., Rohde, P., Seeley, J. R., & Baldwin, C. (2001). Gender differences in suicide attempts from adolescence to young adulthood. Journal of the American Academy of Child and Adolescent Psychiatry, 40, 427.

Styron, W. (1990). Darkness visible: A memoir of madness. New York: Vintage.

Thayer, R. E. (1996). The origin of everyday moods. New York: Oxford University.

Young, J. E., & Klosko, J. S. (1993). Reinventing your life: How to break free of negative life patterns. New York: Dutton.

SUPPLEMENTARY 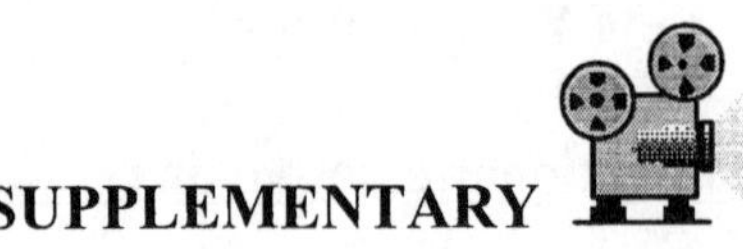 VIDEO RESOURCES FOR CHAPTER SEVEN

Abnormal psychology, inside/out, vol. 1. (*available through your International Thomson Learning representative).* This volume presents an interview with a patient named Barbara, who is experiencing a major depressive episode. Barbara notes that she was depressed most of her life, beginning in high school when she had a headache that lasted for one and one-half years. She describes her current dissatisfaction with her appearance, sleep disturbances, overeating while depressed, and problems with social withdrawal. Barbara was diagnosed with unipolar depression, without psychosis. (11 min)

The second segment presents the case of Mary, who was diagnosed with bipolar depression with psychotic symptoms. During the first interview Mary is experiencing a depressive episode, whereas during the second interview she is in the midst of a manic episode. (15 min)

Abnormal psychology, inside/out, vol. 2. (*available through your International Thomson Learning representative).* A segment on this tape provides an overview of the characteristics of MDD, including an interview with a female client who describes her experience when she is in the midst of a major depressive episode. The female client also talks about her decision to commit suicide. A related segment, titled "Feeling Bad," also covers the feelings that accompany Major Depression, whereas the segment "Feeling Better After Treatment," presents an interview with a female client that describes the stigma she experiences with MDD, how her life improved with treatment, and the importance of asking for help. (7 min)

Antidepressant agents. (Insight Media: 2162 Broadway, New York, NY 10024/ (800)-233-9910). This video examines the causes and manifestations of depression. It considers neurotransmitters and receptors in the brain; presents theories related to how medication provides relief from depression; and examines the three categories of antidepressant agents — tricyclic agents, selective serotonin reuptake inhibitors, and monoamine oxidase inhibitors. (23 min)

Breaking the dark horse: A family copes with manic depression. (Fanlight Productions, 1-800-937-4113). The video presents a story of a woman with manic depression and how it affects her family and friends. (32 min)

CBT for depressed adolescents. (Insight Media: 2162 Broadway, New York, NY 10024/ (800)-233-9910). This three-part video presents cognitive behavioral intervention for adolescents with depression. It reviews the theoretical basis for cognitive behavioral treatment (CBT) and then provides illustrative vignettes. Finally, it discusses potential difficulties encountered when using CBT with adolescents and their families. (130 min)

CNN today: Abnormal psychology, vol. 1. (*available through your International Thomson Learning representative).* The segment titled "Mood Disorders: Depression Alternative" discusses alternative methods to treat depression (e.g. acupuncture, herbal remedies such as St. Johns Wort). Discusses the lack of research regarding herbal solutions and includes testimonials of women who found symptom relief using alternative herbal methods. (2 min 31 sec)

A second segment titled, "Electroconvulsive Therapy (ECT)," describes the nature and use of ECT as a treatment for severe depression, particularly when all other treatment approaches fail. This segment describes some of the controversy and misunderstandings surrounding the use of ECT. (3 min 20 sec)

A third segment titled, "Depression Treatment," describes the nature of bipolar depression, including the high risk of suicide associated with this condition. American Psychiatric Association Guidelines are discussed in the context of treatment. (2 min 5 sec)

Demonstration of the cognitive therapy of depression. (Insight Media: 2162 Broadway, New York, NY 10024/ (800)-233-9910). Aaron Beck, one of the major proponents of cognitive theory and developer of the Beck Depression Inventory, demonstrates his method of cognitive therapy of depression in this interview with a depressed and suicidal woman. The tape illustrates how to conceptualize a patient in a cognitive framework. (40 min)

Depression and manic depression. (Insight Media: 2162 Broadway, New York, NY 10024/ (800)-233-9910). Explaining that many cases of clinical depression remain untreated due to issues of stigma and fear, this video explores the relationship between untreated depression and suicide, using as examples the depressions of such well-known public figures as Mike Wallace and Kay Redfield Jamison. (28 min)

Four lives: A portrait of manic-depression. (Insight Media: 2162 Broadway, New York, NY 10024/ (800)-233-9910). This video explores the psychological effects of bipolar affective disorder by examining four patients. Psychiatrists discuss the history and treatment of each patient, describing the rapid mood swings from depression to mania and considering common manifestations of these moods. The program also examines the uses of ECT, lithium treatment, and psychotherapy. (60 min)

Girl interrupted. (Hollywood Film; Drama). This film, set in the 1960s, illustrates a compelling true story of a woman who attempted suicide and subsequently self-committed to a mental institution. The range of psychopathology of the characters, including the depiction of treatment and life in a mental institution during the 1960s, is outstanding. This film nicely illustrates depression, suicide, but may be useful for personality disorders, schizophrenia, and ethical and legal issues as well.

It's a wonderful life. (Hollywood Film; Drama). A Christmas tradition. This film presents Jimmy Stewart who responds to the stress of life in Bedford Falls by attempting suicide.

Life upside down. (Hollywood Film; Drama). French film about an ordinary young man who becomes increasingly detached from the world. He is eventually hospitalized and treated, but without much success.

Ordinary people. (Hollywood Film; Drama). This film deals with depression, suicide, and family pathology and presents a sympathetic portrayal of a psychiatrist who probably meets DSM-IV-TR criteria for PTSD and depression.

Psychopharmacology for the 21st Century: Antidepressants. (Insight Media: 2162 Broadway, New York, NY 10024/ (800)-233-9910). In this program, Joel Holiner provides an in-depth overview of antidepressants, reviewing their efficacies, dosages, and side effects. He discusses uses of tricyclics, heterocyclics, lithium, and MAOIs for treating depression, anxiety, social phobia, bulimia, and OCD. He also presents recommendations for antidepressant use during pregnancy and highlights the advantages of the newest SSRIs, including Luvox and Celexa, the latest SS -Norepinephrine reuptake inhibitor. (30 min)

The choice of a lifetime. (Fanlight Productions, 1-800-937-4113). This disturbing, but ultimately inspiring, film is told from the point of view of six people, ages 21 to 73, who stepped back from the brink of suicide. In candid interviews, they examine the circumstances that led to their despair, the forces that stopped them, and the methods of healing they discovered, including therapy, support groups, spirituality, and artistic expression. (53 min)

The depressed child. (Insight Media: 2162 Broadway, New York, NY 10024/ (800)-233-9910). Seven percent of children and 27 percent of adolescents meet the criteria for major depressive disorder. If left undiagnosed, depression can have negative long-term effects or lead to suicide. This video examines the problem of youth depression and discusses such treatment options as counseling and antidepressant medications. (25 min)

The hospital. (Hollywood Film; Comedy/Drama). George C. Scott depicts a suicidal physician.

The Mosquito Coast. (Hollywood Film; Adventure). Harrison Ford plays an eccentric American inventor who flees the U.S. for Central America because of his paranoia. His behavior throughout the film is bipolar, and certainly manic.

Treatment strategies for the management of chronic depression. (Insight Media: 2162 Broadway, New York, NY 10024/ (800)-233-9910). An estimated five percent of depression victims suffer from lifelong, chronic depression. This program explores how outcomes may be complicated by co-morbid psychiatric and medical conditions, as well as chronic stressors. It discusses the diagnosis of chronic depression and presents management strategies and challenges for the clinician. HSTN. (90 min)

INTERNET 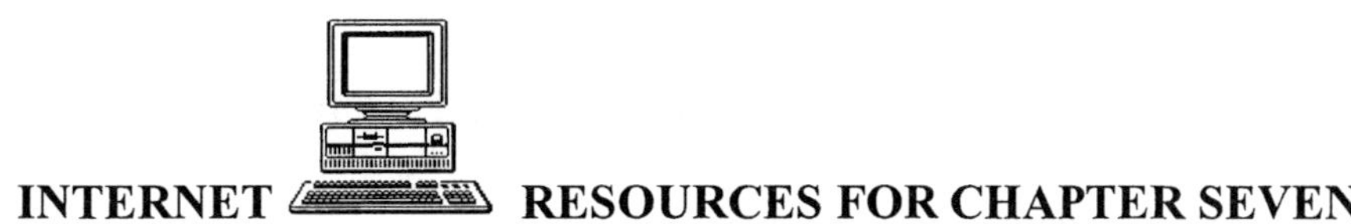 RESOURCES FOR CHAPTER SEVEN

Bipolar Disorder
http://www.mentalhealth.com/p20-grp.html
Internet Mental Health provides this informative web page; information on other disorders are provided as well.

Clinical Depression Screening Test
http://sandbox.xerox.com/pair/cw/testing.html
General Hospital, an "ongoing art and information project of the artist team Margaret Crane/Jon Winet, which looks at mental health and society" developed this online depression examination.

Cyclothymia
http://www.mentalhealth.com/dis/p20-md03.html
Internet Mental Health provides this informative web page; information on other disorders are provided as well.

Depression Central
http://www.psycom.net/depression.central.html
Dr. Ivan's Depression Central offers links to several sites on mood disorders, including sites for books, videos, research, diagnosis, and treatment.

Dysthymia
http://www.mentalhealth.com/p20-grp.html
Internet Mental Health provides this informative web page; information on other disorders are provided as well.

Facts about Women and Depression
http://www.nimh.nih.gov/HealthInformation/depwomen.cfm
An NIMH web page, containing many facts regarding women and mental health.

Major Depressive Disorder
http://www.mentalhealth.com/p20-grp.html
Internet Mental Health provides this informative web page; information on other disorders is provided as well.

Depression and Bipolar Support Alliance
http://www.dbsalliance.org/
Provides a number of links and resources related to mood disorders.

Psychology Information Online
http://www.psychologyinfo.com/depression/index.html

A useful resource to information about the nature of mood disorders, including links to other related sites.

Suicide Resources at the National Institute of Mental Health
http://www.nimh.nih.gov/SuicidePrevention/index.cfm

This NIMH site has several useful bits of information related to suicide and depression, including information on the nature of suicide and data on its prevalence and incidence.

WARNING SIGNS OF DEPRESSION

The following signs and symptoms are considered indicators of depression if they persist for a period of more than two weeks.

- Feeling sad or empty most of the day, nearly every day
- Reduced interest and pleasure in activities
- Significant unintentional weight loss or gain or a change in appetite
- Over or under sleeping
- Feeling worthless, hopeless, and/or inappropriately guilty
- Recurrent thoughts of death or suicide

WARNING SIGNS OF CHILDHOOD DEPRESSION

The following signs and symptoms are considered indicators of depression i they persist for a period of more than two weeks.

- Persistent sadness and hopelessness
- Withdrawal from friends and activities once enjoyed
- Increased irritability or agitation
- Missed school or poor school performance
- Changes in eating and sleeping habits
- Indecision, lack of concentration or forgetfulness
- Poor self-esteem or guilt
- Frequent physical complaints, such as headaches and stomachaches
- Lack of enthusiasm, low energy or motivation
- Drug and/or alcohol abuse
- Recurring thoughts of death or suicide

WARNING SIGNS OF BIPOLAR DISORDER

Increased Energy
- Decreased Sleep, Little Fatigue
- An Increase in Activities
- Restlessness

Speech Disruptions
- Rapid, Pressured Speech
- Incoherent Speech, Clang Associations

Impaired Judgment
- Lack of Insight
- Inappropriate Humor and Behaviors
- Impulsive Behaviors
- Financial Extravagance
- Grandiose Thinking

Increased or Decreased Sexuality

Changes in Thought Patterns
- Distractibility
- Creative Thinking
- Flight of Ideas
- Disorientation
- Disjointed Thinking
- Racing Thoughts

Changes in Mood
- Irritability
- Excitability
- Hostility
- Feelings of Exhilaration

Changes in Perceptions
- Inflated Self-Esteem
- Hallucinations
- Paranoia
- Increased Religious Activities

WARNING SIGNS OF MANIA AND HYPOMANIA

- Insomnia or difficulty sleeping
- Writing pressure
- Others seem slow
- Irritability or surges of energy
- Making lots of plans
- Flight of Ideas
- Pressured speech
- Poor judgment and/or inappropriate behavior
- Increased alcohol consumption
- Spending too much money
- Very productive
- Taking too many responsibilities
- Feeling superior
- Increased creativity
- Dangerous driving
- Unnecessary phone calls
- More sensitive than usual
- Increased appetite and sexual activity
- Noises louder than usual
- Doing several things at once
- Inability to concentrate
- Friends notice behavior change
- Difficulty staying still
- Sociable and thrill seeking
- Anxious and wound-up

WARNING SIGNS FOR SUICIDE (GENERAL)

- Verbal suicide threats or statements
- Previous suicide attempt
- Risk-taking behavior, reckless behavior
- Final arrangements -- giving away prized possessions, making peace, tying up loose ends
- Neglect of academic work and/or personal appearance
- Separation from loved ones or significant others
- Themes in writing or art about death, depression or suicide
- Talk of wanting to die
- Chronic depression; prolonged grief after a loss
- Unusual purchases -- gun, rope, medications; gathering of pills or poisons
- Unusual sadness, discouragement and loneliness
- Unexpected happiness (sudden happiness following prolonged depression)
- Physical complaints, hyperactivity, substance abuse, aggressiveness

DSM-IV-TR Criteria for Major Depressive Episode Criteria A

A. Five (or more) of the following symptoms have been present during the same 2-week period and represent a change from previous functioning; at least one of the symptoms is either

1. depressed mood or
2. loss of interest or pleasure.

Note: Do not include symptoms that are clearly due to a general medical condition, or mood-incongruent delusions or hallucinations.

1. depressed mood most of the day, nearly every day, as indicated by either subjective report (e.g., feels sad or empty) or observation made by others (e.g., appears tearful). Note: In children and adolescents, can be irritable mood.
2. markedly diminished interest or pleasure in all, or almost all, activities most of the day, nearly every day (as indicated by either subjective account or observation made by others)
3. significant weight loss when not dieting or weight gain (e.g., a change of more than 5% of body weight in a month), or decrease or increase in appetite nearly every day. Note: In children, consider failure to make expected weight gains.
4. Insomnia or Hypersomnia nearly every day
5. psychomotor agitation or retardation nearly every day (observable by others, not merely subjective feelings of restlessness or being slowed down)
6. fatigue or loss of energy nearly every day
7. feelings of worthlessness or excessive or inappropriate guilt (which may be delusional) nearly every day (not merely self-reproach or guilt about being sick)
8. diminished ability to think or concentrate, or indecisiveness, nearly every day (either by subjective account or as observed by others)
9. recurrent thoughts of death (not just fear of dying), recurrent suicidal ideation without a specific plan, or a suicide attempt or a specific plan for committing suicide

DSM-IV-TR Criteria for Major Depressive Episode Criteria B, C, D, and E

B. The symptoms do not meet criteria for a Mixed Episode.

C. The symptoms cause clinically significant distress or impairment in social, occupational, or other important areas of functioning.

D. The symptoms are not due to the direct physiological effects of a substance (e.g., a drug of abuse, a medication) or a general medical condition (e.g., hypothyroidism).

E. The symptoms are not better accounted for by Bereavement, i.e., after the loss of a loved one, the symptoms persist for longer than 2 months or are characterized by marked functional impairment, morbid preoccupation with worthlessness, suicidal ideation, psychotic symptoms, or psychomotor retardation.

DSM-IV-TR Criteria for Major Depressive Disorder, Recurrent

A. Presence of two or more Major Depressive Episodes.
Note: To be considered separate episodes, there must be an interval of at least 2 consecutive months in which criteria are not met for a Major Depressive Episode.

B. The Major Depressive Episodes are not better accounted for by Schizoaffective Disorder and are not superimposed on Schizophrenia, Schizophreniform Disorder, Delusional Disorder, or Psychotic Disorder Not Otherwise Specified.

C. There has never been a Manic Episode, a Mixed Episode, or a Hypomanic Episode. Note: This exclusion does not apply if all of the manic-like, mixed-like, or hypomanic-like episodes are substance or treatment induced or are due to the direct physiological effects of a general medical condition.

Specify (for current or most recent episode):

Severity/Psychotic/Remission Specifiers
Chronic
With Catatonic Features
With Melancholic Features
With Atypical Features
With Postpartum Onset

Specify:

Longitudinal Course Specifiers (With and Without Interepisode Recovery)
With Seasonal Pattern

DSM-IV-TR Criteria for Major Depressive Disorder, Single Episode

A. Presence of a single Major Depressive Episode.

B. The Major Depressive Episode is not better accounted for by Schizoaffective Disorder and is not superimposed on Schizophrenia, Schizophreniform Disorder, Delusional Disorder, or Psychotic Disorder Not Otherwise Specified.

C. There has never been a Manic Episode, a Mixed Episode, or a Hypomanic Episode. Note: This exclusion does not apply if all of the manic-like, mixed-like, or hypomanic-like episodes are substance or treatment induced or are due to the direct physiological effects of a general medical condition.

Specify (for current or most recent episode):

Severity/Psychotic/Remission Specifiers
Chronic
With Catatonic Features
With Melancholic Features
With Atypical Features
With Postpartum Onset

DSM-IV-TR Criteria for Dysthymic Disorder Criteria A, B, C, and D

A. Depressed mood for most of the day, for more days than not, as indicated either by subjective account or observation by others, for at least 2 years. Note: In children and adolescents, mood can be irritable and duration must be at least 1 year.

B. Presence, while depressed, of two (or more) of the following:

1. poor appetite or overeating
2. Insomnia or Hypersomnia
3. low energy or fatigue
4. low self-esteem
5. poor concentration or difficulty making decisions
6. feelings of hopelessness

C. During the 2-year period (1 year for children or adolescents) of the disturbance, the person has never been without the symptoms in Criteria A and B for more than 2 months at a time.

D. No Major Depressive Episode has been present during the first 2 years of the disturbance (1 year for children and adolescents); i.e., the disturbance is not better accounted for by chronic Major Depressive Disorder, or Major Depressive Disorder, In Partial Remission.

Note: There may have been a previous Major Depressive Episode provided there was a full remission (no significant signs or symptoms for 2 months) before development of the Dysthymic Disorder. In addition, after the initial 2 years (1 year in children or adolescents) of Dysthymic Disorder, there may be superimposed episodes of Major Depressive Disorder, in which case both diagnoses may be given when the criteria are met for a Major Depressive Episode.

Transparency 7-6

DSM-IV-TR Criteria for Dysthymic Disorder Criteria E, F, G, and H

E. There has never been a Manic Episode, a Mixed Episode, or a Hypomanic Episode, and criteria have never been met for Cyclothymic Disorder.

F. The disturbance does not occur exclusively during the course of a chronic Psychotic Disorder, such as Schizophrenia or Delusional Disorder.

G. The symptoms are not due to the direct physiological effects of a substance (e.g., a drug of abuse, a medication) or a general medical condition (e.g., hypothyroidism).

H. The symptoms cause clinically significant distress or impairment in social, occupational, or other important areas of functioning.

Specify if:
- **Early Onset**: if onset is before age 21 years
- **Late Onset**: if onset is age 21 years or older

Specify (for most recent 2 years of Dysthymic Disorder):
- **With Atypical Features**

DSM-IV-TR Criteria for Manic Episode

A. A distinct period of abnormally and persistently elevated, expansive, or irritable mood, lasting at least 1 week (or any duration if hospitalization is necessary).

B. During the period of mood disturbance, three (or more) of the following symptoms have persisted (four if the mood is only irritable) and have been present to a significant degree:

1. inflated self-esteem or grandiosity
2. decreased need for sleep (e.g., feels rested after only 3 hours of sleep)
3. more talkative than usual or pressure to keep talking
4. flight of ideas or subjective experience that thoughts are racing
5. distractibility (i.e., attention too easily drawn to unimportant or irrelevant external stimuli)
6. increase in goal-directed activity (either socially, at work or school, or sexually) or psychomotor agitation
7. excessive involvement in pleasurable activities that have a high potential for painful consequences (e.g., engaging in unrestrained buying sprees, sexual indiscretions, or foolish business investments)

C. The symptoms do not meet criteria for a Mixed Episode.

D. The mood disturbance is sufficiently severe to cause marked impairment in occupational functioning or in usual social activities or relationships with others, or to necessitate hospitalization to prevent harm to self or others, or there are psychotic features.

E. The symptoms are not due to the direct physiological effects of a substance (e.g., a drug of abuse, a medication, or other treatment) or a general medical condition (e.g., hyperthyroidism).

Note: Manic-like episodes that are clearly caused by somatic antidepressant treatment (e.g., medication, electroconvulsive therapy, light therapy) should not count toward a diagnosis of Bipolar I Disorder.

DSM-IV-TR Criteria for Severity/Psychotic/Remission Specifiers for Current (or most recent) Manic Episode

Note: Code in fifth digit. Can be applied to a Manic Episode in Bipolar I Disorder only if it is the most recent type of mood episode.

.x1--**Mild**: Minimum symptom criteria are met for a Manic Episode.
.x2--**Moderate**: Extreme increase in activity or impairment in judgment.
.x3--**Severe Without Psychotic Features**: Almost continual supervision required to prevent physical harm to self or others.
.x4--**Severe With Psychotic Features**: Delusions or hallucinations. If possible, specify whether the psychotic features are mood-congruent or mood-incongruent:

Mood-Congruent Psychotic Features: Delusions or hallucinations whose content is entirely consistent with the typical manic themes of inflated worth, power, knowledge, identity, or special relationship to a deity or famous person.

Mood-Incongruent Psychotic Features: Delusions or hallucinations whose content does not involve typical manic themes of inflated worth, power, knowledge, identity, or special relationship to a deity or famous person. Included are such symptoms as persecutory delusions (not directly related to grandiose ideas or themes), thought insertion, and delusions of being controlled.

.x5--**In Partial Remission**: Symptoms of a Manic Episode are present but full criteria are not met, or there is a period without any significant symptoms of a Manic Episode lasting less than 2 months following the end of the Manic Episode.

.x6--**In Full Remission**: During the past 2 months no significant signs or symptoms of the disturbance were present.

.x0--**Unspecified**.

DSM-IV-TR Criteria for a Hypomanic Episode

A. A distinct period of persistently elevated, expansive, or irritable mood, lasting throughout at least 4 days, that is clearly different from the usual nondepressed mood.

B. During the period of mood disturbance, three (or more) of the following symptoms have persisted (four if the mood is only irritable) and have been present to a significant degree:

1. inflated self-esteem or grandiosity
2. decreased need for sleep (e.g., feels rested after only 3 hours of sleep)
3. more talkative than usual or pressure to keep talking
4. flight of ideas or subjective experience that thoughts are racing
5. distractibility (i.e., attention too easily drawn to unimportant or irrelevant external stimuli)
6. increase in goal-directed activity (either socially, at work or school, or sexually) or psychomotor agitation
7. excessive involvement in pleasurable activities that have a high potential for painful consequences (c.g., thc pcrson cngagcs in unrestrained buying sprees, sexual indiscretions, or foolish business investments)

C. The episode is associated with an unequivocal change in functioning that is uncharacteristic of the person when not symptomatic.

D. The disturbance in mood and the change in functioning are observable by others.

E. The episode is not severe enough to cause marked impairment in social or occupational functioning, or to necessitate hospitalization, and there are no psychotic features.

F. The symptoms are not due to the direct physiological effects of a substance (e.g., a drug of abuse, a medication, or other treatment) or a general medical condition (e.g., hyperthyroidism).

Note: Hypomanic-like episodes that are clearly caused by somatic antidepressant treatment (e.g., medication, electroconvulsive therapy, light therapy) should not count toward a diagnosis of Bipolar II Disorder.

DSM-IV-TR Criteria for Bipolar I Disorder, Single Manic Episode

A. Presence of only one Manic Episode and no past Major Depressive Episodes.

Note: Recurrence is defined as either a change in polarity from depression or an interval of at least 2 months without manic symptoms.

B. The Manic Episode is not better accounted for by Schizoaffective Disorder and is not superimposed on Schizophrenia, Schizophreniform Disorder, Delusional Disorder, or Psychotic Disorder Not Otherwise Specified.

Specify if:

Mixed: if symptoms meet criteria for a Mixed Episode

Specify (for current or most recent episode):

Severity/Psychotic/Remission Specifiers
With Catatonic Features
With Postpartum Onset

DSM-IV-TR Criteria for Bipolar I Disorder, Most Recent Episode Hypomanic

A. Currently (or most recently) in a Hypomanic Episode.

B. There has previously been at least one Manic Episode or Mixed Episode.

C. The mood symptoms cause clinically significant distress or impairment in social, occupational, or other important areas of functioning.

D. The mood episodes in Criteria A and B are not better accounted for by Schizoaffective Disorder and are not superimposed on Schizophrenia, Schizophreniform Disorder, Delusional Disorder, or Psychotic Disorder Not Otherwise Specified.

Specify:

Longitudinal Course Specifiers (With and Without Interepisode Recovery
With Seasonal Pattern (applies only to the pattern of Major Depressive Episodes)
With Rapid Cycling

DSM-IV-TR Criteria for Bipolar I Disorder, Most Recent Episode Manic

A. Currently (or most recently) in a Manic Episode.

B. There has previously been at least one Major Depressive Episode, Manic Episode, or Mixed Episode.

C. The mood episodes in Criteria A and B are not better accounted for by Schizoaffective Disorder and are not superimposed on Schizophrenia, Schizophreniform Disorder, Delusional Disorder, or Psychotic Disorder Not Otherwise Specified.

Specify (for current or most recent episode):

Severity/Psychotic/Remission Specifiers
With Catatonic Features
With Postpartum Onset

Specify:

Longitudinal Course Specifiers (With and Without Interepisode Recovery)
With Seasonal Pattern (applies only to the pattern of Major Depressive Episodes)
With Rapid Cycling

DSM-IV-TR Criteria for Bipolar I Disorder, Most Recent Episode Mixed

A. Currently (or most recently) in a Mixed Episode.

B. There has previously been at least one Major Depressive Episode, Manic Episode, or Mixed Episode.

C. The mood episodes in Criteria A and B are not better accounted for by Schizoaffective Disorder and are not superimposed on Schizophrenia, Schizophreniform Disorder, Delusional Disorder, or Psychotic Disorder Not Otherwise Specified.

Specify (for current or most recent episode):

Severity/Psychotic/Remission Specifiers
With Catatonic Features
With Postpartum Onset

Specify:

Longitudinal Course Specifiers (With and Without Interepisode Recovery)
With Seasonal Pattern (applies only to the pattern of Major Depressive Episodes)
With Rapid Cycling

DSM-IV-TR Criteria for Bipolar I Disorder, Most Recent Episode Depressed

A. Currently (or most recently) in a Major Depressive Episode.

B. There has previously been at least one Manic Episode or Mixed Episode.

C. The mood episodes in Criteria A and B are not better accounted for by Schizoaffective Disorder and are not superimposed on Schizophrenia, Schizophreniform Disorder, Delusional Disorder, or Psychotic Disorder Not Otherwise Specified.

Specify (for current or most recent episode):

Severity/Psychotic/Remission Specifiers
Chronic
With Catatonic Features
With Melancholic Features
With Atypical Features
With Postpartum Onset

Specify:

Longitudinal Course Specifiers (With and Without Interepisode Recovery)
With Seasonal Pattern (applies only to the pattern of Major Depressive Episodes)
With Rapid Cycling

Transparency 7-15

DSM-IV-TR Criteria for Bipolar I Disorder, Most Recent Episode Unspecified

A. Criteria, except for duration, are currently (or most recently) met for a Manic, a Hypomanic, a Mixed, or a Major Depressive Episode.

B. There has previously been at least one Manic Episode or Mixed Episode.

C. The mood symptoms cause clinically significant distress or impairment in social, occupational, or other important areas of functioning.

D. The mood symptoms in Criteria A and B are not better accounted for by Schizoaffective Disorder and are not superimposed on Schizophrenia, Schizophreniform Disorder, Delusional Disorder, or Psychotic Disorder Not Otherwise Specified.

E. The mood symptoms in Criteria A and B are not due to the direct physiological effects of a substance (e.g., a drug of abuse, a medication, or other treatment) or a general medical condition (e.g., hyperthyroidism).

Specify:

Longitudinal Course Specifiers (With and Without Interepisode Recovery)
With Seasonal Pattern (applies only to the pattern of Major Depressive Episodes)
With Rapid Cycling

DSM-IV-TR Criteria for Bipolar II Disorder

A. Presence (or history) of one or more Major Depressive Episodes.

B. Presence (or history) of at least one Hypomanic Episode.

C. There has never been a Manic Episode or a Mixed Episode.

D. The mood symptoms in Criteria A and B are not better accounted for by Schizoaffective Disorder and are not superimposed on Schizophrenia, Schizophreniform Disorder, Delusional Disorder, or Psychotic Disorder Not Otherwise Specified.

E. The symptoms cause clinically significant distress or impairment in social, occupational, or other important areas of functioning.

Specify current or most recent episode:

Hypomanic: if currently (or most recently) in a Hypomanic Episode
Depressed: if currently (or most recently) in a Major Depressive Episode

Specify (for current or most recent Major Depressive Episode only if it is the most recent type of mood episode):

Severity/Psychotic/Remission Specifiers
Chronic
With Catatonic Features
With Melancholic Features
With Atypical Features
With Postpartum Onset

Specify:

Longitudinal Course Specifiers (With and Without Interepisode Recovery)
With Seasonal Pattern (applies only to the pattern of Major Depressive Episodes)
With Rapid Cycling

DSM-IV-TR Criteria for Cyclothymic Disorder

A. For at least 2 years, the presence of numerous periods with hypomanic symptoms (see p. 338) and numerous periods with depressive symptoms that do not meet criteria for a Major Depressive Episode. Note: In children and adolescents, the duration must be at least 1 year.

B. During the above 2-year period (1 year in children and adolescents), the person has not been without the symptoms in Criterion A for more than 2 months at a time.

C. No Major Depressive Episode, Manic Episode, or Mixed Episode has been present during the first 2 years of the disturbance.

Note: After the initial 2 years (1 year in children and adolescents) of Cyclothymic Disorder, there may be superimposed Manic or Mixed Episodes (in which case both Bipolar I Disorder and Cyclothymic Disorder may be diagnosed) or Major Depressive Episodes (in which case both Bipolar II Disorder and Cyclothymic Disorder may be diagnosed).

D. The symptoms in Criterion A are not better accounted for by Schizoaffective Disorder and are not superimposed on Schizophrenia, Schizophreniform Disorder, Delusional Disorder, or Psychotic Disorder Not Otherwise Specified.

E. The symptoms are not due to the direct physiological effects of a substance (e.g., a drug of abuse, a medication) or a general medical condition (e.g., hyperthyroidism).

F. The symptoms cause clinically significant distress or impairment in social, occupational, or other important areas of functioning.

CHAPTER EIGHT

EATING AND SLEEP DISORDERS

LEARNING OBJECTIVES

1. Describe the clinical manifestations of bulimia nervosa and anorexia nervosa, including important etiologic, diagnostic, and phenomenologic similarities and differences between them.
2. Describe the medical complications associated with bulimia and anorexia nervosa.
3. Compare and contrast the symptoms and psychological features of binge eating disorder and bulimia, and be able to elucidate the core features of rumination disorder, pica, and feeding disorder.
4. Describe the possible social, psychological, and neurobiological causes of eating disorders.
5. Compare the use of medications with psychological therapies for the treatment of eating disorders.
6. Differentiate the core features of dyssomnias from those of parasomnias.
7. Identify the critical diagnostic features of each of the major sleep disorders.
8. Describe the nature of REM and non-REM periods of sleep and how they relate to the parasomnias.
9. Be able to describe the basic operation of the brain and endocrine function that regulate circadian rhythms and the sleep-wake cycle.
10. Describe how medical and psychological treatments are used for the treatment of many sleeping disorders and the role of good sleep hygiene in the prevention of sleep disorders.

OUTLINE

I. Major Types of Eating Disorders
   A. The prevalence of eating disorders is substantially increasing in the Western world, where the problems appear to be culture-specific. However, recent research suggests that rates of eating disorders are increasing in other regions as well, particularly Japan and Hong Kong. Most cases of severe eating disorders are found in young, affluent, white females in competitive environments. Unlike other psychological disorders, the causes of eating disorders have a large sociocultural component.
      1. In **bulimia nervosa**, out of control eating episodes, or binges, are followed by self-induced vomiting, excessive laxative use, or other attempts to purge (get rid of) the food.
      2. In **anorexia nervosa**, eating is restricted to minimal amounts of food, such that body weight can drop to dangerously low levels.
      3. The central characteristic of these related disorders is an overwhelming, all-encompassing drive to be thin.

4. As many as 20% of anorexics die as a result of their disorder, with about 50% of deaths resulting from suicide. The mortality rate from eating disorders is the highest for any psychological disorder, even depression.
5. Eating disorders appeared for the first time as a separate group in the DSM-IV.
6. **Obesity** is not an official disorder in the DSM, but is thought to be one of the most dangerous epidemics confronting public health authorities, as up to 65% of adults in the United States are overweight and 30% meet criteria for obesity. The more overweight someone is at a given height, the greater the risks to health.

B. **Bulimia nervosa** is one of the most prevalent psychological disorders on college campuses. The textbook illustrates bulimia nervosa with the case of Phoebe.

1. The hallmark of bulimia nervosa is **binge eating**. A **binge** is defined as "*a larger amount of food than most people would eat under the circumstances.*" A binge is also marked by uncontrollability, with an average binge consisting largely of junk food.. Actual caloric intake for binges varies significantly from person to person.
2. In addition, persons with bulimia attempt to **compensate** for binge eating and potential weight gain by engaging in **purging techniques**. Common techniques include self-induced vomiting immediately after eating, laxative abuse, and diuretics (i.e., drugs that result in loss of fluids though greatly increased frequency of urination). Some persons with bulimia exercise excessively, whereas others fast.
3. Bulimia is subtyped in the DSM-IV-TR as either **purging or nonpurging types**.
    a. The nonpurging type is quite rare, accounting for 6-8% of patients with bulimia.
    b. No differences between subtypes are evident in severity of psychopathology, frequency of binge episodes, or prevalence of major depression and panic disorder.
4. Purging is an inefficient method to reduce weight and caloric intake as vomiting reduces about 50% of the calories just consumed; laxatives and related methods have little effect on weight.
5. In addition to binging and purging, bulimics show an over concern with body shape.
6. The following **medical consequences** are associated with chronic bulimia of the purging type:
    a. Salivary gland enlargement causes by repeated vomiting. The result is a chubby facial appearance.
    b. Erosion of dental enamel on the inner surface of the front teeth.
    c. May produce an electrolyte imbalance (i.e., disruption of sodium and potassium levels) which, in turn, can lead to potentially fatal cardiac arrhythmia and renal failure.
    d. Intestinal problems resulting from laxative abuse are also potentially serious.

e. Some individuals with bulimia also develop marked calluses on the fingers and backs of hands resulting from efforts to vomit by stimulating the gag reflex.

7. Most bulimics have other comorbid psychological disorders, particularly anxiety, mood disorders, and substance abuse.
8. Most bulimics are within 10% of their normal weight.

C. Persons with **anorexia nervosa**, unlike bulimics, are highly successful at losing weight. Both anorexia and bulimia share a morbid fear of gaining weight and losing control over eating. The major difference is whether the person is successful in losing the weight. The core feature of anorexia nervosa is intense fear of obesity and a relentless and successful pursuit of thinness. This disorder often begins with normal dieting but evolves into an obsessive preoccupation with being thin. Rigorous exercise and dramatic weight loss are seen. The textbook illustrates the clinical features of anorexia nervosa with the case of Julie.

1. Anorexia is less common than bulimia; however, many individuals with bulimia have a history of anorexia.
2. Anorexia often begins in adolescence, particularly in persons who are actually overweight or who otherwise perceives themselves to be overweight.
3. Dramatic weight loss is achieved through severe caloric restriction or by combining caloric restriction and purging.
4. The DSM-IV-TR specifies the following **two subtypes of anorexia nervosa**:
   a. In the **restricting type**, individuals diet to limit caloric intake.
   b. In the **binge-eating-purging type**, persons rely on purging to limit caloric intake. Unlike bulimics, the binge and purge in this subtype involves small amounts of food and the purges occur more consistently. This subtype accounts for about 50% of persons with anorexia nervosa. Few differences exist between the two subtypes on severity of symptoms or personality.
5. Persons with anorexia are never satisfied with weight loss. Typical weight at time of referral is 25-30% below normal, with the DSM-IV-TR requiring only 15% below expected.
6. In addition, this population displays marked disturbances in body image and rarely seeks treatment on their own.
7. **Medical consequences** of anorexia nervosa include the following:
   a. Amenorrhea, or the cessation of menstruation (most common complication).
   b. Other medical consequences include dry skin, brittle hair or nails, sensitivity and intolerance for cold temperatures.
   c. **Lanugo**, or downy hair on the limbs and cheeks, is also common.
   d. Cardiovascular problems (e.g., low blood pressure and heart rate).
   e. Vomiting in anorexia results in similar medical problems as bulimia.
8. Anorexics are often comorbid for anxiety and mood disorders, particularly obsessive compulsive disorder.

D. Persons with **binge eating disorder (BED)** experience marked distress due to binge eating but do not engage in extreme compensatory behaviors. Binge-eating disorder appears in the appendix of the DSM-IV-TR as a potential new disorder requiring further study. Persons with BED are found in weight control programs and show the following characteristics:

1. Such persons show an increased frequency of other comorbid psychological disorders and more psychopathology in general than obese people who do not binge.
2. About 50% of such persons try dieting before resorting to binging, while half start with binging.
3. Like anorexics and bulimics, persons with binge-eating disorder share similar concerns with shape and weight.

E. Additional facts and statistics regarding bulimia and anorexia are as follows:

1. The majority (90% to 95%) of persons with bulimia are female, and most are white from middle to upper-middle class families.
    a. Some male athletes, particularly wrestlers, are a group with more eating disorders.
    b. Bulimia usually develops around 16 to 19 years of age, and as many as 6-8% of college women meet criteria for bulimia nervosa.
    c. Lifetime prevalence for bulimia in the general population is about 1.1% for females, and 0.1% for males, with higher numbers in more urban areas. Once bulimia develops, it tends to be chronic if untreated.
2. The majority (90% to 95%) of persons with anorexia nervosa are also female, and most are white from middle to upper-middle class families. Onset is typically in adolescence, about the age of 13 years.
    a. Anorexia tends to be less prevalent than bulimia.
    b. Anorexia also tends to be more chronic and more resistant to treatment compared to bulimia.

F. Anorexia and bulimia tend to be **highly culture specific** and are found more so in cultures or groups that have become more acculturated or Westernized, particularly in those who identify with Caucasian middle class values. There is a relatively high incidence of purging behavior is some minority groups, particularly in Chippewa women. In traditional Chinese cultures, acne is most often reported as a precipitant for anorexia nervosa than a fear of being fat, and body image disturbance is rare.

G. Anorexia and bulimia are strongly related to **developmental considerations**. Differential patterns of physical development in girls and boys seem to interact with cultural influences to create eating disorders. The ideal is to look tall and muscular for males and prepubertal for females.

H. Several factors, in addition to cultural considerations, have been implicated as causes of anorexia and bulimia.

1. Cultural imperative for thinness directly results in dieting, the first step down the slippery slope toward bulimia and anorexia.
2. Standards of ideal body size change as much as fashion style in clothes. For example, Playboy centerfolds and Miss America contestants have become slightly thinner over the years, suggesting a change in what is considered desirable in terms of body shape and weight. 69% of the Playboy centerfolds and 60% of the Miss America contestants weighed 15% or more below normal weight for their age and height, thus meeting criteria for anorexia.
3. Magazines and the media glorify slenderness. The problem is that today's standards are increasingly difficult to achieve, since the size and weight of the average female has increased over the years with improved nutrition.
4. Dieting and exercise have also increased over the years.
5. Males tend to rate their ideal body weight as heavier than the weight females think is most attractive for men. Women, however, rate their current figures as much heavier than their most attractive, which, in turn, was rated heavier than the ideal. Women also rate the ideal body weight as much lower than what men consider attractive.
6. If members of one's social group resort to extreme dieting or other weight loss techniques, there is a greater chance that others in the group will do the same.
7. Evidence indicates that dietary restraint can lead to preoccupation with food. In a classic WWII semistarvation experiment, it was shown that persons who had their food intake involuntarily restricted became preoccupied with food and eating.

I. The typical **anorexic's family** tends to be successful, hard-driving, concerned with external appearances, and eager to maintain harmony. Family members often deny or ignore conflicts and have communication problems.

J. Eating disorders tend to run in families and seem to have a genetic component. Relatives of patients with eating disorders are 4 to 5 times more likely than the general population to develop eating disorders themselves. It is thought that emotional instability and poor impulse control are inherited. The hypothalamus plays a considerable role in the regulation of eating, and low serotonergic activity is associated with impulsivity and binge-eating specifically.

K. Many females with eating disorders have a diminished sense of personal control and confidence in their abilities and talents. They are also perfectionistic, but more importantly show an intense preoccupation with how they appear to others, and perceive themselves as frauds in the process. Perceptions of body size are also malleable. For example, bulimics tend to rate their body size as larger following a snack compared to non-bulimic controls. Bulimics also experience anxiety before and during snacks, and purging seems to relieve the anxiety via negative reinforcement.

L. **An integrative model** is proposed that emphasizes the following shared characteristics across eating disorders:

1. Share many of the same biological and psychological vulnerabilities as the anxiety and mood disorders, with anxiety and fear focused on becoming overweight.
2. Cultural and social pressures to be thin motivate significant restriction of eating, usually via severe dieting. This coupled with familial pressures to succeed and emphasis on physical appearance, may activate the psychological vulnerability.

M. Only since the 1980s have there been **treatments for bulimia**, whereas less developed **treatments for anorexia** have been around much longer. Here medication and psychological interventions are considered.

1. No medications have been shown effective for the treatment of anorexia nervosa. Effective medications for bulimia are similar to those used for anxiety and mood disorders (i.e., antidepressants). In 1996, the FDA approved the drug Prozac for the treatment of eating disorders. **Antidepressants** can reduce binging and purging; however, antidepressant drugs alone do not have a substantial long-lasting impact on bulimia nervosa.
2. Psychosocial treatments that target a patient's low self-esteem or family interaction problems are largely ineffective for eating disorders. **Cognitive-behavioral therapy (CBT)** targets problematic eating behavior and associated attitudes about body weight and shape, whereas **Interpersonal Psychotherapy (IPT)** focuses on interpersonal relationships and functioning. CBT for bulimia involves education about physical consequences of binge-eating and purging, including adverse effects of dieting. Eating is scheduled, and later cognitive therapy focuses on dysfunctional thoughts and attitudes about body shape, weight, and eating. CBT produces better and more immediate outcomes in the short term; however, CBT and IPT produce comparable results in the long-term.
3. **Psychosocial treatment of binge-eating disorder** follows CBT for bulimia. The central focus here is on binge-eating, and patients who are able to stop binging show the most substantial and lasting weight loss. Self-help programs appear effective and may end up being the first line of treatment for binge-eating disorder.
4. The most important initial goal (and often the easiest goal to meet) in the **treatment of anorexia** involves weight restoration. However, extent of weight gain is a poor predictor of long-term outcome in anorexia. Treatment focuses on dysfunctional attitudes about body shape, and may include focus on anxiety about becoming obese, feelings of uncontrollability over eating, and undue emphasis on thinness as equivalent to self-worth, happiness, and success. Family members are often involved to address dysfunctional communication patterns regarding food and eating, and to set in place a more

structured and enjoyable eating schedule. Attitudes about body shape and image distortion are also addressed in family sessions. Long-term outcome for anorexia is poorer than outcomes for treatment of bulimia.

5. Efforts are being made to **prevent eating disorders**. Such efforts have been successful for high risk females and target the following domains:
    a. Early concern about being overweight. This domain is the most powerful predictor of later eating disorder symptoms.
    b. Emphasis on normality of female weight gain after puberty and that excessive caloric restriction could result in gaining more weight. This domain emphasizes restoration and maintenance of female weight within normal limits.

N. Obesity

1. The prevalence of **obesity** among adults in the U.S. virtually doubled, from 12% in 1991 to 20% in 2000. This condition is associated with increased mortality, and accounted for over 300,000 deaths in the U.S. alone. For adolescents, rates of obesity have tripled in the past 25 years, from 5% to 15%.
2. Between 7% and 15% of obese individuals seeking weight-loss treatment, and as many as 27% of those with extreme obesity, exhibit a disordered eating pattern termed **night eating syndrome**. Such individuals consume a third or more of their daily intake after their evening meal and also get out of bed at least once during the night to have a high-calorie snack.
3. The promotion of an inactive, sedentary lifestyle and the consumption of a high-fat, energy-dense diet is the largest single contributer to the obesity epidemic. Genes are thought to account for about 30% of the equation in the causation of obesity.
4. The treatment of obesity is only moderately successful at the individual level, with somewhat greater long-term evidence for effectiveness in children and adolescents, compared to adults. Treatment for obesity can take the form of self-directed weight-loss programs, commercial self-help programs, professionally directed behavior modification programs, or **bariatric surgery**.

II. Sleep Disorders

A. Humans spend about one-third of their lives asleep, or about 3,000 hours of sleep per year on average. Unfortunately, today most people do not get enough sleep. People who do not get enough sleep report more health problems

B. The limbic system is a region in the brain that is involved with our dream sleep, which is called **rapid eye movement (REM)** sleep. As a brain circuit in the limbic system may also be involved with anxiety, sleep and anxiety may be interrelated. REM sleep also seems related to depression.

C. Sleep disorders are divided into **dyssomnias** and **parasomnias**.

1. Dyssomnias involve difficulties in getting enough sleep, problems in the timing of sleep, and complaints about the quality of sleep.
2. Parasomnias are characterized by abnormal behavioral and physiological events during sleep, such as nightmares and sleepwalking.

D. A **polysomnographic (PSG)** evaluation involves spending one or more nights in a sleep laboratory, while being monitored on a number of measures that include respiration rate and oxygen desaturation (i.e., a measure of airflow), leg movements, brain wave activity as measured by an **electroencephalograph (EEG)**, eye movements as measured by an **electrooculograph (EOG)**, muscle movements as measured by an **electromyography (EMG)**, and heart activity as measured by an **electrocardiogram**. Alternatives to a costly and time consuming sleep assessment include use of an **actigraph**; a device that is able to determine the length and quality of sleep by recording the number of arm movements during sleep.
1. A PSG evaluation includes the amount of time a person sleeps each day, while taking into account the percentage of time the person actually spends asleep (i.e., **sleep efficiency**). Sleep efficiency is calculated by dividing the amount of time sleeping by the amount of time in bed.
2. To determine problematic sleep, a clinician may observe the person's behavior while awake (i.e., **daytime sequelae**).

E. Dyssomnias
1. **Primary Insomnia** is one of the most common sleep disorders and is related to the occurrence of **microsleeps** (i.e., brief periods of sleep lasting several seconds or longer following prolonged periods of little sleep) and **fatal familial insomnia** (i.e., a degenerative brain disorder that produces an inability to sleep and eventually leads to death). Insomnia involves difficulties initiating sleep, difficulties maintaining sleep, and/or nonrestorative sleep. To be considered a disorder, the person must experience discomfort about their sleep. The textbook illustrates insomnia with the case of Sonja.
    a. **Primary insomnia** means that the insomnia is not related to other medical or psychiatric problems.
    b. About one-third of the population report symptoms of insomnia during any given year, and 35% of elderly persons report excessive daytime sleepiness.
    c. Depression, substance abuse disorders, anxiety disorders, and dementia of the Alzheimer's type are all related to decreased total sleep time.
    d. Females report insomnia twice as often as males.
    e. Medical and psychological disorders, including pain and physical discomfort, inactivity during the day, or respiratory problems can contribute to insomnia. Insomnias are sometimes associated with disruption of the biological clock and its control over body temperature. Drop in body temperature is related to sleep, and persons

with insomnia have higher body temperatures than good sleepers. Psychological stress can also disrupt sleep.

   f. Persons with insomnia have unrealistic expectations about how much sleep they need and about how disruptive/disturbed their sleep will be for them.
   g. **An integrative model of insomnia** is proposed where biological vulnerability interacts with sleep stress and other factors (e.g., poor bedtime habits or poor sleep hygiene). Moreover, use of over the counter sleeping pills can result in worse sleep when the medication is withdrawn (i.e., **rebound insomnia**).

2. **Primary hypersomnia** involves problems related to sleeping too much or excessive sleep. The DSM-IV-TR criteria for hypersomnia include excessive sleepiness but also the subjective impression of this as a problem. Such persons often sleep through the night and appear rested upon awakening, but complain of being excessively tired throughout the day. Similar complaints are found in persons suffering from **sleep apnea**. About 39% of persons with hypersomnia have a family history of the disorder. The textbook illustrates primary hypersomnia with the case of Ann.
3. **Narcolepsy** involves daytime sleepiness, but also **cataplexy** (i.e., a sudden loss of muscle tone while awake lasting several seconds to several minutes) that can range from slight weakness in the facial muscles to complete physical collapse. Cataplexic attacks are usually precipitated by strong emotion and involve a sudden onset into the REM period of sleep. Persons with narcolepsy move from a state of being awake right into a state of REM sleep; a state of sleep where input to the muscles is inhibited.
   a. Persons with narcolepsy commonly report **sleep paralysis** (i.e., a brief period after awakening when they can't move or speak). Sleep paralysis is often frightening for those who go through it.
   b. **Hypnagogic hallucinations** (i.e., vivid and often terrifyingly realistic sensory experiences that begin at sleep onset) are also common.
   c. Narcolepsy is rare, occurring in .03% to .16% of the population and is equally distributed between females and males. Onset is usually during adolescence.
   d. Cataplexy, hypnagogic hallucinations, and sleep paralysis often decrease on their own over time. Daytime sleepiness does not improve with age.
   e. Narcolepsy in dogs appears associated with a cluster of genes on chromosome number 6, and may be an autosomal recessive trait.
4. **Breathing-related sleep disorders** involve sleepiness during the day or disrupted sleep at night. Persons whose breathing is interrupted during sleep experience numerous brief arousals throughout the night and do not feel rested even after normal amounts of sleep. **Sleep apnea** involves restricted airflow and/or brief periods (i.e., 10-30 seconds) where breathing ceases completely. Sleep apnea is most common in males and occurs in 10% to 20% of the population. Persons with sleep apnea are minimally aware of such breathing problems; however, loud snoring is one sign of sleep apnea, as are heavy

sweating during the night, morning headaches, and episodes of falling asleep during the day (i.e., sleep attacks).

   a. **Obstructive sleep apnea (OSA)** occurs when airflow stops despite continued activity of the respiratory system. All such persons snore at night, and obesity and increasing age are often associated with this form of apnea.
   b. **Central sleep apnea (CSA)** involves complete cessation of respiratory activity for brief periods of time and is associated with central nervous system disorders such as cerebral vascular disease, head trauma, and degenerative disorders. Persons with CSA, unlike those with OSA, wake up frequently during the night and do not tend to report excessive daytime sleepiness.
   c. **Mixed sleep apnea (MSA)** is a combination of both OSA and CSA

5. **Circadian rhythm sleep disorders** are characterized by disturbed sleep (i.e., either insomnia or excessive sleepiness during the day) brought on by the brain's inability to synchronize its sleep patterns with the current patterns of day and night.
   a. **Circadian rhythms** are self-regulated and do not match our 24-hour day clock.
   b. The **suprachiasmatic nucleus** (i.e., the brain's biological clock) is responsible for keeping us in synch with the outside world. This nucleus located in the hypothalamus and connected to pathways from our eyes is sensitive to changes in light. Changes in light reset the biological clock each day. The hormone **melatonin** also contributes to the setting of our biological clocks. Melatonin is produced by the pineal gland in response to darkness, but not light. Both light and melatonin help set our biological clock.
   c. Circadian rhythm disorders include the **jet lag type** (i.e., problems in sleep caused by rapidly crossing multiple time zones). Persons with jet lag report difficulty going to sleep and feelings of fatigue during the day. **Shift work type** sleep problems are associated with work schedules.
   d. Several circadian rhythm disorders also seem to arise from within the person experiencing the problem; however, they are not included in the DSM-IV. For example, extreme night owls (i.e., people who stay up late and sleep late) may have a problem known as **delayed sleep phase type**. People with **advanced sleep phase type** of circadian rhythm disorder are early to bed and early to rise, with sleep advances or earlier than normal bed time.
6. The following **medical interventions** are available as treatments for dyssomnias:
   a. The most common treatment for insomnia are prescription (i.e., **benzodiazepines** such as Halcion and Dalmane). The drawbacks of medications for insomnia include excessive sleepiness produced by benzodiazepines, dependence on medications, and rebound insomnia.

Medications for insomnia are not recommended as a long-term solution.

   b. Prescription medications for **hypersomnia and narcolepsy** include a stimulant such as **methylphenidate** (i.e., Ritalin), or **amphetamine** or modafinil. Cataplexy is usually treated with antidepressant medication because such medications suppress REM or dream sleep.
   c. **Treatment of breathing-related sleep disorders** focus on improved breathing during sleep and may involve weight loss, medications (i.e., those that help stimulate breathing such as medroxyprogesterone or tricyclics antidepressants), or mechanical devices that are aimed to reposition either the tongue or jaw during sleep.
   d. Generally, medication as a primary treatment is usually not recommended.
   e. **Treatment of circadian rhythm disorders** usually involve either **phase delays** (i.e., moving bedtime later) or **phase advances** (i.e., moving bedtime earlier). Phase delays are generally easier to implement than phase advances. A more recent treatment involves the use of **bright light** to trick the brain into readjusting its biological clock (i.e., greater than 2,500 lux; a normal household light is about 250 lux).

7. The following **psychological treatments** are available for dyssomnias:
   a. Relaxation treatments may help reduce tension related to being able to sleep at night.
   b. For adult sleep problems, **stimulus control procedures** are recommended. Such procedures involve instructions to use the bedroom only for sleeping/sex, not for work or other anxiety-provoking activities, and/or sleep restriction (i.e., limit sleep time per night), and confronting unrealistic expectations about sleep.
   c. For children, treatment often involves setting regular bedtime routines (e.g., bath, story, bed).
   d. Research suggests that combining short-term use of medication with other types of interventions may be most efficacious in the treatment of insomnia; however, treatment research with other dyssomnias is virtually nonexistent.
8. Many dyssomnias can be prevented by better **sleep hygiene** (i.e., changes in daily lifestyle and daytime functioning). Sleep hygiene includes the following:
   a. Setting a regular sleep and wake time.
   b. Avoiding use of caffeine and nicotine.
   c. Educating parents and others about normal sleep and sleep behavior.
   d. Eating a balanced diet.
   e. Going to bed when sleepy and getting out of bed if unable to sleep within 15 minutes.
   f. Reducing noise, stimulation, and temperature in the bedroom.

F. Parasomnias and their treatment

1. **Parasomnias** are not problems with sleep itself, but abnormal events that occur either during sleep or during the twilight time between sleeping and waking. Such events include sleep walking, sleep talking, nightmares, teeth grinding.
2. Parasomnias are of two types:
    a. Those that occur during rapid eye movement (REM) sleep.
    b. Those that occur during non-rapid eye movement sleep (NREM).
3. **Nightmares** occur during REM or dream sleep, and involves dreams that are so distressful and disturbing that they interfere with daily life functioning and interrupt sleep. Nightmares often awaken the sleeper, and are common in children, but not adults (i.e., only 5-10% of adults). We still know little about why people have nightmares and how to treat them.
4. **Sleep terrors** involvepanic-like symptoms during NREM sleep. Sleep terrors are more common in children than adults. Sleep terrors often begin with a piercing scream, and the child appears extremely upset, often sweating, and shows a rapid heartbeat. During the terrors, the child cannot be easily awakened, and most children have no memory of them the next day. Treatment usually involves a wait-and-see posture. If the problem is severe and persists over long periods, antidepressants (i.e., imipramine) or benzodiazepines are recommended. Scheduled awakenings involving the parent awakening the child prior to the regular sleep terror is effective in eliminating such episodes over the long term.
5. **Sleepwalking (i.e., somnambulism)** occurs during NREM sleep, usually during the first few hours while the person is in the deep stages of sleep. DSM-IV-TR criteria require that the person leave the bed. Waking the person during the episode is often difficult, and waking a sleepwalker is not considered dangerous. Sleepwalking is primarily a problem during childhood; though some adults are affected.
    a. A related disorder, **nocturnal eating syndrome**, involves person eating while they are still asleep.

OVERALL SUMMARY

This chapter outlines the major characteristics of eating disorders, particularly bulimia nervosa and anorexia nervosa, and includes discussion of related eating disorders such as binge-eating disorder, rumination disorder, pica, and feeding disorder. Etiological, developmental, and cultural factors that impinge upon these problems are described. In addition, treatment procedures are discussed, including cognitive-behavioral approaches, family and interpersonal therapy, and pharmacotherapy. Additionally, this chapter also provides an overview of the key features of sleep disorders (i.e., dyssomnias and parasomnias) and their assessment, and includes discussion of available medical and psychological treatments. Biological, psychological, and cultural influences on sleep and sleep behavior are also discussed.

KEY TERMS

Anorexia nervosa (p. 257)
Bariatric Surgery (p.282)
Binge (p. 257)
Binge-eating disorder (p. 264)
Breathing-related sleep disorders (p. 289)
Bulimia nervosa (p. 257)
Circadian rhythm sleep disorders (p. 290)
Dyssomnias (p. 284)
Hypersomnia (p. 287)
Microsleeps (p. 284)
Narcolepsy (p. 288)
Nightmares (p. 294)
Night eating syndrome (p.280)
Obesity (p.258)
Parasomnias (p. 284)
Polysomnographic (PSG) evaluation (p. 284)
Primary insomnia (p. 284)
Purging techniques (p. 260)
Rapid eye movement (REM) sleep (p. 283)
Rebound insomnia (p. 287)
Sleep apnea (p. 288)
Sleep efficiency (SE) (p. 284)
Sleep terrors (p. 295)
Sleepwalking (p. 295)

INFOTRAC KEY TERM EXERCISES

Each exercise is linked to key terms from the Wadsworth InfoTrac on-line searchable database. Key terms must be entered exactly as written.

Exercise 1: **Alien Abduction or a Case of Hypnagogic Hallucinations?**
Article: A71563256
Citation: (A Psychological Case Study of 'Demon and 'Alien' Visitation). Andrew D. Reisner
Skeptical Inquirer, March 2001 v25 i2 p46

This InfoTrac article describes the case of John, a 36-year-old employed, married man who misinterpreted hypnagogic and hypnopompic hallucinations as visitations by demons and aliens. He came close to suicide, and even considered killing his family. The article provides an alternative account of alien abduction. After reading this article, you are to address the following points: (a) describe John's history briefly, (b) apply a multidimensional approach (as outlined in the section of textbook chapter dealing with sleep disorders) to understanding factors that contributed to the onset and maintenance of John's sleep difficulties, and (c) describe the author's alternative explanations for John's apparent alien abduction experiences. Limit your answer to 3-5 typed double-spaced pages.

Exercise 2: Developing an Integrative Psychological Model of Bulimia
Key Term: *Bulimia, Psychological Aspects*

Your textbook presents a multidimensional integrative model of bulimia nervosa that includes biological, psychological, social, and cultural factors. Here, your task is to review the InfoTrac article(s) on the psychological risk factors associated with bulimia nervosa, and based on what you have read, to construct your own model of the psychological causes and maintaining factors of bulimic behavior. You should depict your model in a schematic or drawing. Be sure to provide a brief narrative that describes and supports the hypothesized relations among the psychological risk factors and behaviors associated with bulimia in your model. Limit your answer to 3-5 typed double-spaced pages.

Exercise 3: Should you Sleep on it?: Does Sleep Improve Memory
Key Term: *Sleep, Memory*

Sleep is thought to be restorative, both physically and mentally. Increasingly, researchers are also learning that sleep is important in regulating your ability to remember and to learn. Review the InfoTrac article(s) on sleep and memory, and present a review of what is known about how sleep and memory are related. In your answer, be sure to cover what is known about sleep and its affects on memory by including biological, psychological, experiential, and social domains. Finally, based on what you have read, what practical recommendations would you make for others so that they could get the most out of the memory boosting effects of sleep. Limit your answer to 3-5 typed double-spaced pages.

Exercise 4 (Future Trend): Facing the Obesity Epidemic

Rates of obesity are reaching epidemic proportions. Moreover, obesity is on verge of surpassing smoking as the number one cause of preventable death. Yet, there are relatively few good psychosocial interventions for obesity. Most individuals are successful losing some weight, only to regain it later. Here, you may wish to describe the nature of obesity in more detail, including issues regarding whether obesity belongs in the DSM-IV-TR. Illustrate how psychological and behavioral life style factors contribute to obesity. Below are links to help facilitate a discussion of this issue, including a link with a Body Mass Index Calculator (http://www.cdc.gov/nccdphp/dnpa/bmi/index.htm). You may have students calculate their own BMI in class. You will likely find that most of your students have BMIs that put them in the obese range.

http://www.obesity.org/
http://www.cdc.gov/nccdphp/dnpa/obesity/
http://www.cdc.gov/nccdphp/dnpa/bmi/index.htm
http://www.surgeongeneral.gov/topics/obesity/default.htm

CLASSROOM ACTIVITIES, DEMONSTRATIONS, AND LECTURE TOPICS

1. **Activity: Food and Weight Diary.** While lecturing on eating disorders, you could ask your students to keep a food and weight diary. Ask your students to record every item they eat and the time of day each item is eaten. Also, they should weigh in several times a day and record

their weight. This exercise is designed to illustrate how people diagnosed with eating disorders can become consumed with food and weight. Moreover, this exercise will force your students to think about their food intake and weight consistently every day; a feature that is similar to what persons with eating disorders do. Students may be told about a client who used to carry a scale in the trunk of her car and would have to pull off the road to weigh herself periodically if she was taking long trips. Before doing an exercise like this, however, acknowledge that some students may already be struggling with similar food and weight issues and need not do the exercise if it is too stressful for them.

2. **Activity: Food Preferences are Predominantly Socialized.** Our preferences for certain foods over others is heavily influenced by culture, socialization, and experience. Such factors often exert a control of what we eat and avoid eating more so than simple biological need for nutrition and sustenance. To illustrate this concept, choose two foods that would be appropriate to eat depending on the time of day of your class. One food should be something that students would eat if they could, while the other food should be a food that would satisfy the body's need for calories and nutrition, but that students would not prefer. For example, for a class meeting around noon, I give students the option of a nice slice of pizza or a bowl of oatmeal with a few prunes. Bringing food samples to class can make the exercise more effective. Ask students what food they prefer and why? In the example above, most students will overwhelming select the slice of cheese pizza. Use this exercise as a springboard to talk about social and cultural factors, including the media, that influence eating behavior, including poor eating habits.

3. **Activity: Rating Your Body Size.** The text discusses the study by Fallon and Rosen (1985) which found that males rated their current body size, ideal body size, and body size they figured would be most attractive to the opposite sex as approximately equal. They also found, however, that women rated their current figure as much heavier than the most attractive body size, which was in turn rated heavier than the ideal. In addition, females' judgment of an ideal female body weight was less than the weight males thought most attractive. You can easily demonstrate this phenomenon in your class by administering the nine figure drawing (designed by Stunkard, Sorenson, & Schulsinger, 1980) to your students.

   Again, the four questions that you should ask your students to identify is:
   a. What figure most approximates your current figure?
   b. What figure represents what you would like to look like (ideal figure)?
   c. What figure do you think would be most attractive to the opposite sex?
   d. What figure of the opposite sex do you find most attractive?

   You can tabulate your results and present them to the class. This exercise exposes students to research methodology used in this field, while stimulating student interest by getting them actively involved in determining the results!

4. **Video Activity: CNN Today, Abnormal Psychology, Vol. 1.** Present the segment titled "Eating Disorders" in your class. This segment presents cases of women with eating disorders such as bulimia and binge eating, and discusses how eating disorders affect men

and women of all ages. Ask students in your class if they can differentiate important differences between bulimic women and those with binge-eating problems.

5. **Activity: Assessing Sleep Habits.** The following exercise is designed to enable students to assess their sleeping habits and need for a midday nap. Instruct your students to keep a self-assessment log on their sleeping habits for two weeks using the attached record. Give your students the following instructions:

   a. *Week #1:* Take a 20-30 minute nap every day and record how you feel each morning. If you find you cannot nap, just rest quietly. Set the alarm just in case you fall asleep. Also, record the time you go to bed at night, how long it takes you to fall asleep, how many times you awake during the night, and how you feel in the morning.

   b. *Week #2:* Take no naps and keep your sleep record as above. At the conclusion of this week, compare how you feel in the morning and during the day with and without napping. Do naps make a difference to you? Write a paragraph about your previous napping history and how you feel naps affect you after this two-week experiment.

   Source Information. Mayo Clinic Health Letter, December, 1993.

6. **Activity: Dream Diaries.** This activity promises to be quite interesting. Approximately 2 weeks before the chapter on sleep disorders is discussed, tell your class to start keeping a dream diary. Encourage students to keep a pad of paper and pencil near their bed so they can write down any memory of a dream upon waking up. After 2 weeks of keeping the diary, tell students to break up into groups and discuss one or two of their dreams with the other group members. The other students in the group should be instructed to give an interpretation of the dream (Freudian, Jungian, or their own). Although some students may prefer discussing their dreams with friends or other students, prepare yourself to be asked by many what the "true" meaning or interpretation of a particular dream is. This exercise often leads to interesting discussions of learned fears, symbolic meanings of dreams, Freudian psychoanalysis, and how activities during daytime can influence the nature and content of sleep and dreaming.

SUPPLEMENTARY READING MATERIAL FOR CHAPTER EIGHT

(= These sources can be found on "*Infotrac, the online library*" provided by Wadsworth and Brooks/Cole Publishing.)

Anderson, G. H., & Kennedy, S. H. (Eds.) (1992). The biology of feast and famine: Relevance to eating disorders. New York: Academic.

Bruno, F. (1997) Get a good night's sleep. New York: Macmillan.

Cartmill, M. (1998). Animal minds, animal dreams. Natural History, 107, 16(5).

Cooper, R. (Ed.) (1994). Sleep. New York: Chapman and Hall Medical.

Durand, V. M. (1998). Sleep better!: A guide to improving sleep for children with special needs. Baltimore, MD: Paul H. Brookes Publishing.

Fairburn, C. G., & Wilson, G. T. (Eds.) (1993). Binge eating: Nature, assessment, and treatment. New York: Guilford.

Fichter, M. M. (Ed.) (1993). Bulimia nervosa: Basic research, diagnosis and therapy. Chichester, England: Wiley.

Garner, D. M., & Garfinkel, P. E. (Eds.) (1985). Handbook of psychotherapy for anorexia nervosa and bulimia. New York: Guilford.

Hagan, M. M., Whitworth, R. H., & Moss, D. E. (1999). Semistarvation-associated eating behaviors among college binge eaters: A preliminary description and assessment Scale. Behavioral Medicine, 25, 125.

Kryger, M. H., Roth, T., & Dement, W. C. (Eds.) (1989). Principles and practice of sleep medicine. Philadelphia: Saunders.

Maas, J. (1998). Power sleep. New York: Villard.

Moorcroft, W. H. (1993). Sleep, dreaming, and sleep disorders: An introduction. Landham, MD: University Press of America.

Nickell, J. (1998). Alien abductions as sleep-related phenomena. Skeptical Inquirer, 22, 16(3).

Perl, J. (1993). Sleep right in five nights: A clear and effective guide for conquering insomnia. New York: William Morrow and Company.

Rosenfeld, D. S., & Elhajjar, A. J. (1998). Sleepsex: A variant of sleepwalking.. Archives of Sexual Behavior, 27, 269(10).

Williams, R. L., Karacan, I., & Moore, L. A. (Eds.) (1988). Sleep disorders: Diagnosis and treatment. New York: Wiley.

SUPPLEMENTARY 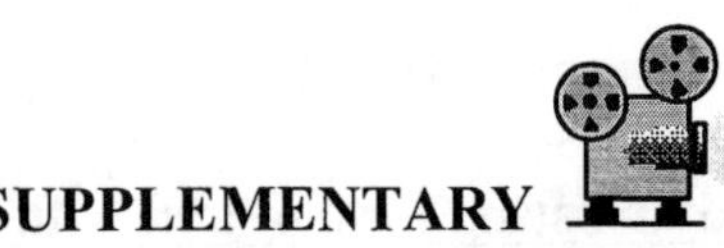 VIDEO RESOURCES FOR CHAPTER EIGHT

CNN today: Abnormal psychology, vol. 1. (*available through your International Thomson Learning representative).* In the segment titled "Eating and Sleep Disorders: Hollywood Thin," celebrities discuss the pressures to remain thin. This segment also includes discussion of the prevalence of eating disorders. (3 min)

A second segment, titled "Eating Disorders," presents cases of women with eating disorders such as bulimia and binge eating, and discusses how eating disorders affect men and women of all ages. A social worker specializing in eating disorders talks about her experiences. (2 min, 44 sec)

Dying to be thin. (Insight Media: 2162 Broadway, New York, NY 10024/ (800)-233-9910). Presenting statistics on the prevalence of eating disorders in America, this video reveals that there are many more sufferers than the stereotypical adolescent girls who starve themselves in emulation of media images of hollow-cheeked fashion models. It explores the psychological aspects of the diseases, considers the damage malnourishment does to the body, and examines effective therapies. (60 min)

Eating disorders. (Fanlight Productions, 1-800-937-4113). The eating disorders anorexia and bulimia have traditionally been thought to affect only young, white women; this program stresses their growing impact on men and on non-whites as well. The stories of several individuals who have dealt with severe eating disorders highlight the fact that this illness is not just about food, but about struggling with the loss of emotional control. (28 min)

Freud's interpretation of dreams. (Insight Media: 2162 Broadway, New York, NY 10024/ (800)-233-9910). The publication of Interpretation of Dreams revolutionized the way people look at their hopes, fears, and fantasies. Using a unique series of dream-sequence reenactments, this video examines what Freud termed "the royal road of the unconscious," probing the meaning of dreams and what they reflect. (23 min)

Mental health/illness. (Insight Media: 2162 Broadway, New York, NY 10024/ (800)-233-9910). Although the direct relationship between psychological health and physical health has long been recognized, there is still a great deal of misinformation and even social stigma surrounding mental illness. This video examines the epidemiology of mental disorders and the treatment approaches emerging from research into the biology of these diseases. It focuses on the diagnosis and treatment of depression, a leading illness worldwide and bulimia, which affects primarily teenagers and young adults. (30 min)

Narcolepsy. (Fanlight Productions, 1-800-937-4113). This film presents the experiences of three individuals whose lives and relationships have been disrupted by narcolepsy. Intertwined with their compelling stories, it offers solid, comprehensive scientific information about this disorder. (25 min)

Shadows and lies: The unseen battle of eating disorders. (Fanlight Productions, 1-800-937-4113). This powerful and honest documentary profiles four women who are working themselves free from the deadly grip of eating disorders, and from the overwhelming physical and psychological complications associated with these disorders. (30 min)

Sleep disorders: Their effects and treatments. (Insight Media: 2162 Broadway, New York, NY 10024/ (800)-233-9910). Lack of sleep is a serious health hazard, increasing susceptibility to colds and viral infections. This program explains such causes of sleeplessness as insomnia, sleep apnea, narcolepsy, restless legs, and sleep timing disturbances. Sleep experts provide tips on how to fall asleep, manage night shifts, travel across time zones, and help infants and young children sleep through the night. (28 min)

Teaching about anorexia nervosa. (Insight Media: 2162 Broadway, New York, NY 10024/ (800)-233-9910). This three-volume set describes the condition of anorexia nervosa. It features interviews with three patients, one of whom has successfully recovered. It also includes commentary of a dietician and presents a dramatization of the development and treatment of anorexia in a college student named Lizzie. (116 min total)

The biology of sleep. (Insight Media: 2162 Broadway, New York, NY 10024/ (800)-233-9910). Featuring the commentary of a noted sleep expert, this video addresses the biology of sleep, revealing why sleep patterns differ so dramatically among human beings and showing how sleep changes throughout the life span. (30 min)

When food is the enemy: Eating disorders. (Insight Media: 2162 Broadway, New York, NY 10024/ (800)-233-9910). Examining the symptoms and complications of such major eating disorders as anorexia, bulimia, and binge eating, this video reveals self-perception as the key underlying issue for sufferers. It explains the seriousness of these dysfunctions, addresses the complexities of recovery, and features the commentary of experts and patients regarding causes and current methods of treatment. (15 min)

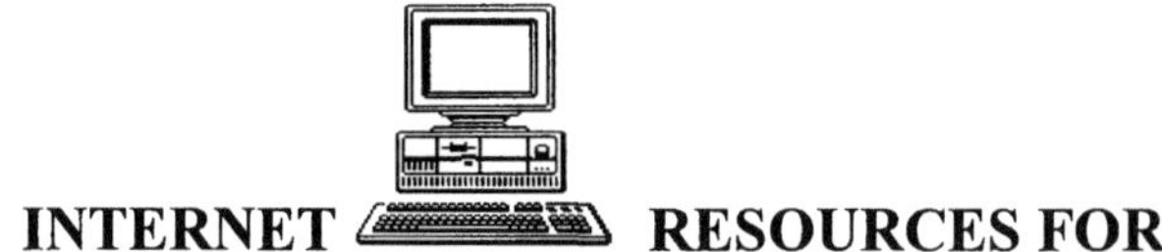

INTERNET RESOURCES FOR CHAPTER EIGHT

Academy for Eating Disorders
http://www.aedweb.org/newwebsite/index.htm

The Academy for Eating Disorders is a multidisciplinary professional organization focusing on Anorexia Nervosa, Bulimia Nervosa, Binge Eating Disorder and related disorders. This site provides some useful links and information related to eating disorders and their treatment.

American Anorexia/Bulimia Association, Inc.
http://www.aabainc.org/

This web page provides much information on anorexia, bulimia, and compulsive eating; it also provides questions to ask potential therapists regarding treatment modalities, hospitalization, length of treatment, and other relevant issues.

American Sleep Apnea Association
http://www.sleepapnea.org/

Information on the phenomenology, assessment, and treatment of sleep apnea.

Children and Sleep Disorders
http://www.stanford.edu/~dement/children.html

Information on numerous sleep disorders that affect children, including infant apnea, sleepwalking, nightmares, and sleep terrors.

MedlinePlus: Sleep Disorders
http://www.nlm.nih.gov/medlineplus/sleepdisorders.html

Excellent resource for current research and links related to sleep disorders.

National Association of Anorexia Nervosa and Associated Disorders (ANAD)
http://www.anad.org/

ANAD is the oldest national non-profit organization helping eating disorder victims and their families. In addition to its free hotline counseling, ANAD operates an international network of support groups for sufferers and families, and offers referrals to health care professionals, who treat eating disorders, across the U.S. and in fifteen other countries. This site contains useful information and links.

National Sleep Foundation
http://www.sleepfoundation.org/

The National Sleep Foundation is a nonprofit organization devoted to raising funds and awareness about the importance of sleep for health and productivity. Answers to questions regarding sleep disorders and proper sleep hygiene can be found here.

SleepDisorders.Com
http://www.sleepdisorders.com/

An excellent megasite containing information and links related to sleep disorders.

SleepNet Web Page
http://www.Sleepnet.com/

This is a great starting place for finding sleep information on the internet. Contains links to other sleep-related web pages.

Sleep, Dreams, and Wakefulness
http://ura1195-6.univ-lyon1.fr/index_e.html

This web page contains 20 articles on topics such as sleep-waking cycle mechanisms, dreams and paradoxical sleep, and sleep/wake disorders.

The Something Fishy Website on Eating Disorders
http://www.something-fishy.org/

This web page is a potpourri of information devoted to eating disorders, including treatments, prevention, and issues for men with eating disorders.

WARNING SIGNS OF SLEEP DISORDERS

- Consistent failure to get enough sleep, or sleep is not restful
- Consistently feeling tired upon waking and/or waking with a headache
- Feelings of chronic tiredness and fatigue during the day
- Struggling to stay awake while driving, or when doing something passive (e.g., watching TV)
- Difficulties concentrating at work or school
- Co-workers, friends, or family members commenting on sleepiness
- Showing a slowed or unusually delayed response to stimuli or events
- Difficulty remembering things or difficulty in controlling emotions
- Feeling the need to nap several times a day
- Others have pointed out that you snore often or cease breathing during sleep

WARNING SIGNS OF ANOREXIA/BULIMIA

- Dramatic weight loss in a relatively short period of time
- Wearing big/baggy clothes or dressing in layers to hide body shape and size
- Obsession with weight/complaints of weight problems
- Obsession with calories, fat content of foods, and exercise
- Frequent trips to the bathroom immediately following meals
- Visible food restriction and self-starvation and/or binging or purging
- Use of diet pills, laxatives, ipecac syrup, or enemas
- Isolation and fear of eating around and with others
- Unusual food rituals (e.g., shifting the food around on the plate to look eaten)
- Hiding food in strange places
- Flushing uneaten food down the toilet (can cause sewage problems)
- Vague or secretive eating patterns
- Preoccupation with thoughts of food, weight, and/or cooking
- Self-defeating statements after food consumption
- Hair loss and/or pale or "grey" skin appearance
- Dizziness, headaches, low blood pressure, constipation, or incontinence
- Frequent soar throats and/or swollen glands
- Perfectionistic personality, low self-esteem and/or feelings of worthlessness
- Complaints of often feeling cold
- Loss of menstrual cycle and/or loss of sexual desire or promiscuous sex
- Bruised or callused knuckles; bloodshot or bleeding in the eyes; light bruising under the eyes and on the cheeks
- Mood swings (e.g., depression, fatigue)
- Insomnia and/or poor sleeping habits

WARNING SIGNS OF BINGE-EATING DISORDER

- Rapid weight gain or obesity
- Constant weight fluctuations
- Frequently eats an abnormal amount of food in a short period of time (usually less than two hours), but does not use methods to purge food
- Fear of not being able to control eating, and while eating, not being able to stop
- Isolation (i.e., fear of eating around and with others)
- Chronic dieting on a variety of popular diet plans
- Holding the belief that life will be better if they can lose weight
- Hiding food in strange places (closets, cabinets, suitcases, under the bed) to eat at a later time
- Hoarding food (especially high calorie/junk food)
- Vague or secretive eating patterns (e.g., eating late at night)
- Self-defeating statements after food consumption
- Blaming failure in social and professional community on weight
- Holding the belief that food is one's only friend
- Frequently feeling out of breath after relatively light activities
- Excessive sweating, high blood pressure, and/or cholesterol
- Leg and joint pain, weight gain
- Decreased mobility due to weight gain

DSM-IV-TR Criteria for Anorexia Nervosa

A. Refusal to maintain body weight at or above a minimally normal weight for age and height (e.g., weight loss leading to maintenance of body weight less than 85% of that expected; or failure to make expected weight gain during period of growth, leading to body weight less than 85% of that expected).

B. Intense fear of gaining weight or becoming fat, even though underweight.

C. Disturbance in the way in which one's body weight or shape is experienced, undue influence of body weight or shape on self-evaluation, or denial of the seriousness of the current low body weight.

D. In postmenarcheal females, amenorrhea, i.e., the absence of at least three consecutive menstrual cycles. (A woman is considered to have amenorrhea if her periods occur only following hormone, e.g., estrogen, administration.)

Specify type:

Restricting Type: during the current episode of Anorexia Nervosa, the person has not regularly engaged in binge-eating or purging behavior (i.e., self-induced vomiting or the misuse of laxatives, diuretics, or enemas)

Binge-Eating/Purging Type: during the current episode of Anorexia Nervosa, the person has regularly engaged in binge-eating or purging behavior (i.e., self-induced vomiting or the misuse of laxatives, diuretics, or enemas)

DSM-IV-TR Criteria for Bulimia Nervosa

A. Recurrent episodes of binge eating. An episode of binge eating is characterized by both of the following:

1. eating, in a discrete period of time (e.g., within any 2-hour period), an amount of food that is definitely larger than most people would eat during a similar period of time and under similar circumstances
2. a sense of lack of control over eating during the episode (e.g., a feeling that one cannot stop eating or control what or how much one is eating)

B. Recurrent inappropriate compensatory behavior in order to prevent weight gain such as self-induced vomiting; misuse of laxatives, diuretics, enemas, or other medications; fasting; or excessive exercise.

C. The binge eating and inappropriate compensatory behaviors both occur, on average, at least twice a week for 3 months.

D. Self-evaluation is unduly influenced by body shape and weight.

E. The disturbance does not occur exclusively during episodes of Anorexia Nervosa.

Specify type:

Purging Type: during the current episode of Bulimia Nervosa, the person has regularly engaged in self-induced vomiting or the misuse of laxatives, diuretics, or enemas

Nonpurging Type: during the current episode of Bulimia Nervosa, the person has used other inappropriate compensatory behaviors, such as fasting or excessive exercise, but has not regularly engaged in self-induced vomiting or the misuse of laxatives, diuretics, or enemas

DSM-IV-TR Criteria for Binge-Eating Disorder

A. Recurrent episodes of binge eating. An episode is characterized by:
   1. Eating a larger amount of food than normal during a short period of time (within any two hour period)
   2. A sense of lack of control over eating during the binge episode (i.e. the feeling that one cannot stop eating).

B. Binge eating episodes are associated with three or more of the following:
   1. Eating until feeling uncomfortably full
   2. Eating large amounts of food when not physically hungry
   3. Eating much more rapidly than normal
   4. Eating alone because you are embarrassed by how much you're eating
   5. Feeling disgusted, depressed, or guilty after overeating

C. Marked distress regarding binge eating is present

D. Binge eating occurs, on average, at least 2 days a week for six months

E. The binge eating is not associated with the regular use of inappropriate compensatory behavior (i.e. purging, excessive exercise, etc.) and does not occur exclusively during the course of bulimia nervosa or anorexia nervosa.

DSM-IV-TR Criteria for Pica

A. Persistent eating of nonnutritive substances for a period of at least 1 month.

B. The eating of nonnutritive substances is inappropriate to the developmental level.

C. The eating behavior is not part of a culturally sanctioned practice.

D. If the eating behavior occurs exclusively during the course of another mental disorder (e.g., Mental Retardation, Pervasive Developmental Disorder, Schizophrenia), it is sufficiently severe to warrant independent clinical attention.

DSM-IV-TR Criteria for Rumination Disorder

A. Repeated regurgitation and rechewing of food for a period of at least 1 month following a period of normal functioning.

B. The behavior is not due to an associated gastrointestinal or other general medical condition (e.g., esophageal reflux).

C. The behavior does not occur exclusively during the course of Anorexia Nervosa or Bulimia Nervosa. If the symptoms occur exclusively during the course of Mental Retardation or a Pervasive Developmental Disorders, they are sufficiently severe to warrant independent clinical attention.

DSM-IV-TR Criteria for Feeding Disorder of Infancy or Early Childhood

A. Feeding disturbance as manifested by persistent failure to eat adequately with significant failure to gain weight or significant loss of weight over at least 1 month

B. The disturbance is not due to an associated gastrointestinal or other general medical condition (e.g., esophageal reflux).

C. The disturbance is not better accounted for by another mental disorder (e.g., Rumination Disorder) or by lack of available food.

D. The onset is before age 6 years.

DSM-IV-TR Criteria for Primary Insomnia

A. The predominant complaint is difficulty initiating or maintaining sleep, or nonrestorative sleep, for at least 1 month.

B. The sleep disturbance (or associated daytime fatigue) causes clinically significant distress or impairment in social, occupational, or other important areas of functioning.

C. The sleep disturbance does not occur exclusively during the course of Narcolepsy, Breathing-Related Sleep Disorder, Circadian Rhythm Sleep Disorder, or a Parasomnia.

D. The disturbance does not occur exclusively during the course of another mental disorder (e.g., Major Depressive Disorder, Generalized Anxiety Disorder, a Delirium).

E. The disturbance is not due to the direct physiological effects of a substance (e.g., a drug of abuse, a medication) or a general medical condition.

DSM-IV-TR Criteria for Insomnia Related to Axis I or Axis II Disorder

A. The predominant complaint is difficulty initiating or maintaining sleep, or nonrestorative sleep, for at least 1 month that is associated with daytime fatigue or impaired daytime functioning.

B. The sleep disturbance (or daytime sequelae) causes clinically significant distress or impairment in social, occupational, or other important areas of functioning.

C. The insomnia is judged to be related to another Axis I or Axis II disorder (e.g., Major Depressive Disorder, Generalized Anxiety Disorder, Adjustment Disorder With Anxiety), but is sufficiently severe to warrant independent clinical attention.

D. The disturbance is not better accounted for by another Sleep Disorder (e.g., Narcolepsy, Breathing-Related Sleep Disorder, a Parasomnia).

E. The disturbance is not due to the direct physiological effects of a substance (e.g., a drug of abuse, a medication) or a general medical condition.

DSM-IV-TR Criteria for Primary Hypersomnia

A. The predominant complaint is excessive sleepiness for at least 1 month (or less if recurrent) as evidenced by either prolonged sleep episodes or daytime sleep episodes that occur almost daily.

B. The excessive sleepiness causes clinically significant distress or impairment in social, occupational, or other important areas of functioning.

C. The excessive sleepiness is not better accounted for by Insomnia and does not occur exclusively during the course of another Sleep Disorder (e.g., Narcolepsy, Breathing-Related Sleep Disorder, Circadian Rhythm Sleep Disorder, or a Parasomnia) and cannot be accounted for by an inadequate amount of sleep.

D. The disturbance does not occur exclusively during the course of another mental disorder.

E. The disturbance is not due to the direct physiological effects of a substance (e.g., a drug of abuse, a medication) or a general medical condition.

Specify if:

Recurrent: if there are periods of excessive sleepiness that last at least 3 days occurring several times a year for at least 2 years.

DSM-IV-TR Criteria for Hypersomnia Related to Axis I or Axis II Disorder

A. The predominant complaint is excessive sleepiness for at least 1 month as evidenced by either prolonged sleep episodes or daytime sleep episodes that occur almost daily.

B. The excessive sleepiness causes clinically significant distress or impairment in social, occupational, or other important areas of functioning.

C. The hypersomnia is judged to be related to another Axis I or Axis II disorder (e.g., Major Depressive Disorder, Dysthymic Disorder), but is sufficiently severe to warrant independent clinical attention.

D. The disturbance is not better accounted for by another Sleep Disorder (e.g., Narcolepsy, Breathing-Related Sleep Disorder, a Parasomnia) or by an inadequate amount of sleep.

E. The disturbance is not due to the direct physiological effects of a substance (e.g., a drug of abuse, a medication) or a general medical condition.

DSM-IV-TR Criteria for Narcolepsy

A. Irresistible attacks of refreshing sleep that occur daily over at least 3 months.

B. The presence of one or both of the following:
   1. cataplexy (i.e., brief episodes of sudden bilateral loss of muscle tone, most often in association with intense emotion)
   2. recurrent intrusions of elements of rapid eye movement (REM) sleep into the transition between sleep and wakefulness, as manifested by either hypnopompic or hypnagogic hallucinations or sleep paralysis at the beginning or end of sleep episodes

C. The disturbance is not due to the direct physiological effects of a substance (e.g., a drug of abuse, a medication) or another general medical condition.

DSM-IV-TR Criteria for Breathing-Related Sleep Disorder

A. Sleep disruption, leading to excessive sleepiness or insomnia, that is judged to be due to a sleep-related breathing condition (e.g., obstructive or central sleep apnea syndrome or central alveolar hypoventilation syndrome).

B. The disturbance is not better accounted for by another mental disorder and is not due to the direct physiological effects of a substance (e.g., a drug of abuse, a medication) or another general medical condition (other than a breathing-related disorder).

Coding note: Also code sleep-related breathing disorder on Axis III.

DSM-IV-TR Criteria for Circadian Rhythm Sleep Disorder

A. A persistent or recurrent pattern of sleep disruption leading to excessive sleepiness or insomnia that is due to a mismatch between the sleep-wake schedule required by a person's environment and his or her circadian sleep-wake pattern.

B. The sleep disturbance causes clinically significant distress or impairment in social, occupational, or other important areas of functioning.

C. The disturbance does not occur exclusively during the course of another Sleep Disorder or other mental disorder.

D. The disturbance is not due to the direct physiological effects of a substance (e.g., a drug of abuse, a medication) or a general medical condition.

Specify type:

Delayed Sleep Phase Type: a persistent pattern of late sleep onset and late awakening times, with an inability to fall asleep and awaken at a desired earlier time

Jet Lag Type: sleepiness and alertness that occur at an inappropriate time of day relative to local time, occurring after repeated travel across more than one time zone

Shift Work Type: insomnia during the major sleep period or excessive sleepiness during the major awake period associated with night shift work or frequently changing shift work

Unspecified Type

DSM-IV-TR Criteria for Sleepwalking Disorder

A. Repeated episodes of rising from bed during sleep and walking about, usually occurring during the first third of the major sleep episode.

B. While sleepwalking, the person has a blank, staring face, is relatively unresponsive to the efforts of others to communicate with him or her, and can be awakened only with great difficulty.

C. On awakening (either from the sleepwalking episode or the next morning), the person has amnesia for the episode.

D. Within several minutes after awakening from the sleepwalking episode, there is no impairment of mental activity or behavior (although there may initially be a short period of confusion or disorientation).

E. The sleepwalking causes clinically significant distress or impairment in social, occupational, or other important areas of functioning.

F. The disturbance is not due to the direct physiological effects of a substance (e.g., a drug of abuse, a medication) or a general medical condition.

DSM-IV-TR Criteria for Nightmare Disorder

A. Repeated awakenings from the major sleep period or naps with detailed recall of extended and extremely frightening dreams, usually involving threats to survival, security, or self-esteem. The awakenings generally occur during the second half of the sleep period.

B. On awakening from the frightening dreams, the person rapidly becomes oriented and alert (in contrast to the confusion and disorientation seen in Sleep Terror Disorder and some forms of epilepsy).

C. The dream experience, or the sleep disturbance resulting from the awakening, causes clinically significant distress or impairment in social, occupational, or other important areas of functioning.

D. The nightmares do not occur exclusively during the course of another mental disorder (e.g., a Delirium, Posttraumatic Stress Disorder) and are not due to the direct physiological effects of a substance (e.g., a drug of abuse, a medication) or a general medical condition.

Transparency 8-16

DSM-IV-TR Criteria for Sleep Terror Disorder

A. Recurrent episodes of abrupt awakening from sleep, usually occurring during the first third of the major sleep episode and beginning with a panicky scream.

B. Intense fear and signs of autonomic arousal, such as tachycardia, rapid breathing, and sweating, during each episode.

C. Relative unresponsiveness to efforts of others to comfort the person during the episode.

D. No detailed dream is recalled and there is amnesia for the episode.

E. The episodes cause clinically significant distress or impairment in social, occupational, or other important areas of functioning.

F. The disturbance is not due to the direct physiological effects of a substance (e.g., a drug of abuse, a medication) or a general medical condition.

CHAPTER NINE

PHYSICAL DISORDERS AND HEALTH PSYCHOLOGY

LEARNING OBJECTIVES

1. Describe the fields of behavioral medicine and health psychology, and outline points of overlap and differences in approach.
2. Describe the nature of stress, the general adaptation syndrome proposed by Selye, and how stress affects physiological and psychological systems.
3. Discuss how psychological factors (e.g., perceived control, personality, mood, and social support) affect immune system functioning.
4. Identify the relationship between immune system function, stress, and physical disorders.
5. Describe the cardiovascular system and how stress contributes to cardiovascular disease.
6. Define acute and chronic pain and their potential causes and maintaining factors.
7. Describe the relation between stress and AIDS, cancer, and chronic fatigue syndrome.
9. Describe the use of biofeedback and progressive muscle relaxation as treatments for stress-related disorders.
10. Identify some procedures and strategies used in stress management, and prevention and intervention programs.

OUTLINE

I. Psychological and Social Factors that Influence Health
   A. At present, some of the major contributing factors to illness and death are psychological and behavioral. The textbook illustrates this fact using an example of the relation between genital herpes and stress. The recurrence of genital herpes may be lessened if one engages in stress control procedures. This chapter is concerned with the relations between psychological and social factors on medical illness and disease.
      1. The DSM-IV-TR codes physical disorders on Axis III and recognizes that psychological factors can affect medical conditions.

   B. Health and health-related behavior
      1. The contribution of psychosocial factors to the etiology and treatment of physical disorders is being studied in several areas, including diabetes, and immune system functioning such as in AIDS. This involves the interdisciplinary field of **behavioral medicine**, or the application of knowledge derived from behavioral science to the prevention, diagnosis, and treatment of medical problems. In addition, the non-interdisciplinary field of **health psychology** is considered a subfield of behavioral medicine that addresses psychological factors important in the promotion and maintenance of health, including improvements in health care systems and health policy formulation.

2. Psychological and social factors influence health in two distinct ways:
    a. Psychological and social factors can affect the basic biological processes that lead to illness and disease.
    b. Long-standing behavior patterns may put people at risk to develop certain physical diseases
3. AIDS is an example of a disease that is influenced by psychological (i.e., stress) and behavioral patterns (i.e., life-style risk behaviors).
4. As many as 50% of all deaths from the 10 leading causes of death in the United States can be traced to life-style behaviors (e.g., smoking, poor eating, lack of exercise, insufficient injury control such as not wearing seat belts).

C. The nature of stress

1. **Stress** is the psychological factor that has received the greatest amount of attention. Hans Selye's early experimental work with rats led to the area of study known as stress physiology. Selye noted that daily injection of substances to rats was sufficiently stressful to cause ulcers and atrophy of the immune system tissue.
2. The term **stress** is referred to in this chapter as a *physiological response of an individual to a stressor*. Selye theorized that the body progressed through the following stages in response to sustained stress (**general adaptation syndrome**).
    a. The first phase represents a type of *alarm response* to immediate threat or danger.
    b. With ongoing stress, the body advances to a second stage of *resistance*. Coping mechanisms are mobilized in this stage.
    c. Finally, if the stress is too intense or lasts too long, the body enters a third stage of *exhaustion*; a stage where permanent damage or death may occur.

D. Stress activates the sympathetic branch of the autonomic nervous system (i.e., fight or flight), including the **HPA axis**. In addition to changes in the flow of neurotransmitters under stress, much attention has focused on the endocrine system's neuromodulators or neuropeptides which act very much like neurotransmitters in carrying the brain's messages to various parts of the body.

1. **Corticotropin releasing factor (CRF)** is secreted by the hypothalamus and stimulates the pituitary gland, which in turn, activates the adrenal gland to produce corticosteroids such as the hormone **cortisol**. Cortisol and other related hormones are known as **stress hormones**.
2. The HPA axis is closely related to the limbic system. The limbic system contains the **hippocampus**. This structure is involved in emotional memories and is very responsive to cortisol. When the hippocampus is stimulated during HPA activity, it helps to turn off the body's stress response.
    a. The study of this feedback loop is important because changes in these areas can significantly impact mental and physical health.
    b. For example, work with primates has shown that increased levels of cortisol in response to chronic stress may kill nerve cells in the

hippocampus, thereby diminishing the body's ability to stop the stress response cycle, including memory functioning. Similar processes occur in humans (e.g., persons with PTSD).

E. Contributions to the stress response

1. **Psychological and social factors** profoundly influence stress physiology. For example, work with baboons indicates that high levels of cortisol correlate with low social status.
    a. The most likely explanation is excess secretion of CRF by the hypothalamus in subordinate animals combined with a diminished sensitivity of the pituitary gland. Thus, the body system is less efficient in stopping the stress response.
    b. Subordinate baboons also have fewer circulating lymphocytes (white blood cells) than dominant males – a sign of immune system suppression.
    c. The primary benefit conferred on the dominant males seems to be predictability and controllability, with stability and controllability together being the most important factors.

F. Stress, anxiety, depression, and excitement

1. Stressful life events combined with psychological vulnerabilities are important in psychological and physical disorders and the same holds for the relation between emotional disorders and physical disorders.
    a. Males who develop psychological disorders such as depression or anxiety or who are highly stressed are more likely to develop chronic illness. These individuals have higher mortality rates than males who are free from psychological disorders. Thus, the same type of stress that contributes to psychological disorders may also contribute to the later development of physical disorders.
    b. The underlying physiology of stress, anxiety, depression, and excitement may be similar, but psychological factors (e.g., sense of control, **self-efficacy**) seem to differ and lead to different feelings.

G. Stress and the immune response

1. The relation between stress (e.g., tests) and increased risk of infection (e.g., respiratory) is well established. This relation is mediated by the **immune system**, which protects the body from any foreign materials that may enter it. Stress affects immune system function rapidly.
2. This is a good point to ask students whether they notice any relation between when they are stressed and their susceptibility to illness (e.g., during final exams).

H. The immune system identifies and eliminates foreign materials, called **antigens** and consists of two main parts:

1. The **humoral branch**, which operates in the blood and other bodily fluids.
2. The **cellular branch**, which protects against viral and parasitic infections.

3. White blood cells (i.e., **leukocytes**) are the primary agents of the immune system.
4. Types of leukocytes include:
   a. **Macrophages**, which are considered the body's first line of defense. These cells surround identifiable antigens and destroy them. They also signal lymphocytes.
   b. **Lymphocytes** consist of two groups: B and T cells.
5. **B cells** operate within the humoral part of the immune system, release molecules that seek out antigens in the blood and other bodily fluids so as to neutralize them, and produce highly specific molecules called **immunoglobins** that act as antibodies. After the antigens are neutralized, **memory B cells** are created so that the next time the antigen is encountered, the immune system response will be faster. This process accounts for the success of inoculations.
6. **T cells** operate in the cellular branch of the immune system and do not produce antibodies.
   a. One subgroup, **killer T cells** directly destroy viral infections and cancerous processes, and subsequently produce **memory T cells** to speed future response to the same antigen.
   b. **T4 cells** (i.e., **helper T cells**) enhance the immune system response by signaling **B cells** to produce antibodies and by telling other T cells to destroy the antigen.
   c. **Suppressor T cells** suppress the production of antibodies by B cells when they are no longer needed.
   d. Too many T4 cells lead the immune system to be overreactive and contribute to it attacking the body's normal cells rather than antigens (e.g., **autoimmune diseases** such as **rheumatoid arthritis**). Too many suppressor T cells make the body susceptible to invasion by antigens. Human immunodeficiency virus (HIV) directly attacks T helper cells, thereby weakening the immune system and causing AIDS.
7. There are many connections between the nervous system and the immune system. Nerve endings exist in immune system tissues such as the thymus, lymph nodes, and bone marrow. **Psychoneuroimmunology (PNI)** is an area that studies psychological influences on the neurological response and its relation with immune system response. Examples include the previously described direct connection between the brain (CNS) and HPA axis (hormonal) and the immune system.

II. Psychosocial Contributions to Physical Disorders

A. **AIDS** has become the highest priority in our public health system. In 2000, the total number of people living with HIV was estimated to be about 34.3 million. In South Africa, between 15% and 36% of all adults are believed to be HIV positive.

1. The course of AIDS and **AIDS-related complex** (i.e., HIV infection followed by minor health problems such as weight loss, fever, and night sweats) is variable, and the diagnosis is not made until severe physical illness is present (e.g., pneumocystis pneumonia, cancer, dementia, wasting syndrome).

a. Median time from initial infection to the development of full-blown AIDS is estimated to range from 7.3 to 10 years or more.
b. Most people with AIDS die within 1 year of diagnosis, whereas 15% survive 5 years or longer.

2. Investigators have identified a group of people who have been exposed repeatedly to the AIDS virus but have not contracted the disease. Resistance to AIDS in such cases is believed to be due, in large part, to the strength of the cellular branch of their immune systems. Efforts to boost the strength of the immune system may help prevent AIDS.
3. Stress of learning one has HIV or AIDS can be devastating. **Stress reduction programs** appear to lessen anxiety and depression associated with learning one has HIV, while increasing immune system functioning as measured by T-helper, inducer (CD4), and natural killer (NK) cells, and reductions in antibodies for two herpes viruses that are closely related to HIV.
    1. Two-year follow-up showed less disease progression in the stress reduction group. Similar results have been shown for symptomatic HIV and AIDS patients in response to a cognitive-behavioral stress reduction program.
    2. Generally, higher levels of stress and low social support are associated with faster progression of HIV and AIDS.

B. **Cancer** is also influenced by psychosocial factors. This link, in turn, has led to the growing field of **psychoncology**. **Oncology** means the study of cancer.

1. Persons with breast cancer who received psychosocial treatment consisting of coping and stress management techniques live twice as long on average (i.e., about 3 years) as persons who do not receive this form of intervention.
    a. It is believed that such interventions work by fostering better health habits, closer adherence to medical treatment, and enhanced social adjustment and coping; all of which improve endocrine functioning in response to stress and thereby enhance immune system functioning.
    b. Perceived lack of control, inadequate coping responses, overwhelming stressful life events, use of inappropriate coping responses (i.e., denial) seem to contribute, in part, to the development of cancer.
2. Psychological factors are also implicated in addressing nausea, including conditioned nausea, associated with **chemotherapy treatment**. Such reactions usually begin by the fourth or fifth treatment and slowly escalate in severity.
    a. Between 18% and 50% of patients report development of conditioned nausea, which can lead to refusal to continue with chemotherapy regimens.
    b. Relaxation and graduated exposure to cues that trigger conditioned nausea can diminish or eliminate the response.
3. Psychological factors are also involved in the treatment and recovery from cancer in children. Stress and anxiety associated with painful cancer treatments can have detrimental effects on the disease process.

a. Psychological interventions with child cancer patients include pain and stress management procedures, breathing exercises, information about the procedures, and rehearsal of the procedures with dolls.

C. **Cardiovascular problems** involve parts of the cardiovascular system, comprised of the heart, blood vessels, and mechanisms for regulating their function. This system is also intricately involved in alarm responses to threat or danger. Problems in the cardiovascular system include **strokes** (i.e., **cerebral vascular accidents**), or temporary blockages of blood vessels that cause brain damage and loss of functioning. Also, persons with **Raynaud's disease** lose circulation and suffer pain and feelings of coldness. Cardiovascular problems that are receiving the most attention are hypertension and coronary heart disease. The textbook presents the case of John to illustrate the concepts.

D. **Hypertension** (i.e., high blood pressure) is a major risk factor for stroke, heart disease, and kidney disease. This risk is derived from constriction of blood vessels. This, in turn, causes the heart to work harder to force blood to all parts of the body. The result, in turn, is increased pressure. Hypertension results in wear and tear of the blood vessels, leading to cardiovascular disease. Most cases of hypertension have no verifiable physical cause, and are therefore labeled **essential hypertension**.

1. **High blood pressure** is in excess of 160 over 95, with values of 140/90 or above considered borderline and cause for concern. As an instructor you should note that, since the publication of the text, new guidelines have been proposed for hypertension. For instance, "prehypertension" – describes people with blood pressures between 120-139 millimeters of mercury over 80-89 mm Hg. Those in the prehypertension range are at higher risk than those with lower blood pressures and are much more likely to move into the hypertension range where medication is required.
    a. **Systolic blood pressure** (top number) is represented by the first value and indicates the pressure when the heart is pumping blood.
    b. The second value (bottom number) is **diastolic blood pressure**, and represents the pressure between beats when the heart is at rest. Elevations of diastolic pressure are more worrisome in terms of risk of disease.
2. About 20% of all adults between the ages of 25 and 74 suffer from essential hypertension, and African Americans are twice as likely to develop hypertension as whites. Hypertension also runs in families and the biological vulnerability for hypertension is easy to activate.
3. Neurobiological causes of hypertension are linked to the autonomic nervous system and mechanisms regulating sodium in the kidneys, both of which are important in regulating blood pressure.
    a. Activation of the sympathetic branch of the ANS constricts blood vessels, resulting in more vascular resistance against circulation (i.e., elevations in blood pressure). Such activation is closely related to

stress. Retaining too much salt increases blood volume and raises blood pressure.

4. Psychological factors in hypertension are not simply hostility or repressed hostility, but the frequency one experiences anger and hostility.

E. **Coronary heart disease (CHD)** is a blockage of the arteries supplying blood to the heart muscle or myocardium.

1. **Angina pectoris** is chest pain resulting from partial obstruction of the arteries.
2. **Arteriosclerosis** is the accumulation of artery plaque (i.e., fatty substances) that causes an obstruction.
3. **Ischemia** is the term for deficiency of blood supply to a body part caused by a narrowing of the arteries because of too much plaque.
4. **Myocardial infarction** (i.e., heart attack) refers to the death of heart tissue when a supplying artery is occluded. Genetic factors impinge upon CHD etiology.
5. Stress, anxiety, and anger, combined with poor coping skills and low social support, are implicated in coronary heart disease. Stress reduction procedures have been shown to prevent future heart attacks.
    a. Clusters of behaviors may place one at risk for CHD include the classic **Type A** behavior pattern, marked by excessive competitive drive, time pressure, accelerated activity, and anger outbursts.
    b. **Type B** behavior is the opposite of Type A. People with Type A behavior are twice as likely to develop CHD as people with Type B. Yet, more recent studies do not support the relation between Type A and coronary heart disease.
    c. Sociocultural differences appear to mediate these findings, and other studies have not replicated earlier results.
6. The primary Type A behavior associated with CHD is **anger**, including experience of high levels of **negative affect**.

F. **Chronic pain** and pain account for most physician visits and represents a huge cost to the health care system.

1. Two types of clinical pain are delineated in the textbook:
    a. **Acute pain** typically follows an injury and often disappears once the injury heals or is effectively treated (usually within one month).
    b. **Chronic pain** may begin with an acute episode but does not decrease over time, even with healing or treatment. Typically, chronic pain is experienced in the muscles, joints, or tendons, particularly the lower back, but may include vascular or other areas such as the head.
2. Clinicians distinguish between the **subjective experience** (termed "pain") as reported by the patient, and the **overt manifestations** of this experience (termed "pain behaviors"). Pain behaviors include changing the way one sits or walks, continually complaining about pain to others, grimacing, and most importantly, avoiding activities such as work or recreational pursuits. Emotional suffering may or may not accompany pain.

3. The severity of chronic pain does not predict one's reaction to it. Instead, **psychological factors** mediate this reaction. These factors are the same ones that are implicated in the stress response and other negative emotional states.
    a. The core psychological factor seems to be the person's general sense of control over the situation (i.e., whether the person can deal with pain and its consequences in an effective and meaningful way).
    b. Positive psychological factors are associated with active attempts to cope, such as exercise and other regimens, as opposed to suffering and passivity.
    c. Generally, a profile of negative emotion (e.g., anxiety or depression), poor coping skills, low social support, and the possibility of being compensated for pain through disability claims predict most types of chronic pain.
    d. **Phantom limb pain** illustrates how pain can be disconnected from disease or injury. Evidence suggests that changes in the sensory cortex of the brain may contribute to this phenomenon.
4. **Social factors** also influence the experience of pain. Social forms of pain behavior, such as verbal complaints, facial expressions, and obvious limps or other symptoms, may result in persons who were once critical and demanding now becoming more caring and sympathetic. This phenomenon is referred to as **operant control of pain behavior** because the behavior is under the control of social consequences.
    a. Positive social support, however, may reduce stress associated with pain and injury and promote more adaptive coping and a sense of control.
5. The **gate control theory** of pain incorporates both psychological and physical factors. According to this theory, nerve impulses from painful stimuli make their way to the spinal column that, in turn, controls the flow of pain stimulation to the brain. The **dorsal horns** of the spinal column acts as a gate to transmit sensations of pain if the stimulation is intense. Small fibers tend to open the gate, thereby increasing the transmission of painful stimuli, whereas large fibers tend to close this gate. The brain sends signals back down the spinal cord that may affect the gating mechanism. Strong negative emotions from the brain seem to potentiate the gating and signals of intense pain.
6. **Endogenous opiods**, similar to other opiod substances such as heroin and morphine, seem to exist in the body and are called **endorphins** or **enkephalins** and act very much like neurotransmitters. Endogenous opiods are distributed widely throughout the body and may be influenced by feelings of self-efficacy.
7. **Males and females** seem to experience different types of pain.
    a. Females suffer migraine headaches, arthritis, carpal tunnel syndrome, and temporomandibular joint pain (i.e., TMJ) more so than males.
    b. Males experience more cardiac pain and backache than females.
    c. The female neurochemistry may be based on an **estrogen-dependent neuronal system**; a system that has evolved to cope with pain associated with reproductive activity.

G. **Chronic fatigue syndrome** (originally termed **neurasthenia,** meaning lack of nerve strength) refers to those displaying lack of energy, marked fatigue, pain, and low-grade fever.

1. Neurasthenia disappeared in the early 20th century in Western cultures, but is still the most prevalent form of psychopathology in China. Now chronic fatigue syndrome is spreading rapidly throughout the Western world.
2. Originally this condition was attributed to viral infection, specifically **Epstein-Barr virus**, immune system dysfunction, exposure to toxins, or clinical depression. No evidence exists to support such causes. The causes of chronic fatigue syndrome remain unknown.
3. Chronic fatigue syndrome is more common in females. This condition associated with achievement-oriented lifestyles coupled with a periods of extreme stress and/or acute illness.
4. The symptoms of fatigue, pain, and inability to function are misinterpreted as a continuing disease that is worsened by continued activity. This, in turn, results in behavioral avoidance, helplessness, depression, and frustration.
5. Pharmacological treatment is not effective for chronic fatigue syndrome; however, **cognitive-behavioral treatment** involving procedures to increase activity, regulate periods of rest, address problematic cognitions, relaxation skills and breathing exercises, seem to help diminish fatigue and improve overall level of functioning.

III. Psychosocial Treatment of Physical Disorders

A. **Biofeedback** is a process of making patients aware of specific physiological functions that they would not ordinarily notice consciously (e.g., heart rate, blood pressure, muscle tension, EEG rhythms, and blood flow). It is used to teach patients ways of controlling such reactions directly. This is accomplished by connecting a person to physiological monitoring equipment to make the physiological response visible or audible. The person then learns to control different physiological responses. Lack of practice may explain why humans can discriminate changes in autonomic activity despite usually being so poor at doing so.

1. Biofeedback is used for persons suffering from physical disorders or stress-related conditions, such as hypertension and headache.
2. Biofeedback is equally as effective and long-lasting as teaching people to relax in the treatment of headache.

B. Several varieties of **relaxation and meditation procedures** have been used alone, or in combination with other procedures, to treat physical disorders and pain in pain patients. Generally, relaxation procedures have positive effects on headaches, hypertension, and acute and chronic pain, although the results are relatively modest. Relaxation and meditation are almost always part of a comprehensive pain-management program.

1. **Progressive muscle relaxation** is designed to increase awareness of bodily tension and to counteract this tension by relaxing specific muscle groups. Often this is accomplished by teaching clients to tense and release muscle groups.

2. **Autogenic relaxation training** involves focusing attention on tense muscle groups and blood flow as well as self-suggestion.
3. **Transcendental meditation (TM)** involves focusing attention on a repeated syllable or the **mantra**.
4. A more specific version of TM is the **relaxation response**, or repeating a word to eliminate distraction and induce calm.

C. A **comprehensive stress management** program may involve teaching the person to closely monitor stress and identify significant daily and major life stressors; teaching the person to note bodily and cognitive events related to stress; teaching the person deep muscle relaxation; use of cognitive therapy to address exaggerating negative thinking and unrealistic thoughts about stress and their lives; developing new coping strategies such as time management and assertiveness training.
   a. Data suggest that a comprehensive program is better than individual components alone in the treatment of chronic pain, tension headaches, and cancer pain.

D. Chronic reliance on analgesic medications may lessen the efficacy of comprehensive treatment programs for headache. In addition, psychological treatment seems to reduce drug consumption and may reduce the amount of medication needed for hypertension.

E. **Denial or lack of optimism** has many negative effects, including the neglect of symptom variations and pursuit of treatment.
1. Most mental health professionals work to eliminate denial because it may have negative effects on treatment. However, denial may not always be unhealthy, particularly during the initial stressful phase where one learns they may have a serious condition. Here denial may allow a person time to develop coping strategies.
2. Lower levels of corticosteroids may also be found in persons undergoing denial. The value of denial as a coping mechanism may depend on timing.

F. Modifying Behaviors to Promote Health
1. Many **lifestyle practices** contribute to physical disorders, including unhealthy eating and exercise habits, smoking and alcohol use. Many of these behaviors contribute directly to diseases and physical disorders that are among the leading causes of death, including coronary heart disease, cancer, accidents, cirrhosis of the liver, and respiratory disease such as influenza and pneumonia (both of which are related to smoking and stress).
2. **Injuries** are the leading cause of death for people 1 to 45, and loss of productivity due to injury is greater from injuries than from the other three leading causes of death (i.e., heart disease, cancer, and stroke).
   a. Psychological variables mediate virtually all factors that lead to injury.
   b. Efforts to prevent injuries in children include teaching about fire and escape from fire, how to identify and report emergencies, how to safely

cross streets and ride bicycles, and how to handle cuts. Repeatedly warning children or others is ineffective in preventing injuries. Teaching skills about injury prevention is best.

3. **AIDS** represents a disease that is due exclusively to life-style behaviors and is highly preventable. One of the most successful behavior change programs was carried out in San Francisco. Such programs teach safe sex practices and foster a sense of self-efficacy and control over sexual behavior.
4. **China** has one of the most tobacco-addicted populations in the world. Approximately 250 million people in China are habitual smokers; a number that equals the entire population of the United States.
    a. Using children as agents of change in their families, researchers have developed an anti-smoking campaign in schools. Children took home antismoking literature and questionnaires for their fathers, and wrote letters to their fathers asking them to quit smoking.
    b. About 12% of fathers in the intervention group quit smoking for 6 months.
5. The **Stanford three community study** is one of the best-known and most successful efforts to reduce risk factors for disease.
    a. Three communities were studied in central California, and the target was reducing the risk for coronary heart disease, with a focus on smoking, high blood pressure, diet, and weight reduction.
    b. Results were successful in reducing risk for coronary heart disease, with the greatest benefit from those who also received face-to-face contact with a mental health provider.

OVERALL SUMMARY

This chapter outlines the primary psychological and social factors that influence the development and maintenance of several physical disorders. Specifically, the psychological effects of stress on the immune system and related diseases are described. In addition, lifestyle practices that place one at risk for certain physical disorders are discussed. Finally, both limited and comprehensive psychosocial treatment and prevention efforts for these problems are delineated.

KEY TERMS

Acute pain (p. 319)
AIDS-related complex (ARC) (p. 312)
Antigens (p. 310)
Autoimmune disease (p. 311)
Behavioral medicine (p. 305)
Biofeedback (p. 324)
Cancer (p. 313)
Cardiovascular disease (p. 315)
Chronic fatigue syndrome (p. 322)
Chronic pain (p. 319)

Coronary heart disease (CHD) (p. 317)
Endogenous opiods (p. 321)
Essential hypertension (p. 316)
General adaptation syndrome (p. 306)
Health psychology (p. 305)
Hypertension (p. 316)
Immune system (p. 309)
Psychoncology (p. 287)
Psychoneuroimmunology (PNI) (p. 311)
Relaxation response (p. 325)
Rheumatoid arthritis (p. 311)
Self-efficacy (p. 309)
Stress (p. 306)
Stroke / Cerebral vascular accident (CVA) (p. 315)
Type A behavior pattern (p. 318)
Type B behavior pattern (p. 318)

INFOTRAC KEY TERM EXERCISES

Each exercise is linked to key terms from the Wadsworth InfoTrac on-line searchable database. Key terms must be entered exactly as written.

Exercise 1: **Mindfulness-Based Stress Reduction: The New Wave Toward Heathy Living**
Article: A106224321
Citation: (Integrating mindfulness-based stress reduction). Kathryn Proulx. Holistic Nursing Practice, July-August 2003 v17 i4 p201(8)

Mindfulness and other meditative techniques pre-date psychology as a formal discipline, and yet are becoming increasingly popular in psychology and allied medical professions. What is new about such procedures within psychology is there systematic development, manualization, and inclusion in empirically-supported psychosocial interventions. John Kabatt-Zinn and colleagues have developed an intervention program for stress-related problems known as Mindfulness-Based Stress Reduction (MBSR). This InfoTrac article describes MBSR and studies that have been conducted to test its efficacy. You are to read this article, and answer the following questions: (a) what is mindfulness?, (b) what is MBSR?, (c) based on available studies, what is MBSR helpful for?, and (d) relate the MBSR approach with the chapter discussion about stress and illness. Based on what you read in the text and the article, can you see any benefits for using MBSR in behavioral medicine and health psychology? Limit your answer to 3-5 typed double-spaced pages.

Exercise 2: **The Nature and Treatment of Phantom Limb Pain**
Key Term: *Phantom Limb Pain*

Phantom limb pain is a curious phenomenon whereby a person experiences mild-to-severe pain in a limb that was removed during surgery. Yet, until recently, little was known about the biological underpinnings of phantom limb pain, including how to effectively treat it. Your task is to review the InfoTrac article(s) on the biological and psychological factors that contribute to phantom limb pain and to devise a comprehensive psychosocial intervention program in light of what you learn. Your intervention program should address the components of phantom limb phenomena that are related to the persistence of pain. That is, back up the components of your program with evidence and information gleaned from what you read. Try to be creative and limit your answer to 3-5 typed double-spaced pages.

Exercise 3: Is Chronic Fatigue Syndrome a Somatoform Disorder in Disguise?
Key Term: *Chronic Fatigue Syndrome*

Chronic fatigue syndrome (CFS) is a little understood condition that affects females more often than males. CFS shares many similarities with the somatoform disorders, namely hypochondriasis and somatization disorder. Assume that you are an expert on CFS and that you have been invited to join a task force responsible for developing the next edition of the *Diagnostic and Statistical Manual of Mental Disorders, 5th edition.* The committee members would like you to evaluate whether CFS is simply hypochondriasis or somatization disorder, or a separate disorder in its own right. Your task is to prepare your arguments for the meeting in light of reviewing the InfoTrac article(s) on CFS and in the context of your past reading about somatoform disorders. You should address what is known about CFS, including similarities and differences with hypochondriasis and somatization disorder. Finally, take a stand in light of what you have read – should CFS be considered as a disorder in its own right for the DSM-V?, or does it belong with the somatoform disorders? Limit your answer to 3-5 typed double-spaced pages.

Exercise 4 (Future Trend): Managed Behavioral Health Care and the Future of Psychology

The text authors rightly point out that many of the leading and most costly diseases are, either directly or indirectly, the result of behavioral and psychological factors. Managed behavioral health care companies are increasingly recognizing this too, and are looking for evidence showing that psychosocial interventions help offset medical costs. For instance, a psychologists trained in behavioral medicine might show that a stress reduction program results in fewer physician visits and less utilization of expensive medical procedures relative to treatment as usual. This may be a good time to introduce students to managed behavioral health care, and psychology's evolving role in such contexts. The links below represent some useful stating points.

http://www.cdc.gov/nchs/
http://www.fenichel.com/Managed2.html
http://www.psychologyinfo.com/consumers/commoncomplaints.html
http://www.division42.org/StEC/articles/transition/crossroads.html
http://www.institute-shot.com/managed_mental_health_care.htm

CLASSROOM ACTIVITIES, DEMONSTRATIONS, AND LECTURE TOPICS

1. **Activity: Stress Log.** This exercise is designed to help students gain an awareness of the stress they experience in their life and how they react to the stress. Have students keep a record of their stress for one week using a "Stress Log" (this should consist of a table with separate columns for date, time, brief description of the stressful event, and their bodily, cognitive, and overt behavioral reactions). Instruct your students to try and complete their

records once or twice a day and include the event they perceived as stressful, regardless how small the event and their reactions. Have them review and turn in their records at the end of the week. Ask them to respond verbally or in writing to the following:

a. What did you notice about the sources of your stress and the patterns of stress that you experienced?
b. Are there situations or people that seem to precipitate considerable stress for you?
c. What patterns, if any, do you notice in the way you respond to the stressors you experienced?
d. How did this activity impact you, particularly regarding your perceptions about, and reactions to, stress?
e. What changes would you like to make in your coping methods?

2. **Activity: How Do You Cope With Stress?** To help students gain more specific insight into how they attempt to cope with stress, distribute HANDOUT 9.1 and ask them to complete it. After they have finished, you should remind them that no strategy assures a person of positive results and every strategy has some potential for having a positive effect in certain situations. According to some researchers, however, strategies that involve active methods of planning and coping and that focus on the positive tend to be associated with reduced anxiety and higher self-esteem. Such strategies as giving up, trying to hurt others, blaming oneself, and overindulgence tend to be less constructive ways of coping.

    Source Information. Knight, S., Vail-Smith, K., Jenkins, L., Phillips, J., Evans, L., & Brown, K. (1994). How Do You Adapt/Cope With Stress? Instructor's resource manual for Williams and Knight's healthy for life: Wellness and the art of living. Pacific Grove, CA: Brooks/Cole.

3. **Activity: Assessing the Type A Personality.** The text describes the differences between Type A and Type B personalities. Students can gain some insight into whether they are Type A or B by completing HANDOUT 9.2. After they have answered all of the questions, tell them the questionnaire was designed to explore Type A characteristics. Remind them that Type A is characterized by time urgency, competitiveness, and being hurried and driven by deadlines. This questionnaire is not diagnostic of that problem but, if they answered yes to several items, they may want to consider the possibility of Type A behavior as a potential pattern that may present health problems. If they answered yes to item 19 and also have strong, recurrent feelings of hostility and anger, they may be especially prone to health problems.

    Source Information. Knight, S., Vail-Smith, K., Jenkins, L., Phillips, J., Evans, L., and Brown, K. (1994). How Do You Adapt/Cope With Stress? Instructor's resource manual for Williams and Knight's healthy for life: Wellness and the art of living. Pacific Grove, CA: Brooks/Cole.

4. **Activity: Discussion of the Relation Between Health, Stress, and Use of Alcohol and Other Drugs.** Exam time is often a source of stress and typically the incidence of viral and bacterial infection rises predictably on campuses during exam periods. Many students also drink alcohol, smoke cigarettes, or experiment with other drugs. Ask

students whether they have noted any relation between school stress and the likelihood of getting sick, whether they remain sick longer under times of stress, and whether they use alcohol or other recreational drugs more often during times of stress. You may use this as an opportunity to talk about adaptive ways to reduce stress and boost immunity, and how many drugs actually weaken our body's ability to fight stress and illness.

5. **Video Activity: Identifying Psychological and Behavioral Risks Associated With HIV/AIDS.** Present the segment titled "HIV/AIDS" (from Abnormal Psychology Inside/Out, vol 2). This segment presents an interview with an HIV positive male who discusses overcoming the challenges of his illness, including how his life has changed since he was diagnosed. After discussing stress and risk factors associated with physical disorders and disease, ask your students to identify both psychological and behavioral risk factors in this client, including positive health promoting factors. Use this activity as a springboard for discussion about developing comprehensive prevention and treatment programs for HIV/AIDS.

HANDOUT 9.1

How Do You Adapt/Cope With Stress?

People adapt to or cope with stress in a variety of ways. Individuals tend to use their personal adaptation/coping styles fairly consistently, across situations. Which of the following is consistent with your style? Circle the question numbers that are true of you.

In the face of stressful situations, I tend to.....

1. Take some kind of action to try to solve the problem
2. Try to strategize about possible actions to take
3. Make time to consider my options and do some planning
4. Make myself wait for an opportune or right time to do something about it
5. Find out what other people would do in a similar situation
6. Talk to and get emotional support from others about my problem
7. Try to focus on the positive aspects of what is happening
8. Accept what is happening and learn to live with it
9. Seek guidance from God or my higher power
10. Get upset and vent my emotions
11. Deny a problem exists and refuse to believe it is happening
12. Give up trying to get what I want
13. Try to take my mind off the problem by turning to work or other activities
14. Use alcohol or other drugs to avoid thinking about the problem
15. Indulge myself by means of food, drugs, spending money, etc.

HANDOUT 9.2

What are Your Usual Reactions?

Take a minute to respond yes or no to the following statements:

___1. When I stop at a red light while driving, I find it difficult to patiently wait for the light to turn green.

___2. When I talk to other people, I find myself finishing their sentences for them.

___3. I often find myself trying to do several things at once (like reading while I eat).

___4. I have difficulty relaxing.

___5. I cannot sit still long enough to watch one program on television.

___6. I am often involved in too many projects at once.

___7. I tend to overextend myself.

___8. People tell me that I am a fast talker, eater, and walker.

___9. I cannot stand waiting in lines.

___10. I am very competitive.

___11. I am frequently angry and frustrated.

___12. When I am driving, I usually race through yellow lights and often speed.

___13. In order to enjoy sports or playing games, I need to win.

___14. I never seem to have enough time.

___15. I often eat "on the run."

___16. I am not a patient person.

___17. I get upset with people who drive, move, talk, or think slowly.

___18. People tell me that if I do not slow down, I'm going to get an ulcer, high blood pressure, or have a heart attack.

___19. I probably have Type A behavior.

SUPPLEMENTARY READING MATERIAL FOR CHAPTER NINE

(= These sources can be found on "*Infotrac, the online library*" provided by Wadsworth and Brooks/Cole Publishing.)

Anderson, B., Anderson, B., & DeProsse, C. (1989). Controlled longitudinal study of women with cancer. Journal of Consulting and Clinical Psychology, 57, 692-697.

Blanchard, E. B. (1989). Non-drug treatments for essential hypertension. New York: Pergamon.

Blanchard, E. B., & Epstein, L. H. (1978). A biofeedback primer. Reading, MA: Addison-Wesley.

Duckro, P. N., Richardson, W. D., & Marshall, J. E. (1995). Taking control of your headaches. New York: Guilford.

Fried, R. (1993). The psychology and physiology of breathing: In behavioral medicine, clinical psychology, and psychiatry. New York: Plenum.

Goodheart, C. D., & Lansing, M. H. (1997). Treating people with chronic disease: A psychological guide. Washington, DC: American Psychological Association.

Hayes, S. C., Bissett, R. T., Korn, Z., Zettle, R. D., Rosenfarb, I. S., Cooper, L. D., & Grundt, A. M. (1999). The impact of acceptance versus control rationales on pain tolerance. The Psychological Record, 49, 33(1).

McGrath, P. (1999). Posttraumatic stress and the experience of cancer: A literature review. The Journal of Rehabilitation, 65, 17.

Pedersen, P. K., & Hoffman-Goetz, L. (2000). Exercise and the immune system: Regulation, integration, and adaptation. Physiological Reviews, 80, 1055.

Resnick, R. J., & Rosensky, R. H. (1996). Health psychology through the life span: Practice and research opportunities. Washington, DC: American Psychological Association.

Robertson-Ritchie, H. (2001). Toward a new definition of chronic fatigue syndrome. The Western Journal of Medicine, 174, 241.

Selye, H. (1976). Stress in health and disease. Woburn, MA: Butterworth.

Schneiderman, N., Antoni, M. H., Saab, P. G., & Ironson, G. (2001). Health psychology: Psychosocial and biobehavioral aspects of chronic disease management. Annual Review of Psychology, 555.

Strube, M. J. (Ed.) (1991). Type A behavior. Newbury Park, CA: Sage.

Watson, M. (Ed.) (1991). Cancer patient care: Psychosocial treatment methods. New York: Cambridge University Press.

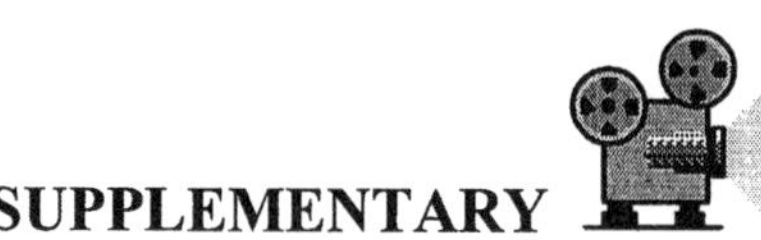

SUPPLEMENTARY VIDEO RESOURCES FOR CHAPTER NINE

Abnormal psychology inside/out, vol 2. (*available through your International Thomson Learning representative).* The segment on "HIV/AIDS" presents an interview with an HIV positive male who discusses overcoming the challenges of his illness, including how his life has changed since he was diagnosed. (4 min)

A second segment, titled "The Role of Social Support," presents the male client described above, who describes the role of social support in his ability to cope with HIV and AIDS. (2 min)

Blue. (Hollywood Film; Drama). British filmmaker Derek Jarman's last film; he died from AIDS shortly after the movie was completed. Jarman reviews his life and analyzes the ways in which his life has been affected by his disease.

Cancer treatment. (Fanlight Productions, 1-800-937-4113). This program follows several people through the process of chemotherapy or radiation treatments, explaining how they work and their side effects, as well as the emotional ups and downs which all patients experience. (28 min)

CNN today: Abnormal psychology, vol. 1. (*available through your International Thomson Learning representative).* The segment titled "Physical Disorders and Health Psychology: Stressful Heart," presents relaxation methods (e.g., yoga and meditation) to help with stress management and describes the relation between stress and the heart. (2:06 min)

Finding your way. (Fanlight Productions, 1-800-937-4113). Behavioral techniques for coping with the discomfort or pain of cancer treatment. (22 min)

Health, stress, and coping. (Insight Media: 2162 Broadway, New York, NY 10024/ (800)-233-9910). This program explores a range of stressors from everyday tension to post-traumatic stress disorder. Case studies illuminate the link between psychology and biology in understanding stress. Norman Cousins discusses the relationship between stress and physical illness, Hans Selye's General Adaptation Syndrome (GAS), and strategies for coping with stress and illness. (30 min)

Lives in balance. (Insight Media: 2162 Broadway, New York, NY 10024/ (800)-233-9910). Explaining that unrelieved stress can result in serious health problems, this program explores a variety of approaches for helping individuals cope with stress. It points out that while stress is an inevitable consequence of modern life and many people are subject to similar stresses, individuals often react very differently to the same set of stress-inducing circumstances. (30 min)

Managing stress, anxiety, and frustration. (Insight Media: 2162 Broadway, New York, NY 10024/ (800)-233-9910). This video defines stress, analyzes its causes and effects, and teaches techniques for managing it. It explains the physiological bases for stress-related illnesses and contrasts ineffective means of coping with positive steps. (60 min)

Marvin's room. (Hollywood Film; Drama). A compelling look at the ways in which chronic illness affects caregivers and families.

My left foot. (Hollywood Film; Biography). Life story of Christy Brown, an Irish writer, who overcomes cerebral palsy.

Pain management. (Fanlight Productions, 1-800-937-4113). From The Dr. is in series. This video offers an overview of the causes of pain and how it can be effectively managed if it cannot be cured. (28 min)

Psychobiology of stress. (Insight Media: 2162 Broadway, New York, NY 10024/ (800)-233-9910). This video probes how the brain controls stress response through nervous, hormonal, and adrenal regulation. The changes in the body in response to stress are examined. The video also shows how to break unhealthy patterns. (10 min)

Stress, health, and you. (Time-Life Films/Video). Includes discussion by Hans Selye and Richard Rahe, including suggestions for handling stress. (18 min)

Tell them you're fine. (Fanlight Productions, 1-800-937-4113). Three young people with cancer confront the day-to-day realities of coping with the impact of the disease, with therapy, and with the attitudes of family, friends and co-workers. (17 min)

Whose life is it anyway? (Hollywood Film; Drama). Richard Dreyfuss depicts a sculptor who was paralyzed below the neck from a car crash and who argues for the right to die.

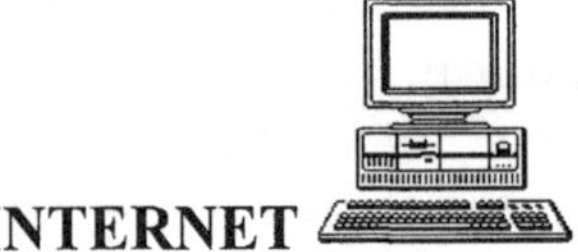

INTERNET RESOURCES FOR CHAPTER NINE

American Academy of Pain Management
http://www.aapainmanage.org/
This site provides information and links related to the management of acute and chronic pain.

Health Psychology & Rehabilitation
http://www.healthpsych.com/
This web site provides information on research and viewpoints on the practice of health psychology in medical and rehabilitation settings.

High Blood Pressure
http://www.nhlbi.nih.gov/hbp/index.html

A useful National Institute of Health site about the assessment, prevention, and treatment of high blood pressure.

History of Pain Management
http://www.library.ucla.edu/libraries/biomed/his/bonica/index.html

Excellent resource for information related to past and present theories and conceptions of pain and pain management.

MedlinePlus: Chronic Fatigue Syndrome
http://www.nlm.nih.gov/medlineplus/chronicfatiguesyndrome.html

A useful source of scholarly information about chronic fatigue syndrome.

National Institute of Psychosocial Oncology
http://www.psycho-oncology.net/

This site provides information and links related to the psychological and medical care of cancer patients.

Pain.Com
http://www.pain.com/

A megasite of information and links to information about pain and pain management.

Society for Behavioral Medicine
http://www.sbmweb.org/

A scholarly organization devoted to the science and practice of behavioral medicine.

Stress Management: Review and Principles
http://www.unl.edu/stress/mgmt/

This web site presents the core concepts of stress management education. It has been used
as the Body of Knowledge for Certification in Stress Management Education.

The American Heart Association
http://www.amhrt.org

This is the American Heart Association's official web site, providing information on books, support groups, educational materials, diets, fact sheets, research and more on heart disease, stroke, and related conditions.

WARNING SIGNS OF STRESS

- Increased irritability
- Difficulty sleeping, awakening early, or excessive sleeping
- Loss of energy or zest for life
- Becoming increasingly isolated
- Feeling out of control, engaging in uncharacteristic actions or emotions (crying a lot, becoming shrill, focusing on petty things)
- Drinking too many caffeinated beverages or relying too much on nicotine and alcohol, sleeping pills and other medications
- Changes in the body's normal functioning (e.g., a pounding 0
- Denying physical or psychological symptoms (e.g., “There's nothing wrong with taking slccping pills cvcry night," or "Anybody would bc dcprcsscd in my situation.")
- Handling family members less gently or considerately than is customary
- Entertaining suicidal thoughts

DSM-IV-TR Criteria for Psychological Factors Affecting Medical Condition

A. A general medical condition (coded on Axis III) is present.

B. Psychological factors adversely affect the general medical condition in one of the following ways:

1. The factors have influenced the course of the general medical condition as shown by a close temporal association between the psychological factors and the development or exacerbation of, or delayed recovery from, the general medical condition
2. The factors interfere with the treatment of the general medical condition
3. The factors constitute additional health risks for the individual
4. Stress-related physiological responses precipitate or exacerbate symptoms of the general medical condition

Choose name based on the nature of the psychological factors (if more than one factor is present, indicate the most prominent):

Mental Disorder Affecting...[Indicate the General Medical Condition] (e.g., an Axis I disorder such as Major Depressive Disorder delaying recovery from a myocardial infarction)
Psychological Symptoms Affecting...[Indicate the General Medical Condition] (e.g., depressive symptoms delaying recovery from surgery; anxiety exacerbating asthma)
Personality Traits or Coping Style Affecting...[Indicate the General Medical Condition] (e.g., pathological denial of the need for surgery in a patient with cancer; hostile, pressured behavior contributing to cardiovascular disease)
Maladaptive Health Behaviors Affecting...[Indicate the General Medical Condition] (e.g., overeating; lack of exercise; unsafe sex)
Stress-Related Physiological Response Affecting...[Indicate the General Medical Condition] (e.g., stress-related exacerbations of ulcer, hypertension, arrhythmia, or tension headache)
Other or Unspecified Psychological Factors Affecting...[Indicate the General Medical Condition] (e.g., interpersonal, cultural, or religious factors)

CHAPTER TEN

SEXUAL AND GENDER IDENTITY DISORDERS

LEARNING OBJECTIVES

1. Describe how sociocultural factors influence what are considered "normal" sexual behaviors.
2. Illustrate important similarities and differences between males and females with regard to sexual behavior and attitudes.
3. Describe research related to the biological, psychological, and social influences on homosexuality, including evidence supporting the genetic component of homosexual patterns of sexual arousal.
4. Understand the relation between aging and sexual behavior.
5. Describe the defining clinical features, causes, and treatment of gender identity disorder. Also be able to distinguish gender identity disorder from transvestic fetishism.
6. Define sexual dysfunction and describe how sexual dysfunctions are organized around the sexual response cycle.
7. Describe the defining clinical features and known causes of sexual dysfunctions, including important gender differences.
8. Describe psychosocial and medical treatments for sexual dysfunctions, including what is known about their efficacy.
9. Identity the common clinical features of each of the different paraphilias.
10. Explain what is known about the causes of paraphilias.
11. Describe the important differences in patterns of sexual arousal between perpetrators of incest and pedophiles, and similarly between rapists and sadistic rapists.
12. Describe available psychosocial and drug treatments for paraphilias, including what is known about their efficacy.

OUTLINE

I. What is Normal Sexuality?

A. With males, vaginal intercourse is a nearly universal experience. About three-fourths of men also engage in oral sex, whereas only one-fifth engage in anal sex. Approximately 23.3% of males report having sex with 20 or more partners, whereas 70% report only one sexual partner during the previous year. More males report engaging in heterosexual sex, only 2.3% report engaging in homosexual sex, with 1.1% engaging in exclusively homosexual activity. Similar results have been reported in Britain and France.

B. **Sexual risk** behavior is alarmingly high in college samples and young adults. For example, though regular condom use has increased from 12% in 1975 to 41% in 1989, more than half of sexually active college-age women practice unprotected sex.

C. **Elderly** samples generally report an active sex life. Decreases in sexual activity among the elderly is generally correlated with decreases in mobility, disease processes and use of medication, and normal aging that slows various vasocongestive responses that are part of sexual arousal.

D. The following are known **gender differences** in sexual behavior:

1. A greater percentage of males than females engage in masturbatory behavior. Among those who do masturbate, the frequency is three times greater for males than females. Masturbation is the largest gender difference in sexuality and is unrelated to later sexual functioning.
2. Males also show a more permissive attitude regarding premarital sex than females; though this gap is shrinking.
3. Males tend to approve of premarital intercourse in the context of a committed relationship slightly more so than females.
4. Number of sexual partners and frequency of intercourse are slightly greater for males compared to females.
5. Females tend to desire more demonstrations of love and intimacy during sex compared to males who focus more on the arousal aspects of sex.
6. No gender differences exist with regard to homosexuality (generally acceptable), the experience of sexual satisfaction, or attitudes about masturbation (generally accepting).
7. Regarding **sexual self-schemas** (or core beliefs about sexual aspects of one's self), females tend to report the experience of passionate and romantic feelings as an integral part of their sexuality; however, a substantial number of females hold an embarrassed, conservative, or self-conscious schema that can conflict with more positive aspects of sexual attitudes. Males do not report such negative core beliefs.

E. **Cultural differences** exist in sexual practices. For example, the Sambia in New Guinea believe that semen is essential for growth and development in young boys and that it is not produced naturally. Young boys at age 7 engage in oral sex with other male teenagers in the tribe to gain semen. Only oral sex is permitted, while masturbation is forbidden in this tribe. In addition, premarital sex is accepted in many societies but not others. Subcultural differences are also apparent in Western countries.

F. The **development of sexual orientation** is complex. Homosexuality runs in families and concordance rates for homosexuality are higher for monozygotic than dizygotic twins. Though the media often concludes that sexual orientation has a biological cause, no studies have confirmed singular biological causation. There may be many pathways to the development of heterosexuality and homosexuality, and no one factor can predict outcome.

1. **Bem** proposed that persons inherit a temperament to behave in a certain way that later interacts with environmental factors to produce sexual orientation.

The result is that the opposite sex becomes more **exotic** to the extent that the individual engages in typical male or female behaviors and social patterns.

2. Moreover, about 50% of monozygotic twins with exactly the same genetic structure and same environment did not have the same sexual orientation.
3. Biology is best thought of as setting limits on the development of sexual orientation.

II. Gender Identity Disorder

A. **Gender identity disorder (GID)** or **transsexualism** refers to cases where a person's physical/biological gender is inconsistent with his/her sense of identity as a male or female. Gender identity disorder is rare, with males showing this disorder more often than females. Persons with this disorder feel trapped in a body of the wrong sex, whereas persons with **transvestic fetishism** (discussed later) are sexually aroused by wearing clothes associated with the opposite sex. In GID, the primary goal is not sexual, but the desire to live one's life openly in a manner consistent with the opposite gender. Moreover, GID individuals have no physical abnormalities as is the case with intersex individuals (i.e., **hermaphrodites**). GID also is not synonymous with homosexual arousal patterns (e.g., a male homosexual who sometimes behaves effeminately), but rather is independent of them. The textbook illustrates gender identity disorder with the case of Joe.

B. There are **no known biological contributions** to the development of GID; though higher levels of testosterone or estrogen at certain critical periods of development might masculinize a female fetus or feminize a male fetus.

1. Some evidence suggests that gender identity firms up between 18 months and 3 years of age and is relatively fixed after that. Gender identity may be something learned at a very young age.

C. **Treatment of gender identity disorder** most commonly involves sex reassignment surgery, and secondarily psychosocial interventions to alter mistaken gender identity itself.

1. To qualify for **sex reassignment surgery**, individuals must live in the opposite-sex role for 1 to 2 years so that they can be sure they want to change sex. Additionally, such persons must be stable psychologically, financially, and socially. Reassignment surgery is irreversible.
    a. In **male-to-female** candidates, hormones are administered to promote gynecomastia (i.e., growth of breasts) and the development of other secondary characteristics. Facial hair is removed via electrolysis, and only later the genitals are removed and a vagina constructed.
    b. For **female-to-male** transsexuals, an artificial penis is constructed via often difficult plastic surgery, and breasts are surgically removed.
    c. Approximately 75% report satisfaction with surgery and good adjustment, with female-to-male conversions adjusting better than male-to-female. 7% of reassignment cases regret surgery.

2. **Treatment of intersex (i.e., hermaphrodites) individuals** involves surgery and hormonal replacement therapy. Such persons may be born with physical characteristics of both sexes. Others have suggested there are actually five sexes: males, females, **herms** (i.e., named after true hermaphrodites or people with both testes and ovaries), **merms** (i.e., persons who are anatomically more male than female, but have some aspects of female genitalia), and **ferms** (i.e., persons with ovaries and aspects of male genitalia). Approximately 17/1000 births (or 1.7%) are intersexed in some form. Current approaches are less likely to opt for surgery immediately after birth is such cases, and instead consider psychological treatment to help the person adapt to their particular anatomy.
3. **Psychosocial interventions** attempt to modify thinking and behaviors to be more consistent with one's biological sex, and involve behavioral rehearsal, modeling, role play, imagery and imaginal reconditioning of sexual interactions and behaviors consistent with one's biological sex. Many look to psychosocial interventions when under distress or confusion, or when surgery is unavailable. Psychosocial interventions can be effective in resolving gender identity disorder; however, few large-scale studies have been conducted.

III. Overview of Sexual Dysfunctions

A. Three stages of the sexual response cycle (i.e., desire, arousal, and orgasm) are associated with specific sexual dysfunctions.

1. Pain may also be associated with sexual functioning.
2. Males and females experience parallel versions of most disorders. Two disorders that are sex specific are premature ejaculation and vaginismus (i.e., painful contractions of the vagina during attempted penetration in females).
3. Sexual dysfunctions may be **lifelong** (i.e., chronic) or **acquired** (i.e., more recent onset after a pattern of normal sexual functioning).
4. Sexual dysfunctions may be **generalized** or **specific**, and may also be due to psychological factors or psychological factors combined with a medical condition (i.e., when the person has demonstrable vascular, hormonal, or an associated physical condition that is known to contribute to sexual dysfunction).
5. As many as 43% of all females and 31% of males suffer from sexual dysfunction, making this class of disorder the most prevalent of any psychological or physical disorder in the United States.
6. As many as 40% of happily married and sexually satisfied males report occasional erectile and ejaculatory difficulties, and 63% of women report occasional dysfunction of arousal or orgasm. Occurrence of such problems does not typically diminish sexual satisfaction.
7. The best predictor of sexual distress among women meeting objective criteria for a sexual dysfunction are deficits in general emotional well-being or emotional relationships with the partner during sexual relations, not lack of lubrication or orgasm.

B. Sexual desire disorders

1. **Hypoactive sexual desire disorder** involves little or no interest in any type of sexual activity. As many as 50% of patients (mostly females) who come to sexuality clinics for help complain of hypoactive sexual desire. Approximately 22% of women and 5% of men suffer from this disorder. Such persons rarely have sexual fantasies, seldom masturbate, and attempt intercourse once a month or less. The textbook illustrates hypoactive sexual desire disorder with Judy and Ira.
2. **Sexual aversion disorder** involves little interest in sex and fear, panic, or disgust related to physical or sexual contact or thoughts. About 10% of males with this disorder report panic attacks during attempted sexual activity, and about 25% of persons with this disorder also meet criteria for panic disorder. The textbook illustrates sexual aversion disorder with the case of Lisa.

C. Sexual arousal disorders

1. Sexual arousal disorders include **male erectile disorder** and **female sexual arousal disorder**. The problem in both cases is not desire, but becoming aroused. Males have difficulty achieving or maintaining an erection, and females experience problems achieving or maintaining adequate lubrication. The outdated and pejorative term for male erectile disorder was impotence, whereas the parallel problem in females was termed frigidity. The textbook illustrates the problem of male erectile disorder with the case of Bill.
   a. Males typically feel more impaired by arousal disorders than females; though it is unusual for a man to be completely unable to achieve an erection.
   b. The prevalence of erectile dysfunction is about 5% in males between 18-59 years of age and the problem increases with age. Erectile disorder is the most common problem for which men seek help.
   c. Prevalence of female arousal disorders is hard to estimate as many women do not consider absence of arousal to be a problem, but it is estimated that 14% of women experience arousal disorder.

D. Orgasm disorders

1. **Inhibited orgasm** (female and male orgasmic disorder) is an inability to achieve orgasm despite adequate sexual desire and arousal. This disorder is rarely seen in men, although **retarded ejaculation** may occur. Males may also exhibit **retrograde ejaculation**, where ejaculatory fluids travel backwards into the bladder.
   a. Inhibited orgasm is the most common complaint of women who seek therapy for sexual problems, as approximately 25% of women report significant difficulty reaching orgasm and only 50% report experiencing regular orgasms during sexual intercourse.
   b. For the disorder, the female must indicate that orgasm *never or almost never* occurs, including distress over the problem. The textbook illustrates inhibited orgasm with the cases of Greta and Will.

2. **Premature ejaculation** is ejaculation occurring well before the man or partner wishes it to. Frequency of premature ejaculation is high, with 21% of all men meeting criteria for premature ejaculation making it the most frequent male sexual dysfunction. It is difficult to define "premature," as adequate time before ejaculation varies widely.
   a. Surveys indicate that many with this problem climax 1 to 2 minutes after penetration, whereas the climax occurs on average between 7 and 10 minutes in persons without this problem.
   b. Perceived lack of control over orgasm is a core psychological dimension of this problem in males.
   c. Premature ejaculation occurs mostly in young, sexually inexperienced men and the problem declines with age. The textbook illustrates premature ejaculation with the case of Gary.

E. Sexual pain disorders involve marked pain during intercourse.

1. **Dyspareunia** (meaning unhappily mated as bedfellows) refers to pain during intercourse in the context of sexual desire and an ability to attain arousal and orgasm. Dyspareunia is diagnosed only if no medical reasons for pain can be found. This condition is rarely seen in clinics, with estimates ranging from 1% to 5% of men and about 10% to 15% of women.
2. **Vaginismus** is more common than dyspareunia and is a female condition whereby the outer third of the vagina undergoes involuntary spasms when intercourse is attempted, and may occur during gynecological exams or when attempting to insert a tampon.
   a. Common sensations include ripping, burning, or tearing during intercourse.
   b. Best estimates suggest that over 5% of women who seek treatment in the United States suffer from this condition, with higher rates in more conservative countries such as Ireland (as high as 42% to 55% of cases). The textbook illustrates vaginismus with the case of Jill.

IV. Assessing Sexual Behavior

A. Sexual behavior is often assessed via interview, medical evaluation, and psychophysiological assessment.

1. During the **interview**, clinicians must demonstrate comfort talking about sexual issues in a language the client can understand. Interview questions may include the following: one's current and past interest in sex, extent of sexual fantasies, frequency of masturbation and sexual intercourse, history of abuse, rape, or negative sexual experiences, problems with erection or orgasm, and pain during intercourse, to name a few. Questionnaires also may be used to supplement interview information.
2. **Medical examinations** are often routine so as to rule out medical causes of sexual dysfunction. Several drugs (e.g., those prescribed for hypertension, anxiety, depression) can disrupt sexual functioning, and so can surgery, hormonal levels, and adequate vascular functioning. Urologists or gynecologists often conduct such evaluations.

3. **Psychophysiological assessment** is used to assess the ability of individuals to become sexually aroused to sexual stimuli while awake, and general arousal while asleep. Most often this form of assessment involves watching erotic videotape or listening to erotic audiotape, while physiological and subjective measures of arousal are assessed. REM sleep in males is associated with erections, and thus **nocturnal penile tumescence (NPT)** is assessed directly, often with a snap gauge (a noninvasive ring that fits around the penis and breaks during erections).
   a. In men, a **penile strain gauge** is used to measure extent of erection via blood flow. Extent to penile rigidity is also assessed.
   b. For women, a **vaginal photoplethysmograh** is inserted by the woman into her vagina, and photo sensors detect blood flow around the vaginal walls during sexual arousal.

V. Causes and Treatment of Sexual Dysfunction
   A. Causes of sexual dysfunction
      1. **Biological contributions** are important to consider as a number of physical and medical conditions can contribute to sexual dysfunction. Examples include neurological diseases, diabetes, kidney disease, vascular disease (particularly arterial insufficiency and venous leakage), and chronic illness (e.g., heart disease).
         a. **Prescription medications** are a major cause of sexual dysfunction (i.e., they interfere with sexual desire and arousal in males and females), particularly antihypertensive medications (e.g., beta blockers, including propranolol), tricyclics, and other antidepressant and anti-anxiety drugs.
         b. Sexual dysfunction is the most widespread side effect of SSRIs, specifically low desire and arousal difficulties.
         c. **Alcohol and other drugs of abuse** (e.g., cocaine, heroin) also can produce widespread sexual dysfunction in users and abusers. **Disinhibition** from alcohol may promote the myth that alcohol facilitates sexual arousal and behavior, but alcohol is a nervous system suppressant. Chronic alcohol use may also lead to neurological, liver, and testicular damage as well as fertility problems.
      2. Historically, **psychological contributions** wrongly focused on anxiety as the main cause of sexual dysfunction. We know that anxiety may increase sexual arousal in certain circumstances such as contingent shock and threat to life. Instead, the critical factor appears to be **distraction**, as this factor interferes with the process of sexual arousal. Two other factors also seem important:
         a. Men and women with sexual dysfunction consistently underestimate their sexual arousal. Normally functioning men show increased sexual arousal during performance demand situations, experience positive affect, are distracted by nonsexual stimuli, and have a good idea of how aroused they are. Men with sexual problems show decreased arousal during performance demand, experience negative affect, are not

distracted by nonsexual stimuli, and are inaccurate with regard to their arousal.

b. **Performance anxiety** has several components: arousal, cognitive processes, and negative affect. Each component feeds on the others in sexual dysfunctions in a vicious positive feedback loop.
   i. **Cognitively**, those with sexual dysfunctions expect the worst and experience sexual situations as negative and unpleasant. They also avoid becoming aware of sexual cues, tend to distract themselves with negative thoughts.
   ii. **Physiologically**, those with sexual dysfunctions underestimate their arousal.
   iii. **Emotionally**, persons with sexual dysfunctions tend to experience sexual situations more negatively and experience negative emotion in the process.

3. **Social and cultural contributions** are important because sexual behavior may result from learning that sexuality is negative and somewhat threatening; a negative set termed **erotophobia**. Erotophobia is believed to be learned in early childhood from families, religious authorities, and others, and seems to predict sexual difficulties later in life. Sexual cues therefore become associated with negative affect. Other social factors may include negative or traumatic sexual experiences that, in turn, appear to make females more likely to develop orgasmic dysfunction later in life. Male victims of early sexual victimization are 3.5 times more likely to report erectile dysfunction than those without such histories. Other factors include:
   a. Marked deterioration in **close interpersonal relationships**, including poor communication and sexual skills.
   b. According to the **script theory of sexual functioning**, persons are guided by scripts reflecting social and cultural expectations. For example, a person with the script that sexuality is potentially dangerous, dirty, or forbidden is more vulnerable to sexual dysfunction later in life. This attitude is evidenced in cultures and religious groups with restrictive attitudes toward sex.
4. A **combination of psychological and physical causes** is usually present in those who develop sexual dysfunctions. For example, socially transmitted negative attitudes about sex may interact with relationship difficulties and predispose one toward performance anxiety and sexual dysfunction. Specific biological predispositions likely play an important role as well.

B. Treatment of sexual dysfunction
   1. Psychosocial treatments
      a. **Education** is a surprisingly simple and effective treatment for a large number of persons who experience sexual dysfunction. The textbook illustrates the role of education about sexual functioning with the case of Carl.
      b. **Masters and Johnson's** treatment approach involves a male and female therapist to intensively facilitate communication in a

dysfunctional couple. Therapy is conducted daily over a two-week period. The program includes the following components:

   i. Basic **education** about sexual functioning, including altering myths, and fostering increased communication between partners.
   ii. The primary goal is to eliminate performance anxiety. This is accomplished by using **sensate focus** and **nondemand pleasuring**, involving exploration of each other's body without intercourse or genital contact. After this phase, the couple moves to genital pleasuring, but with a ban on orgasm and intercourse. Following this, arousal should be established and intercourse may be attempted in parts.
   iii. Subsequent research indicated that one therapist is equally effective as having two therapists, though the results have been difficult to replicate.

c. Most therapies for sexual dysfunction integrate specific procedures in the context of general sex therapy. Examples are as follows:
   i. The **squeeze technique** is often used for persons with premature ejaculation and involves establishing a firm erection and then having the partner squeeze the penis near the top to quickly reduce arousal.
   ii. Lifelong female orgasmic disorder may be treated with explicit training in **masturbatory training procedures**.
   iii. To treat vaginismus, a woman and then a man gradually insert larger and larger dilators into the woman's vagina at the woman's own pace. Penile insertion is then attempted.
   iv. Low sexual desire is treated with standard reeducation and communication procedures involved in sex therapy, with masturbatory training and introduction of erotic material.

2. Medical treatments
   a. Most medical treatments should be combined with psychosocial interventions for optimal effectiveness.
   b. Most medications are designed for male erectile dysfunction, the most popular of which is **Sildenafil** (tradename **Viagra**). Though about 50% to 80% of men with erectile dysfunction benefit from Viagra, 30% or more suffer severe headaches as a side effect, particularly at high doses and reports of sexual satisfaction are not optimal. Cost is about $10 a pill and it is widely prescribed. Use of Viagra for post-menopausal women is disappointing. Yohimbine and testosterone do little to help erectile dysfunction.
   c. Patients may also be taught to inject **vasodilating drugs** (papaverine or prostaglandin) into the penis to produce an erection when they want to have intercourse. These drugs dilate blood vessels, increase blood flow to the penis, and work within 15 minutes. This procedure is somewhat painful, and 50% to 60% of men stop using this treatment after a short

time, with side effects including bruising and development of fibrosis nodules in the penis.

d. Insertion of **penile prostheses** or implants has been a surgical option for male erectile disorder for about 100 years. Prostheses include silicone rods and inflatable cylinders. The newest model of penile prosthetic device is an inflatable rod that contains a pumping device. Surgical implants fall short of restoring pre-surgical sexual functioning or assuring satisfaction in most patients and are used if other treatments fail. **Vascular surgery** may also be done to correct arterial or venous malfunctions.

e. **Vacuum device therapy** works by creating a vacuum in a cylinder that is placed over the penis. The vacuum draws blood into the penis and the blood is thereby trapped by a specially designed ring placed at the base of the penis. About 70% to 100% of users report satisfactory erections.

VI. Paraphilia: Clinical Descriptions

A. **Paraphilias** refer to unusual sexual attractions to inappropriate people such as children or objects such as clothing. As with sexual dysfunctions, it is unusual for an individual to have just one paraphilic pattern of sexual arousal, and it is not uncommon for individuals with paraphilia to suffer from comorbid mood, anxiety, or substance abuse disorders. Some paraphilias are common (e.g., transvestic fetishism) and most are seen more often in males compared to females.

1. **Fetishism** refers to sexual attraction to nonliving objects, usually those that are inanimate or provide a source of specific tactile stimulation. Fetishistic arousal, fantasy, urges, and desires are focused on the object. **Partialism** refers to another source of arousal related to a part of the body, such as the foot, buttocks, or hair; however this attraction is no longer technically classified as a fetish because distinguishing it from more normal patterns of arousal is often difficult.
2. **Voyeurism** is the practice of observing an unsuspecting individual undressing or naked in order to become aroused.
3. **Exhibitionism** refers to sexual arousal and gratification by exposing one's genitals to unsuspecting strangers. The textbook illustrates exhibitionism with the case of Robert and The Lawyer. The thrilling element of risk is an important part of exhibitionism.
4. In **transvestic fetishism**, sexual arousal is strongly associated with the act of dressing in clothes of the opposite sex, or cross-dressing. The textbook illustrates transvestic fetishism with the case of Mr. M. It is not unusual for males who are strongly inclined to dress in female clothes to compensate by associating with macho organizations (e.g., police, fire fighters, paramilitary organizations); though most individuals with this disorder do not show compensatory behaviors. Many wives accept the cross-dressing behavior and many males with this disorder are married.
5. **Sexual sadism and masochism** are associated with either inflicting pain or humiliation (i.e., sadism) or suffering pain and humiliation (i.e., masochism).

a. **Sadistic rape** is different than rape as a crime, in that most rapists do not show patterns of arousal that are paraphilic and many rapists meet criteria for antisocial personality disorder, including engaging in several antisocial and aggressive acts.
b. Some rapists do fit the definitions of paraphilia and are best described as sadists. Non-rapists show normal patterns of arousal to mutually consenting intercourse, but not intercourse involving force. Rapists, however, become aroused to both types of material, and more so with violent sexual and nonsexual material.

6. Persons with **pedophilia** are sexually attracted to children or very young adolescents, whereas attraction to family members who are children is called **incest**. In both cases, the pattern of arousal may include male and/or female children. Victims of pedophilia tend to be young children, and victims of incest tend to be young girls who are beginning to mature physically.
   a. Incestuous males are more aroused to adult women than are males with pedophilia, with the later focusing almost exclusively on children. The textbook illustrates incest with the case of Tony.
   b. Most child molesters are not physically abusive to their victims and often rationalize their behavior as loving the child or teaching the child useful lessons about sexuality. Child molesters almost never consider the psychological damage the victim suffers, including their power over children.
   c. Individuals with pedophilia often rationalize their behavior by engaging in other practices that they consider morally correct or uplifting (e.g., highly religious).
7. Other paraphilias include **telephone scatologia**, or compulsively making obscene telephone calls. **Frotteurism** refers to sexual arousal and gratification through rubbing the body parts on unsuspecting strangers (usually in crowded areas).

B. Paraphilia in women
1. Paraphilia is rarely seen in women, and was thought to be totally absent in women, except for sadomasochistic tendencies. However, in recent years, several cases of pedophilia, exhibitionism, and sadomasochism have been reported in women.

C. Causes of paraphilia are complex and include the following dimensions:
1. Deviant patterns of sexual arousal often occur in the context of other **sexual and social problems**. For example, undesired sexual arousal may be associated with deficiencies in levels of desired arousal with adults.
2. In addition, people with paraphilias may **lack the social skills** needed for meeting and dating persons of the opposite sex; though others also lack such skills and do not engage in paraphilic behavior.
3. **Early sexual experiences and fantasies** seem to play a large etiological role. For example, association of arousal and fantasies over unusual or inappropriate objects may be reinforced via an association with sexual

pleasure via masturbation. In some cases, however, sexual scripts may override these learning processes.

4. Persons with paraphilias display **strong sexual drives** that may produce obsessive-compulsive-like behavior. Acts of suppressing such thoughts and urges may paradoxically results in their greater frequency and urgency, leading the person to act on them in a vicious cycle.

VII. Assessment and Treatment of Paraphilia

A. The assessment of paraphilia often involves psychophysiological procedures to determine patterns of normal and deviate sexual arousal. Important variables to evaluate include the presence of deviant arousal, level of desired arousal to adults, social skills, and the ability to form relationships.

B. Most **psychosocial treatments** for decreasing unwanted sexual arousal are behavioral, and focus on changing associations and contexts from arousing to neutral with regard to unusual or inappropriate sexual objects.

1. **Covert sensitization** is a procedure carried out entirely in the imagination of the patient and involves associating sexually arousing images with the very negative consequences that often bring the patient to therapy in the first place. The textbook returns to the previous case of Tony to illustrate covert sensitization.
2. Many persons with paraphilias require **family/marital therapy** to address deficits and problems in interpersonal relationships.
3. **Orgasmic reconditioning** involves instructing patients to masturbate to their usual fantasies but to substitute more desirable and appropriate fantasy and imagery just before ejaculation or orgasm. Over time, the appropriate fantasy is started earlier in the process.
4. **Coping and relapse prevention** are often important components of treatment, wherein patients are taught to recognize early signs of temptation and to institute one of a number of self-control procedures before their urges become too strong.

C. When implemented by an experienced professional, treatment success using the above psychosocial procedures is 70 to 100%.

1. Men who rape have the lowest success rate among all offenders with a single diagnosis, and individuals with multiple paraphilias have the lowest success rate of any group.
2. The best predictors of treatment failure are a history of unstable social relationships, an unstable employment history, strong denial that a problem exists, a history of multiple victims, and a situation where the offender continues to live with the victim.
3. In general, the recidivism rate is high for persons who commit sexual offenses but do not receive treatment, and most pedophilias run a chronic course with high rates of recurrence.

D. **Drugs** may also be used to treat persons with paraphilia, particularly dangerous sexual offenders who do not respond to alternative treatments, or those in need for a means of temporarily suppressing sexual arousal

1. The most popular drug to treat paraphilias is an **anti-androgen** called **cyproterone acetate**. This drug eliminates sexual desire and fantasy by reducing testosterone levels dramatically; the equivalent of chemical castration. Relapse rates are high following medication discontinuation.
2. A second drug, **medroxyprogesterone acetate** (i.e., **Depo-Provera** in injectable form) also reduces testosterone. Relapse rates are high following medication discontinuation.
3. Triptoretin, is a newer drug that functions much like chemical castration in reducing fantasy and desire by inhibiting gonadotropin secretion in men. This drug is somewhat more effective with long-standing paraphilias than the other drugs mentioned above and includes fewer side effects.

OVERALL SUMMARY

This chapter outlines the primary features of sexual and gender identity disorders, including information regarding normal and deviate sexual behavior and attitudes. Gender identity disorders, sexual dysfunctions, and paraphilias are described, with an emphasis on clinical description, information about known causes, and assessment and treatment approaches (i.e., medical and psychosocial).

KEY TERMS

Covert sensitization (p. 371)
Dyspareunia (p. 353)
Exhibitionism (p. 365)
Female sexual arousal disorder (p. 349)
Female orgasmic disorder (p. 351)
Fetishism (p. 364)
Gender identity disorders (p. 342)
Heterosexual sex (p. 338)
Homosexual sex (p. 338)
Hypoactive sexual desire disorder (p. 348)
Incest (p. 368)
Inhibited orgasm (p. 351)
Male erectile disorder (p. 349)
Male orgasmic disorder (p. 352)
Orgasmic reconditioning (p. 372)
Paraphilias (p. 364)
Pedophilia (p. 368)
Premature ejaculation (p. 352)
Relapse prevention (p. 372)
Sex reassignment surgery (p. 345)
Sexual aversion disorder (p. 349)

Sexual dysfunction (p. 346)
Sexual masochism (p. 366)
Sexual pain disorders (p. 353)
Sexual sadism (p. 366)
Transvestic fetishism (p. 365)
Vaginismus (p. 353)
Voyeurism (p. 365)

INFOTRAC KEY TERM EXERCISES

Each exercise is linked to key terms from the Wadsworth InfoTrac on-line searchable database. Key terms must be entered exactly as written.

Exercise 1: Is Pedophilia a Mental Disorder?
Article: A94690092
Citation: (Is pedophilia a mental disorder?). Richard Green.
Archives of Sexual Behavior, Dec 2002 v31 i6 p467(5)

The DSM-IV considers pedophilia a psychiatric disorder. Yet, it is also a criminal act. This InfoTrac article takes issue with the notion that pedophilia constitutes a psychiatric disorder. Read the article and then answer the following questions: (a) what cross-cultural factors challenge the argument that pedophilia is a psychiatric disorder?, (b) do personality and patterns of adult-child attraction clearly discriminate pedophiles from nonpedophiles, and (c) in light of what you read on this topic in the textbook, how would you respond to the author's argument. Should pedophilia remain in the DSM-IV-TR, or should it be removed much like homosexuality was removed from the DSM not long ago? Limit your answer to 3-5 typed double-spaced pages.

Exercise 2: Why is Sex Not Good Unless it Hurts?: Understanding Sexual Masochism
Key Term: *Sexual Masochism*

Sexual masochism is a paraphilic disorder that involves an experience of pain or humiliation for sexual arousal. This feature alone is somewhat counterintuitive to what we normally think about sexual activity; namely as a completely pleasurable experience. Your task here is to learn about causes and prevalence of this form of sexual activity. When is masochism a disorder? What causes masochism (saying a sadist is not a good answer)? Is pain and humiliation just fun and games, or is it real and does it hurt? And, what suggestions would you offer for persons seeking treatment for this problem? Review the InfoTrac article(s) on this topic and prepare a 3-5 page response.

Exercise 3: The Nature of Sexual Fantasies and Sexual Functioning in Males and Females
Key Term: *Sexual Fantasies*

Sexual fantasy is part of normal and deviant sexual behavior. Yet, sexual fantasy is also often a very private matter that is rarely discussed openly between consenting partners. For this reason, little is known about the nature of the content of sexual fantasy in normal sexual behavior, including information regarding gender differences in sexual fantasy. Your task here is to review the InfoTrac article(s) on this topic and to summarize what is known about the role of sexual fantasy in sexual behavior, including differences (if any) between males and females with regard to the content and extent of sexual fantasy. In your answer, address whether open discussion about sexual fantasy between consenting partners should (or should not) be encouraged and why? Limit your answer to 3-5 typed double-spaced pages.

Exercise 4 (Future Trend): Internet Pornography – A Disorder in the Making?

At suburban Riverdale Public School in New Jersey, a visitor recently posed a question to an eighth-grade class: "Have you seen Internet pornography?" All 42 students raised their hands. According to a study by the Henry J. Kaiser Family Foundation, 70 percent of the nation's 15-to 17-year-olds have looked at Internet pornography, much of it graphically hardcore. Most college students will likely have similarly viewed internet pornography, some quite deliberately and regularly. Some of your students may even feel that they cannot stop doing so. The terms "cyber-compulsive" and "cybersex compulsivity" have been used to describe this tendency and refer to a person who cannot control their use of online pornography. The availability of internet pornography raises a host of issues related to sexuality and mental health. Some individuals, for instance, appear to obsessively and compulsively seek out cybersex, thus raising issues as to whether such behavior constitutes a disorder (e.g., Internet Addiction Disorder – Pornography Type). How viewing pornography affects development of healthy sexuality remains unclear. Some see it as potentially harmful. The range of possible topics for discussion here is large. Students will likely have a range of opinions about whether viewing porn on the internet can be viewed as a psychological disorder. The links below are some good starting points.

http://www.contentwatch.com/learn_center/article.php?id=101
http://allpsych.com/journal/internetaddiction.html
http://www.mentalhelp.net/books/books.php?id=1032&type=de
http://www.studentbmj.com/back_issues/1099/editorials/351.html
http://www.rpi.edu/~anderk4/research.html
http://www.psychiatrictimes.com/p980852.html

CLASSROOM ACTIVITIES, DEMONSTRATIONS, AND LECTURE TOPICS

1. **Activity: Defining Normal Sexual Behavior.** Kite (1990) has developed a classroom exercise that requires students to label specific examples of sexual behaviors either normal or abnormal. Students can work in groups or individually; upon completion of the exercise, you can tabulate the results on the chalkboard or overhead. Ask students if they experienced any difficulty labeling certain behaviors as normal or abnormal. What ultimately influenced their decisions?

   Source Information. Kite, M. E. (1990). Defining normal sexual behavior: A classroom exercise. Teaching of Psychology, 17, 118-119.

2. **Activity: "Normal" Sexual Behavior Case Studies.** To explore definitions of "normal" sexual behavior, you can read or distribute case studies and ask your students to evaluate the behavior. The students may want to work in small discussion groups and then present their group's ideas to the class. Some examples of cases could include:

a. Mr. Jones is a 72-year-old man. He lost his first wife four years ago, but recently began dating another woman. He is concerned because he is "only able to have sex twice a week" and is seeking an intervention that will enhance his sexual performance.
b. Kenny is a 14-year-old boy. Recently, he and his best friend, Rob, have begun mutually masturbating together after school.
c. Sarah is a 28-year-old female. She has been married for 5 years, but has never had an orgasm with her husband. She reports that she is not concerned about not having an orgasm because she finds the sexual contact with her husband pleasurable in other ways.
d. Pat and Jan have been in a monogamous relationship for 8 years. They usually have sex with each other once a week. During their sex, Pat enjoys slapping Jan in the face and Jan enjoys being slapped.

3. **Activity: Quick Classroom Poll.** Ask students for a show of hands in response to the following question: "How many of you ever had diarrhea when you were a teenager?" Most of the class will usually raise their hands fairly quickly. Then ask, "How many of you ever masturbated when you were a teenager?" Note the usual reluctance of hand-raising. Discuss the class response to both questions in the context of why we would rather admit to having experienced a rather awful illness than to having experienced an almost universal healthy sexual experience.

4. **Activity: Student Reflections on Sexual Dysfunctions.** In small groups, ask students to select the sexual difficulties they consider to be the three worst ones to experience. Have them include their reasons for their choices. Share group choices looking for similarities and differences. Can the groups or class agree on the top three worst sexual problems to have, or are there enough differences to make this task impossible? This exercise is useful as a way to show how sexual problems are often idiosyncratic.

5. **Activity: Invite a Sex Therapist as a Guest Speaker.** Obviously, a sex therapist would be a great speaker for this topic. Students could be asked to write anonymous questions or problems they have experienced a week prior to this class. Such questions could then be given to the sex therapist and the therapist could respond to some of them in a generic fashion. Note that students should be informed that the goal is to have the sex therapist respond to real issues, and that participation is voluntary (though all information will be completely anonymous).

6. **Video Activity: Complexity of Sexual Dysfunction – The Case of Clark.** Present the video segment from Abnormal Psychology, Inside/Out Video 1, Vol 1, depicting a client named Clark. Clark suffers from hypoactive sexual desire disorder and male erectile disorder. Ask the students to identify psychological and physical causes of his sexual dysfunctions and their interaction. Have the students offer ideas about what problems they might address with Clark in therapy and in what order.

SUPPLEMENTARY READING MATERIAL FOR CHAPTER TEN

(= These sources can be found on "*Infotrac, the online library*" provided by Wadsworth and Brooks/Cole Publishing.)

Arndt, W. B. (1991). Gender disorders and the paraphilias. Madison, CT: International Universities Press.

Bem, D. J. (2000). Exotic becomes erotic: Interpreting the biological correlates of sexual orientation. Archives of Sexual Behavior, 29, 531.

Davis, C. M., Yarber, W. L., & Davis, S. L. (Eds.) (1988). Sexuality-related measures: A compendium. Lake Mills, IA: Graphic Publishing.

Docter, R. F., & Prince, V. (1997). Transvestism: A survey of 1032 cross-dressers. Archives of Sexual Behavior, 26, 589(17).

McCarthy, B. W. (1988). Male sexual awareness. New York: Caroll and Graf.

McConaghy, N. (1999). Unresolved issues in scientific sexology. Archives of Sexual Behavior, 28, 285.

Rosen, R. C., & Leiblum, S. R. (Eds.) (1992). Erectile disorders: Assessment and treatment. New York: Guilford.

Rowland, D. L., Cooper, S. E., & Schneider. M. (2001). Defining premature ejaculation for experimental and clinical investigations. Archives of Sexual Behavior, 30, 235.

Simons, J. S., Carey, M. P. (2001). Prevalence of sexual dysfunctions: Results from a decade of research. Archives of Sexual Behavior, v30, p177.

Slijper, F. M. E., Drop, S. L. S., Molenaar, J. C., & de Muinck Keizer-Schrama, S. M. P. F. (1998). Long-term psychological evaluation of intersex children. Archives of Sexual Behavior, 27, 125(20).

Wilson, G. D. (1987). Variant sexuality: Research and theory. Baltimore, MD: Johns Hopkins University Press.

Wincze, J. P., & Carey, M. P. (1991). Sexual dysfunction: A guide for assessment and treatment. New York: Guilford.

SUPPLEMENTARY 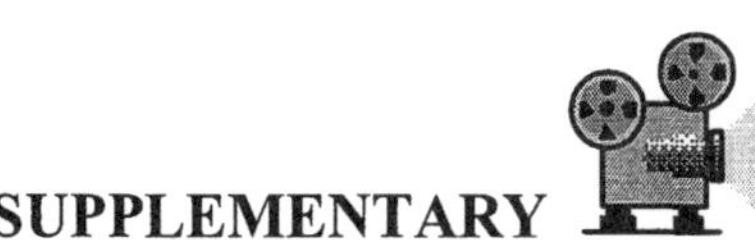 VIDEO RESOURCES FOR CHAPTER TEN

Abnormal psychology inside/out, video 1, vol 1. (*available through your International Thomson Learning representative).* Clark, a male with hypoactive sexual desire disorder and male erectile disorder, is presented. This is an interesting case of a mix of psychological as well as physical causes producing a sexual dysfunction. (15 min)

Abnormal psychology inside/out, vol 2. (*available through your International Thomson Learning representative).* The segment on "Gender Identity Disorder" presents an interview with a woman (who was previously a man), where she describes the process of changing genders, how it felt being raised as a boy as a child, and her difficulties with family, relationships, and rejection. (5 min)

A second related segment, titled "Being Accepted As A Woman," the previous client talks about what it was like living as a woman for one year prior her sex reassignment surgery and her feelings of awkwardness during that transition year. (2 min)

As time goes by. (Fanlight Productions, 1-800-937-4113). Humans are sexual until the very end. The seniors profiled in this video openly share their experiences with love, romance and growing old. (23 min)

Cabaret. (Hollywood Film; Musical/Drama/Dance). This film is about sadomasochism, bisexuality, and the relationship between sex and power.

Claire's knee. (Hollywood Film; Drama). This film depicts a middle-aged man who becomes obsessed with a young girl's knee.

CNN today: Abnormal psychology, vol. 1. (*available through your International Thomson Learning representative).* The segment titled "Sexual and Gender Identity Disorders: Viagra Failures," discusses Viagra and how it does not work with everyone, including other treatment alternatives. (1:87 min)

Fetishes. (Hollywood Film; Documentary). Examines the clients of Pandora's box; an elite club in New York City that caters to the sexual fetishes of clients.

Gender and relationships. (Insight Media: 2162 Broadway, New York, NY 10024/ (800)-233-9910). Explaining why human emotional interactions and attachments are so complex, this video stresses that even the most respected authorities remain uncertain about which factors influence people's feelings of love, affection, and sexual attraction. It examines some of the most beguiling mysteries of the ages: What is love? What makes sexual behavior "normal" or "abnormal"? Do men and women differ in their sexual motives and behavior? (30 min)

Human sexuality (it's personal). (Insight Media: 2162 Broadway, New York, NY 10024/ (800)-233-9910). Sexuality is an integral part of human identity and a primary factor in human behavior. This video explores the development of sexual behavior and considers the range of sexual experience and preference that exists within contemporary human society. It also examines whether fear of the AIDS virus and other sexually transmitted diseases has altered patterns of sexual behavior. (28 min)

Love and death in America: Sexual revolution/AIDS. (Insight Media: 2162 Broadway, New York, NY 10024/ (800)-233-9910). This video tours three decades of shifting American attitudes toward sex. It explores the 1960's break with inhibitions traceable to the nation's Puritan origins, examines the impact of the birth control pill, and discusses the chaos of behavioral codes that followed the advent of AIDS. (50 min)

Pulp fiction. (Hollywood Film; Drama). This film depicts an underworld sadomasochistic den run by two sexual sadists.

Sex, lies, and videotape. (Hollywood Film; Drama). This film depicts an impotent young man who can achieve orgasm only by masturbating while watching videotapes of women whom he has persuaded to share their most intimate details.

Sexual abuse of children: Victims and abusers. (Insight Media: 2162 Broadway, New York, NY 10024/ (800)-233-9910). Featuring candid interviews with therapists, victims, and recovering offenders, this video explores the devastating long-term effects of physical, emotional, and/or sexual abuse on children. (28 min)

The adjuster. (Hollywood Film; Drama). This Canadian film explores voyeurism and exhibitionism.

The crying game. (Hollywood Film; Drama). This film explores homosexuality, transsexualism, interracial sexuality, and the ability of human beings to love one another in the context of an asexual relationship.

The sex history. (Insight Media: 2162 Broadway, New York, NY 10024/ (800)-233-9910). Wardell Pomeroy, co-author of the Kinsey Report, demonstrates his style of taking a sex history, which he developed through taking 35,000 sex histories. Working with two resistant adults, he explains how to gather data, elicit information about sensitive topics, and build a positive rapport. He emphasizes the importance of using clear language, avoiding euphemisms, and being supportive. (60 min)

Transgender revolution. (Insight Media: 2162 Broadway, New York, NY 10024/ (800)-233-9910). This video explores the growing subculture of transsexuality. It interviews both the founder of the transsexual political organization GenderPAC and a neurosurgeon who specializes in sex change operations, and follows the surgical transformation of a man into a woman. (50 min)

Unusual sexual behavior. (Insight Media: 2162 Broadway, New York, NY 10024/ (800)-233-9910). This training video features simulated interviews with six different clients. The clients portrayed include a man who is sexually interested in young boys, a couple whose marriage is threatened because the husband (a transvestite) has decided to "come out," and a man who has an unusual sexual fetish. (66 min)

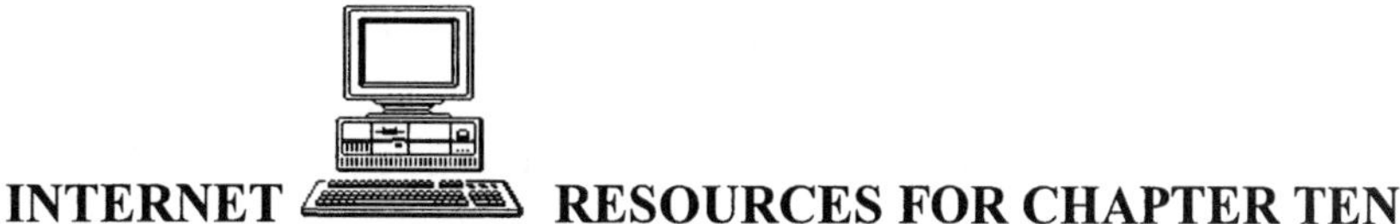

INTERNET RESOURCES FOR CHAPTER TEN

DSM-IV-TR Diagnostic Information
http://www.behavenet.com/

Contains diagnostic criteria for just about all DSM-IV-TR disorders.

HisandHerHealth
http://www.hisandherhealth.com/

Is a highly-credentialed, HON-registered site providing medical information and articles on the causes and treatments of male and female sexual dysfunction, prostate, incontinence, fertility and related issues. The site includes videos, moderated chat rooms, bulletin board, and scheduled chats with a doctor.

Impotence
http://hstat.nlm.nih.gov/hq/Hquest/screen/HquestHome/s/59699

An elaborate description of impotence provided by the National Institutes of Health. Type in the search word "impotence."

Kinsey Institute for Research in Sex, Gender, and Reproduction, Inc.
http://www.indiana.edu/~kinsey/

This is an excellent research website, that includes links to current research publications.

Masters and Johnson
http://www.mastersandjohnson.com/

The web site of Masters and Johnson. Not particularly useful, but informative as to their current research and treatment interests.

Sexual Disorders and Dysfunctions
http://sexuality.about.com/cs/sexualdisorders/index.htm

This is an About.com megasite with links to a variety of topics related to sexual behavior and sexual dysfunctions.

Sexual Health.Com
http://www.sexualhealth.com/

This web site provides useful resources regarding health and sexual behavior, including links to current research and news about available treatments.

Society for the Scientific Study of Sexuality
http://www.ssc.wisc.edu/ssss/

An international organization dedicated to the advancement of knowledge about sexuality. It is the oldest organization of professionals interested in the study of sexuality in the

U.S. This site details the importance of both production of quality research and the clinical educational, and social applications of research related to all aspects of sexuality.

The American Association of Sex Educators, Counselors and Therapists (AASECT)
http://www.aasect.org/

A not-for-profit, interdisciplinary professional organization dedicated to promoting understanding of human sexuality and healthy sexual behavior.

WARNING SIGNS OF SEXUAL DYSFUNCTION

- Occur in women more often than in men
- Often occurs after the age of 30 but may occur prior to that age
- Painful intercourse is a sign of sexual dysfunction
- Old age increases the chance of sexual dysfunction
- May occur in conjunction with cardiovascular disease, depression, diabetes, and general poor health especially in erectile failure
- Alcohol abuse and medications serve as predictors of sexual dysfunction
- Estrogen deprivation especially in postmenopausal women
- Sexual abuse especially before puberty is a significant risk factor for sexual dysfunction
- Emotional or stress-related problems
- Decreased libido
- Delay or absence of an orgasm is a sign of sexual dysfunction
- Inability to attain or maintain vaginal lubrication and swelling response in women
- Inability to attain or maintain an erection in males
- Loss of interest in sexual activity

WARNING SIGNS OF SEXUAL AVERSION DISORDER

- Occurs equally among men and women
- May develop anytime during or after puberty
- Stress, hormonal imbalance, or fatigue
- Emotional distress, ranging from moderate anxiety to strong disgust or fear
- Difficulty in attaining or maintaining intimate relationships
- Devoting excessive energy to other activities such as work or travel
- Neglecting personal hygiene and appearance
- Going to bed unusually early
- Prior traumatic or negative sexual experiences
- Experience of anger, fear, guilt
- Communication problems, lack of affection, power struggles and conflicts, and lack of time together are risk factors
- Lack of feelings of emotional attachment to one's partner

WARNING SIGNS OF DYSPAREUNIA

- More common in females than in males
- May occur any time after puberty
- Not uncommon after menopause in females
- Inadequate lubrication in females
- Lack of sexual arousal and lack of effective stimulation
- Past history of sexual trauma
- Feelings of guilt, or negative attitudes towards sex
- Low estrogen levels
- In men recent reduction in the frequency of sex
- Inadequate foreplay
- Significant pain or discomfort during or after sexual intercourse
- Vaginal spasms in women
- Aggressive or inpatient partner

WARNING SIGNS OF PEDOPHILIA

- Vast majority are males and heterosexual
- Sexual urges geared towards prepubescent child
- Recurrent, intense sexually arousing fantasies with prepubescent chil
- Record of prior sexual conviction
- Lack of intimate partners
- Never being married is a risk factor for pedophilia
- Poor relationship with own mother
- Overly touchy and affectionate with kids
- Being alone with children a lot
- Being a victim of child abuse at a younger age
- Excessive use or abuse of alcohol
- Often accompanied with low self-esteem
- Repeated lying

DSM-IV-TR Criteria for Gender Identity Disorder

A. A strong and persistent cross-gender identification (not merely a desire for any perceived cultural advantages of being the other sex). In children, the disturbance is manifested by four (or more) of the following:

1. repeatedly stated desire to be, or insistence that he or she is, the other sex
2. in boys, preference for cross-dressing or simulating female attire; in girls, insistence on wearing only stereotypical masculine clothing
3. strong and persistent preferences for cross-sex roles in make-believe play or persistent fantasies of being the other sex
4. intense desire to participate in the stereotypical games and pastimes of the other sex
5. strong preference for playmates of the other sex. In adolescents and adults, the disturbance is manifested by symptoms such as a stated desire to be the other sex, frequent passing as the other sex, desire to live or be treated as the other sex, or the conviction that he or she has the typical feelings and reactions of the other sex.

B. Persistent discomfort with his or her sex or sense of inappropriateness in the gender role of that sex. In children, the disturbance is manifested by any of the following: in boys, assertion that his penis or testes are disgusting or will disappear or assertion that it would be better not to have a penis, or aversion toward rough-and-tumble play and rejection of male stereotypical toys, games, and activities; in girls, rejection of urinating in a sitting position, assertion that she has or will grow a penis, or assertion that she does not want to grow breasts or menstruate, or marked aversion toward normative feminine clothing. In adolescents and adults, the disturbance is manifested by symptoms such as preoccupation with getting rid of primary and secondary sex characteristics (e.g., request for hormones, surgery, or other procedures to physically alter sexual characteristics to simulate the other sex) or belief that he or she was born the wrong sex.

C. The disturbance is not concurrent with a physical intersex condition.

D. The disturbance causes clinically significant distress or impairment in social, occupational, or other important areas of functioning.

Specify if (for sexually mature individuals):

Sexually Attracted to Males, **Sexually Attracted to Females**
Sexually Attracted to Both, or **Sexually Attracted to Neither**

DSM-IV-TR Criteria for Hypoactive Sexual Desire Disorde

A. Persistently or recurrently deficient (or absent) sexual fantasies and desire for sexual activity. The judgment of deficiency or absence is made by the clinician, taking into account factors that affect sexual functioning, such as age and the context of the person's life.

B. The disturbance causes marked distress or interpersonal difficulty.

C. The sexual dysfunction is not better accounted for by another Axis I disorder (except another Sexual Dysfunction) and is not due exclusively to the direct physiological effects of a substance (e.g., a drug of abuse, a medication) or a general medical condition.

Specify type:
Lifelong Type
Acquired Type

Specify type:
Generalized Type
Situational Type

Specify:
Due to Psychological Factors
Due to Combined Factors

DSM-IV-TR Criteria for Sexual Aversion Disorder

A. Persistent or recurrent extreme aversion to, and avoidance of, all (or almost all) genital sexual contact with a sexual partner.

B. The disturbance causes marked distress or interpersonal difficulty.

C. The sexual dysfunction is not better accounted for by another Axis I disorder (except another Sexual Dysfunction).

Specify type:
Lifelong Type
Acquired Type

Specify type:
Generalized Type
Situational Type

Specify:
Due to Psychological Factors
Due to Combined Factors

DSM-IV-TR Criteria for Male Erectile Disorder

A. Persistent or recurrent inability to attain, or to maintain until completion of the sexual activity, an adequate erection.

B. The disturbance causes marked distress or interpersonal difficulty.

C. The erectile dysfunction is not better accounted for by another Axis I disorder (other than a Sexual Dysfunction) and is not due exclusively to the direct physiological effects of a substance (e.g., a drug of abuse, a medication) or a general medical condition.

Specify type:
Lifelong Type
Acquired Type

Specify type:
Generalized Type
Situational Type

Specify:
Due to Psychological Factors
Due to Combined Factors

DSM-IV-TR Criteria for Sexual Aversion Disorder

A. Persistent or recurrent inability to attain, or to maintain until completion of the sexual activity, an adequate lubrication-swelling response of sexual excitement.

B. The disturbance causes marked distress or interpersonal difficulty.

C. The sexual dysfunction is not better accounted for by another Axis I disorder (except another Sexual Dysfunction) and is not due exclusively to the direct physiological effects of a substance (e.g., a drug of abuse, a medication) or a general medical condition.

Specify type:
Lifelong Type
Acquired Type

Specify type:
Generalized Type
Situational Type

Specify:
Due to Psychological Factors
Due to Combined Factors

DSM-IV-TR Criteria for Male Orgasmic Disorder

A. Persistent or recurrent delay in, or absence of, orgasm following a normal sexual excitement phase during sexual activity that the clinician, taking into account the person's age, judges to be adequate in focus, intensity, and duration.

B. The disturbance causes marked distress or interpersonal difficulty.

C. The orgasmic dysfunction is not better accounted for by another Axis I disorder (except another Sexual Dysfunction) and is not due exclusively to the direct physiological effects of a substance (e.g., a drug of abuse, a medication) or a general medical condition.

Specify type:
Lifelong Type
Acquired Type

Specify type:
Generalized Type
Situational Type

Specify:
Due to Psychological Factors
Due to Combined Factors

DSM-IV-TR Criteria for Female Orgasmic Disorder

A. Persistent or recurrent delay in, or absence of, orgasm following a normal sexual excitement phase. Women exhibit wide variability in the type or intensity of stimulation that triggers orgasm. The diagnosis of Female Orgasmic Disorder should be based on the clinician's judgment that the woman's orgasmic capacity is less than would be reasonable for her age, sexual experience, and the adequacy of sexual stimulation she receives.

B. The disturbance causes marked distress or interpersonal difficulty.

C. The orgasmic dysfunction is not better accounted for by another Axis I disorder (except another Sexual Dysfunction) and is not due exclusively to the direct physiological effects of a substance (e.g., a drug of abuse, a medication) or a general medical condition.

Specify type:
Lifelong Type
Acquired Type

Specify type:
Generalized Type
Situational Type

Specify:
Due to Psychological Factors
Due to Combined Factors

DSM-IV-TR Criteria for Premature Ejaculation

A. Persistent or recurrent ejaculation with minimal sexual stimulation before, on, or shortly after penetration and before the person wishes it. The clinician must take into account factors that affect duration of the excitement phase, such as age, novelty of the sexual partner or situation, and recent frequency of sexual activity.

B. The disturbance causes marked distress or interpersonal difficulty.

C. The premature ejaculation is not due exclusively to the direct effects of a substance (e.g., withdrawal from opiods).

Specify type:
Lifelong Type
Acquired Type

Specify type:
Generalized Type
Situational Type

Specify:
Due to Psychological Factors
Due to Combined Factors

DSM-IV-TR Criteria for Dyspareunia

A. Recurrent or persistent genital pain associated with sexual intercourse in either a male or a female.

B. The disturbance causes marked distress or interpersonal difficulty.

C. The disturbance is not caused exclusively by Vaginismus or lack of lubrication, is not better accounted for by another Axis I disorder (except another Sexual Dysfunction), and is not due exclusively to the direct physiological effects of a substance (e.g., a drug of abuse, a medication) or a general medical condition or due to combined factors.

Specify type:
- **Lifelong Type**
- **Acquired Type**

Specify type:
- **Generalized Type**
- **Situational Type**

Specify:
- **Due to Psychological Factors**
- **Due to Combined Factors**

DSM-IV-TR Criteria for Vaginismus

A. Recurrent or persistent involuntary spasm of the musculature of the outer third of the vagina that interferes with sexual intercourse.

B. The disturbance causes marked distress or interpersonal difficulty.

C. The disturbance is not better accounted for by another Axis I disorder (e.g., Somatization Disorder) and is not due exclusively to the direct physiological effects of a general medical condition.

Specify type:
Lifelong Type
Acquired Type

Specify type:
Generalized Type
Situational Type

Specify:
Due to Psychological Factors
Due to Combined Factors

DSM-IV-TR Criteria for Fetishism

A. Over a period of at least 6 months, recurrent, intense sexually arousing fantasies, sexual urges, or behaviors involving the use of nonliving objects (e.g., female undergarments).

B. The fantasies, sexual urges, or behaviors cause clinically significant distress or impairment in social, occupational, or other important areas of functioning.

C. The fetish objects are not limited to articles of female clothing used in cross-dressing (as in Transvestic Fetishism) or devices designed for the purpose of tactile genital stimulation (e.g., a vibrator).

DSM-IV-TR Criteria for Voyeurism

A. Over a period of at least 6 months, recurrent, intense sexually arousing fantasies, sexual urges, or behaviors involving the act of observing an unsuspecting person who is naked, in the process of disrobing, or engaging in sexual activity.

B. The person has acted on these urges, or the sexual urges or fantasies cause marked distress or interpersonal difficulty.

DSM-IV-TR Criteria for Exhibitionism

A. Over a period of at least 6 months, recurrent, intense sexually arousing fantasies, sexual urges, or behaviors involving the exposure of one's genitals to an unsuspecting stranger.

B. The person has acted on these urges, or the sexual urges or fantasies cause marked distress or interpersonal difficulty.

DSM-IV-TR Criteria for Transvestic Fetishism

A. Over a period of at least 6 months, in a heterosexual male, recurrent, intense sexually arousing fantasies, sexual urges, or behaviors involving cross-dressing.

B. The fantasies, sexual urges, or behaviors cause clinically significant distress or impairment in social, occupational, or other important areas of functioning.

Specify if:

With Gender Dysphoria: if the person has persistent discomfort with gender role or identity

DSM-IV-TR Criteria for Sexual Sadism

A. Over a period of at least 6 months, recurrent, intense sexually arousing fantasies, sexual urges, or behaviors involving acts (real, not simulated) in which the psychological or physical suffering (including humiliation) of the victim is sexually exciting to the person.

B. The person has acted on these urges, or the sexual urges or fantasies cause marked distress or interpersonal difficulty.

DSM-IV-TR Criteria for Sexual Masochism

A. Over a period of at least 6 months, recurrent, intense sexually arousing fantasies, sexual urges, or behaviors involving the act (real, not simulated) of being humiliated, beaten, bound, or otherwise made to suffer.

B. The fantasies, sexual urges, or behaviors cause clinically significant distress or impairment in social, occupational, or other important areas of functioning.

DSM-IV-TR Criteria for Pedophilia

A. Over a period of at least 6 months, recurrent, intense sexually arousing fantasies, sexual urges, or behaviors involving sexual activity with a prepubescent child or children (generally age 13 years or younger).

B. The person has acted on these urges, or the sexual urges or fantasies cause marked distress or interpersonal difficulty.

C. The person is at least age 16 years and at least 5 years older than the child or children in Criterion A.

Note: Do not include an individual in late adolescence involved in an ongoing sexual relationship with a 12- or 13-year-old.

Specify if:

Sexually Attracted to Males
Sexually Attracted to Females
Sexually Attracted to Both

Specify if:

Limited to Incest

Specify type:

Exclusive Type (attracted only to children)
Nonexclusive Type

Transparency 10-18

DSM-IV-TR Criteria for Frotteurism

A. Over a period of at least 6 months, recurrent, intense sexually arousing fantasies, sexual urges, or behaviors involving touching and rubbing against a non consenting person.

B. The person has acted on these urges, or the sexual urges or fantasies cause marked distress or interpersonal difficulty.

CHAPTER ELEVEN

SUBSTANCE-RELATED AND IMPULSE-CONTROL DISORDERS

LEARNING OBJECTIVES

1. Describe the nature of substance-related disorders and distinguish among substance use, substance intoxication, substance abuse, and substance dependence.
2. Differentiate the signs and symptoms of tolerance from those of withdrawal.
3. Define a psychoactive substance and describe the main classes of psychoactive substances (i.e., depressants, stimulants, opiods, hallucinogens, and other common drugs of abuse).
4. Describe the physiological and psychological effects of alcohol generally and in the context of alcohol use disorders, including what is known about prevalence, course, and cultural and social factors related to their use and abuse.
5. Describe the physiological and psychological effects of sedative, hypnotic, or anxiolytic substances, including what is known about prevalence, course, and cultural and social factors related to their use and abuse.
6. Describe the physiological and psychological effects of stimulants (e.g., amphetamines, cocaine, nicotine, and caffeine), including what is known about prevalence, course, and cultural and social factors related to their use and abuse.
7. Distinguish opiods from hallucinogens, and describe their psychological and physiological effects and patterns of use and abuse.
8. Describe other drugs of abuse and their physiological and psychological effects.
9. Describe the psychological and physiological processes involved in substance dependence, including the role of positive and negative reinforcement, expectancies, and social and cultural factors.
10. Describe the genetic contribution to substance-related disorders, with particular emphasis on alcoholism.
11. Describe the main features of the integrative model of substance-related disorders.
12. Describe the course of substance-use disorders including remission, relapse, and recovery.
13. Discuss various psychological and medical treatments for addictions, and the controversies surrounding abstinence and controlling drinking as a goal of addiction treatment.
14. Understand the role of early prevention and relapse prevention programs, including what is known about their relative effectiveness.

OUTLINE

I. Perspectives on Substance-Related Disorders
   A. In the U.S. use and abuse of drugs and alcohol costs hundreds of billions of dollars each year, kills 500,000 Americans annually, and is implicated in street crime, homelessness, and gang violence. The textbook illustrates the general problems with substance abuse, and particularly **polysubstance use**, with the case of Danny.

B. **Substance-related disorders** involve problems associated with using and abusing drugs that alter patterns of thinking, feeling, and behaving. The term **substance** refers to chemical compounds that are ingested in order to alter mood or behavior, and includes alcohol, nicotine, caffeine.

1. **Psychoactive substances** refers to a broad class of agents that alter mood and/or behavior which are ingested to become intoxicated or high, with abuse of such substances related to dependence and addiction.
2. **Substance use** is simply the ingestion of psychoactive substances on occasion, whereas the physiological reaction to ingested substances (e.g., drunkenness, getting high) is referred to as **substance intoxication**. Intoxication depends on the drug, the amount of the drug ingested, and the person's biological reaction.
3. **Substance abuse** is difficult to define on the basis of amount of substance ingested. According to the DSM-IV-TR, substance abuse is defined on the basis of interference with the user's life.
4. **Substance dependence** is usually described as addiction; though there is considerable disagreement about how to define addiction. Dependence can exist without abuse.
    a. One definition considers addiction as **physiological dependence** on the drug or drugs, thus requiring greater and greater amounts of the drug to experience the same effect (i.e., **tolerance**), while responding physically in a negative way when the substance is not longer ingested (i.e., **withdrawal**).
    b. **Tolerance** and **withdrawal** are physiological reactions to the chemicals ingested. Withdrawal from many substances can cause chills, fever, diarrhea, nausea and vomiting, and aches and pains. LSD and marijuana do not produce symptoms of withdrawal.
    c. Another view focuses on **drug-seeking behaviors** as a measure of dependence. Examples include repeated use of the drug, desperate need to ingest more of the substance, stealing money to buy drugs, standing outside in the freezing cold to smoke, and likelihood that use will resume after a period of abstinence. Such reactions are sometimes referred to in terms of **psychological dependence**, not physiological dependence.
    d. The DSM-IV-TR definition of substance dependence combines the physiological aspects of tolerance and withdrawal with the behavioral and psychological aspects.

II. Diagnostic Issues

A. Early versions of the DSM did not treat alcoholism and drug abuse as disorders, but instead as representing sociopathic personality disturbances. Substance use was seen as a symptom of another problem. The DSM-III was the first to create a separate category for substance-related disorders.

1. The DSM-IV-TR term **substance-related disorders** indicates several subtypes of diagnoses for each substance, including dependence, abuse, intoxication, and/or withdrawal.

2. Symptoms of other disorders can complicate the substance abuse picture significantly. Factors that contribute to comorbidity with substance-related disorders are numerous.

B. Five main categories of substances include the following:
1. **Depressants** result in behavioral sedation and include alcohol, sedative, hypnotic, and anxiolytic drugs belonging to the barbiturates and benzodiazepine classes.
2. **Stimulants** increase alertness and can elevate mood and include amphetamines, cocaine, nicotine, and caffeine.
3. **Opiates** primarily produce analgesia (i.e., reduce pain) and euphoria and include heroin, opium, codeine, and morphine.
4. **Hallucinogens** alter sensory perception and can produce delusions, paranoia, and hallucinations, and including drugs like marijuana and LSD.
5. **Other drugs of abuse** include inhalants, anabolic steroids, and over-the-counter prescription medications. These drugs produce several psychoactive effects.

III. Depressants

A. Depressants primarily decrease central nervous system activity, reduce arousal, and help people to relax. Included in this group are **alcohol** and the **sedative**, **hypnotic**, and **anxiolytic** drugs and those prescribed for insomnia. These substances are among the most likely to produce symptoms of physical dependence, tolerance, and withdrawal.

B. Alcohol use disorders
1. **Although** alcohol is a depressant, its initial effect is stimulation from a depression of inhibitory centers in the brain. Continued drinking depresses other brain areas that interfere with functioning and include impaired motor coordination, slowed reaction time, confusion, ability to make judgments is reduced, and vision and hearing can be negatively affected.
2. Alcohol affects many parts of the body. Small amounts of alcohol are absorbed in the stomach, but most passes directly into the blood stream via the small intestine. The circulatory system distributes alcohol throughout the body, where it contacts every major organ, including the heart and some goes to the lungs where it is exhaled. As alcohol passes through the liver it is broken down or metabolized into carbon dioxide and water. An average person can metabolize 7 to 10 grams of alcohol per hour, or about 1 glass of beer or 1 ounce of 90-proof spirits.
    a. Alcohol tends to influence a number of different neuroreceptor systems such as the **gamma-aminobutyric (GABA) inhibitory system**. When GABA attaches to its receptor, chloride ions enter the cell and desensitize it to the effects of other neurotransmitters. Alcohol reinforces the movement of **chloride ions** to make it difficult for the neuron to fire, thus making it difficult for neurons to

communicate with each other. Alcohol's anti-anxiety effects may result from an interaction with the GABA system.

   b. The **glutamate system** is excitatory in nature, helps neurons fire, and is believed to affect learning and memory. Blackouts, or the loss of memory that occurs with alcohol intoxication, may result from the interaction of alcohol with the glutamate system.
   c. The **serotonin system** is also sensitive to alcohol and this system is known to affect mood, sleep, and eating behavior, including cravings for alcohol.
3. Long-term effects of heavy drinking are often severe. **Withdrawal** from chronic alcohol use includes tremors, and within several hours, nausea and vomiting, anxiety, transient hallucinations, agitation, insomnia, and at its most extreme, **withdrawal delirium** (or **delirium tremens – DTs**). DTs can produce frightening hallucinations and body tremors. Consequences of long-term excessive drinking include liver disease, pancreatitis, cardiovascular disorders, and brain damage.
4. It is not necessarily true that alcohol permanently kills brain cells. Chronic use of alcohol can produce two types of serious brain syndromes:
   a. **Dementia** involves a general loss of intellectual abilities and can result directly from neurotoxicity or poisoning of the brain by excessive amounts of alcohol.
   b. **Wernicke's disease** results in confusion, loss of muscle coordination, and unintelligible speech and is believed to be causes by thiamine deficiency; a vitamin that is metabolized poorly by heavy drinkers.
5. Alcohol also negatively affects prenatal development and can result in **fetal alcohol syndrome (FAS)**; a condition related to a mother drinking while pregnant. FAS is associated with growth retardation, cognitive deficits, behavior problems, and learning difficulties, and characteristic facial features. African-Americans and Apache and Ute Indian women appear at the greatest risk of having children with FAS if they drink while pregnant.
   a. Alcohol is **metabolized** via an enzyme called **alcohol dehydrogenase (ADH)** and three forms of this enzyme have been identified (i.e., beta 1, beta 2, and beta 3 ADH).
   b. Beta 3 ADH is found most frequently in African Americans and is prevalent in children with FAS. This work suggests that FAS may be related to a genetic tendency to have certain enzymes.
6. **Statistics** on alcohol use suggest that most adults in the U.S. characterize themselves as light drinkers or abstainers. Alcohol consumption has declined. However, about 23% of Americans report binge drinking (five or more drinks on the same occasion) in the past month.
   a. Alcohol use during a 1-month period is highest among Caucasian Americans and somewhat lower for Hispanics or those with multi-racial backgrounds.
   b. Males are more likely than females to drink alcohol and are also more likely to drink heavily. 42% of college-age men and women report that they had gone on a binge of heavy drinking at least once in the

preceding two weeks, with men more likely to report multiple binges in the same two-week period.

   c. About 15 million U.S. adults are thought to be alcohol dependent. Among the general population, young (18-29), single males are most likely to be heavy drinkers and to have alcohol use problems.
   d. Many people who abuse alcohol or are dependent on it fluctuate between drinking heavily, drinking "socially" without negative effects, and not drinking at all.
   e. Violence is often associated with alcohol, but alcohol does not cause aggression. Rather it reduces fear associated with punishment and inhibition related to impulse control.
   f. Outside the U.S. rates of alcohol abuse and dependence vary widely.

7. According to **Jellinek's model**, alcohol use and dependence may involve a predictable downward pattern involving the following stages:
   a. First, persons go through the **prealcoholic stage** where few serious consequences to drinking occur.
   b. Second, they move into the **prodromal stage**, where they drink heavily but with few outward signs of a problem.
   c. Third, they move into a **crucial stage** where the person loses control of drinking and has occasional binges.
   d. Lastly, the person enters a **chronic stage** where one's activities surround getting and drinking alcohol.
8. Jellinek's model was based on a flawed research study, and led to the idea that once problems arose with drinking, they would become steadily worse, following a predictable downward pattern so long as the person kept drinking. More recent research suggests that the course of alcohol dependence may be progressive for most people, although the course of alcohol abuse may be more variable. About 20% of those with severe alcohol dependence experience spontaneous remission.

C. Sedative, hypnotic, or anxiolytic substance use disorders

1. **Sedative** (calming), **hypnotic** (sleep-inducing), and **anxiolytic** (anxiety reducing) drugs include **barbiturates** for sleep and **benzodiazepines** to reduce anxiety. These drugs relax muscles but may cause problems similar to alcohol at high doses. **Rohypnol** (i.e., "roofies" or the "date rape drug") gained a following among teenagers in the 1990s because it had the same effect as alcohol but without the telltale odor.
2. Large doses of **barbiturates** produce effects similar to heavy drinking, such as slurred speech, problems in walking, concentration, and working. At extremely high doses, barbiturates relax the diaphragm muscles to the point of death by suffocation. Overdose on barbiturates in a common means of suicide.
3. **Benzodiazepines** likewise produce a calming effect, a pleasant high, reduction of inhibition, similar to effects of alcohol. Continued use of benzodiazepines can result in tolerance and dependence and withdrawal effects are similar to those experienced with alcohol.

4. DSM-IV-TR criteria for sedative, hypnotic, and anxiolytic drug use disorders do not differ much from those for alcohol use disorders. Both include maladaptive behavioral changes such as inappropriate sexual or aggressive behavior, variable moods, impaired judgment and social or occupational functioning.
5. Like alcohol, these drugs affect the **GABA system**, but by a slightly different mechanism. Alcohol combined with any of these drugs can be synergistic and quite dangerous.
6. Since 1960s, use of barbiturates has declined, but benzodiazepine use has increased. Of those seeking treatment for substance-related problems, less than 1% present problems with benzodiazepines, compared to other drugs of abuse.

IV. Stimulants

A. **Stimulants** are the most widely consumed drug in the U.S., and include **caffeine**, **nicotine**, **amphetamines**, and **cocaine**. Amphetamines are manufactured and were used as a treatment for asthma, nasal congestion, and weight loss. Amphetamines are also prescribed for persons with narcolepsy and attention deficit/hyperactivity disorder. Such drugs increase alertness and increase energy.

B. Amphetamine use disorders

1. At low doses, **amphetamines** can produce elation, vigor, reduce fatigue, followed by a crash accompanied by feeling depressed and tired.
2. DSM-IV diagnostic criteria for amphetamine intoxication include significant behavioral symptoms such as euphoria or affective blunting, changes in sociability, interpersonal sensitivity, anxiety, tension, anger, stereotyped behaviors, impaired judgment, and impaired social or occupational functioning.
3. **Physiological symptoms** can include heart rate and blood pressure changes, perspiration or chills, nausea or vomiting, weight loss, muscular weakness, respiratory depression, chest pain, seizures, or coma. The danger of amphetamines and other stimulants are in the negative side effects. Severe intoxication or overdose can cause hallucinations, panic, agitation, and paranoid delusions. Symptoms of withdrawal are similar to depression.
4. Mini-epidemics of designer drugs are not uncommon. For example, an amphetamine called methylene-dioxymethamphetamine was once used as an appetite suppressant; however, recreational use of this drug – called **Ecstasy** – rose sharply in the late 1980s and about 2% of college students report use of this drug.
   a. Ecstasy produces effects like speed, but without the crash. Users report feeling warm and trippy like acid, but without the possibility of a "major freak-out."
   b. A purified crystallized form of amphetamine, called **ice**, is ingested through smoking. This drug causes marked aggressive tendencies and stays in the body longer than cocaine.
   c. Both drugs can involve dependence.

5. Amphetamines stimulate the central nervous system by enhancing norepinephrine and dopamine activity via increasing their release while blocking their reuptake. Too much amphetamine can cause hallucinations and delusions.

C. Cocaine use disorders

1. **Cocaine** replaced amphetamines as the stimulant of choice in the 1970s. Cocaine is derived from the leaves of the coca plant, indigenous to South America. Until 1903, Coca-Cola contained about 60mg of cocaine per 8-ounce serving.
2. Like amphetamines, small amounts of cocaine increases alertness, euphoria, blood pressure and pulse, and causes insomnia and loss of appetite. The effects of cocaine are short-lived.
    a. Cocaine and crack cocaine may adversely affect fetuses and produce crack babies, infants with low birth weight, or disruptions in a baby's biological clock. This picture is complicated by the fact that most cocaine and crack using mothers use several other drugs and often come from disruptive home environments.
3. **Cocaine use** across most age groups has declined over the past decade and a half. About 0.2% of Americans report trying crack.
4. The effects of cocaine resemble that of the amphetamines and tend to block dopamine reuptake. The result is increased stimulation of the dopamine neurons in the pleasure pathway, resulting in the high associated with cocaine use.
5. Many thought that cocaine was not addictive, but we know that this is not the case. Cocaine dependence develops slowly, and typically people only find that they have a growing inability to resist taking more. Few short-term negative effects are noticed initially, but with continued use sleep is disrupted, higher doses are required, and paranoia and other symptoms set it. Cocaine abusers go through patterns of tolerance and withdrawal comparable to abusers of other psychoactive substances.

D. Nicotine use disorders

1. **Nicotine**, named after Jean Nicot who introduced tobacco to the French court in the 16th century, is what gives smoking its pleasurable qualities. About 30% of all Americans smoke, which is down from the 42.4% who were smokers in 1965.
2. DSM-IV-TR does not describe an intoxication pattern for nicotine, but rather includes withdrawal symptoms such as depressed mood, insomnia, irritability, anxiety, difficulty concentrating, restlessness, and increased appetite and weight gain.
3. Nicotine in small doses stimulates the central nervous system, but may also relieve stress and improve mood. It can also cause high blood pressure, heart disease, and cancer. High doses can blur vision, cause confusion, lead to convulsions, and sometimes death.

a. Nicotine enters the bloodstream and the brain 7 to 19 seconds after inhalation. Nicotine stimulates specific **nicotinic acetylcholine receptors** in the midbrain reticular formation and limbic system pleasure pathway. Smokers dose themselves throughout the day to maintain a steady nicotine level in the bloodstream.
b. Overwhelming evidence indicates that nicotine is addictive. In addition, smoking is related to depression, anxiety, and anger. Severe depression occurs more often among people with nicotine dependence.

E. Caffeine use disorders
1. **Caffeine** is called the "gentle stimulant" and is used regularly by 90% of Americans. This drug is found in tea, coffee, cola drinks, and cocoa products. In small doses, caffeine can elevate mood and reduce fatigue, but larger doses can produce jitteriness and insomnia.
2. Regular caffeine use can result in tolerance and dependence. Withdrawal symptoms include headaches, drowsiness, and a generally unpleasant mood.
3. Caffeine's effect on the brain appears to involve the neurotransmitters **adenosine** and to a lesser extent **serotonin**. Caffeine blocks adenosine reuptake.

V. Opiods

A. The word **opiate** refers to the natural chemical in the opium poppy that has a narcotic effect (i.e., relieve pain and induce sleep). The broader term **opiods** refers to a family of substances that include natural opiates, synthetic variations (i.e., methadone, pethidine), and comparable substances that occur naturally in the brain (e.g., enkephalins, beta-endorphins, and dynorphins). **Heroin**, **opium**, **codeine**, and **morphine** are included in this group.
1. Opiates induce euphoria, drowsiness, and slowed breathing. High doses can lead to death if respiration is completely depressed. Opiates are also **analgesics** (i.e., substances that help relieve pain such as morphine).
2. Withdrawal symptoms include excessive yawning, nausea and vomiting, chills, muscle aches, diarrhea, and insomnia that may disrupt work, school, and social functioning. Such symptoms can persist for 1 to 3 days, and withdrawal usually runs its course in about 1 week.
3. Opiate users tend to be secretive, making estimates of prevalence difficult. Because such drugs are usually injected intravenously, users are at increased risk for HIV infection and therefore AIDS.
4. Life of an opiate addict is bleak, with about 28% dying prematurely, with almost half of deaths due to homicide, suicide, and accident, and about 33% of these resulting from overdose.
5. The high comes from activation of the body's natural opiod system that includes enkephalins and endorphins that together provide narcotic effects.

VI. Hallucinogens

A. **Hallucinogens** are substances that change the way the user perceives the world, and may produce delusions, paranoia, hallucinations, and altered sensory perception.

B. Marijuana

1. **Marijuana** was the drug of choice in the 1960s and early 1970s. Marijuana is the name given to the dried parts of the cannabis or hemp plant (**cannabis sativa**). Reactions to marijuana include mood swings, heightened sensory experiences, paranoia, hallucinations, dizziness, and impairment of memory, concentration, impairment in motivation (i.e., **amotivational syndrome**), self-esteem, and interpersonal and occupational relationships. It is not uncommon for someone to report having no reaction to the first use of the drug, and it appears that people can turn off the high if they are sufficiently motivated.
2. Evidence for marijuana tolerance is contradictory, with reports of tolerance in chronic heavy users and reverse tolerance (i.e., regular users experience more pleasure from the drug after repeated use). Major signs of withdrawal do not occur with marijuana, or when they do they are not severe. No evidence exists that marijuana users experience craving and psychological dependence characteristic of other substances.
3. Use of marijuana for **medicinal purposes** is controversial. Marijuana smoke may contain carcinogens and long-term use contributes to diseases such as lung cancer.
4. Most users inhale the drug by smoking it; others use preparations such as hashish. Marijuana contains over 80 types of chemicals called cannabinoids, which are believed to alter mood and behavior. The most common chemical is **tetrahydrocannabinol (THC)**. The brain seems to produce its own version of THC via a neurochemical called **anandamide** (ananda from the Sanskrit word meaning "bliss").

C. LSD and other hallucinogens

1. **LSD** or **d-lysergic acid diethylamide** is the most common hallucinogenic drug and is produced synthetically in laboratories or derived from ergot fungus. This fungus was known in the middle ages to lead to **ergotism**; a condition involving constricted blood flow to the arms or legs, eventually resulting in gangrene and loss of limbs. Another type of illness resulted in convulsions, delirium, and hallucinations. LSD was first produced illegally in the 1960s.
2. Other hallucinogens include **psilocybin** (found in certain species of mushrooms), **lysergic acid amide** (found in the seeds of the morning glory plant), **dimethyltryptamine** (found in the bark of the Virola tree which grows in South and Central America), and **mescaline** (found in the peyote cactus plant).
3. DSM-IV-TR diagnostic criteria for hallucinogen intoxication are similar to those for marijuana and include perceptual changes such as intensification of perceptions, depersonalization, hallucinations, papillary dilation, rapid heart beat, sweating, and blurred vision.

4. Tolerance develops quickly to LSD, psilocybin, and mescaline and repeated use results in the drugs losing their effectiveness. Sensitivity returns after a week or so of complete abstinence from the drug. Withdrawal symptoms are uncommon; however, psychotic reactions are of concern (e.g., people jumping out of windows because they believed they could fly).
5. How LSD and other hallucinogens affect the brain is unclear. Many of such drugs are similar to neurotransmitters. LSD, psilocybin, lysergic acid amide, and DMT (dimethyltryptamine) are similar to serotonin; mescaline resembles norepinephrine; and several other hallucinogens not covered in the textbook resemble acetylcholine.

VII. Other Drugs of Abuse

A. This class does not fit neatly into the previous categories and includes inhalants, steroids, and designer drugs.

B. Inhalants

1. **Inhalants** covers several substances found in volatile solvents and are breathed into the lungs directly. Common inhalants include spray paint, hair spray, paint thinner, gasoline, amyl nitrate, nitrous oxide, nail polish remover, felt-tipped markers, airplane glue, contact cement, spot remover.
2. These drugs are rapidly absorbed into the bloodstream through the lungs and the high resembles alcohol intoxication and includes dizziness, slurred speech, poor coordination, euphoria, and lethargy. Users build up tolerance and withdrawal symptoms (e.g., sleep disturbance, tremors, irritability, nausea) can last 2 to 5 days. Long-term use can damage bone marrow, kidneys, the liver, and the brain.
3. Inhalants are used most often by young males (age 13-15 years) who are economically disadvantaged.

C. Anabolic-androgenic steroids

1. **Steroids** are derived or synthesized from testosterone. Legitimate medical uses of such drugs are for asthma, anemia, breast cancer, and males with inadequate sexual development. The anabolic action of these drugs can produce increased body mass.
2. Steroids can be taken orally or via injection and approximately 2% of males use such drugs illegally at some point in their lives. Users may engage in **cycling** (i.e., administer the drug on a schedule of several weeks or months followed by a break) or **stacking** (i.e., use combinations of several types of steroids).
3. Steroids do not produce a desirable high, but instead enhance performance and body size. Dependence involves the desire to maintain performance gains, not the desire to experience altered emotional or physical states.
4. Long-term use of steroids is related to mood disturbances, and more serious physical consequences may also result.

D. Designer drugs

1. **Designer drugs** refer to a growing group of drugs produced by pharmaceutical companies to target specific diseases or disorders. Ecstasy is part of this group, but belongs with the stimulants. Other such drugs include 3, 4 methelenedioxyethamphetamine (MDEA or "Eve") and 2-(4-Bromo-2, 5-dimethoxy-phenyl)-ethylamine (BDMPEA or "Nexus"). Such drugs heighten auditory and visual perception, sense of taste and touch, and are becoming popular in nightclubs, all-night dance parties (i.e., raves), or large social gatherings of primarily gay men (i.e., circuit parties).
   a. Another drug associated with the club scene is **ketamine** (street name "K," "Special K," or "Cat Valium). This drug is a dissociative anesthetic that produces a sense of detachment and reduced awareness of pain.
   b. Gamma hydroxybutyrate (GHB or "Liquid Ecstasy") is a central nervous system depressant that was marketed in health food stores in the 1980s as a means of stimulating muscle growth. At low doses this drug produces a state of relaxation and increased talkativeness, but at higher doses or in combination with alcohol or other drugs it can result in seizures, respiratory depression, or coma.
2. All of the designer drugs can produce tolerance and dependence.

VIII. Causes of Substance-Related Disorders

A. Biological dimensions: Familial and genetic influences

1. Evidence suggests that substance abuse has a genetic component. Twin, family, and adoption studies indicate that certain people may be genetically vulnerable to drug abuse. Most genetic data on substance abuse comes from research on alcoholism.
   a. Both twin and adoption studies suggest genetic factors play a role in alcoholism, particularly in males.
   b. Two studies have located genes that may influence alcoholism on chromosomes 1, 2, 7, and 11, plus a finding that a gene on chromosome 4 may serve to protect people from becoming alcohol dependent.
   c. The field of functional genomics focuses on how genes work to influence addiction.

B. Biological dimensions: Neurobiological influences

1. The pleasurable experience reported by people who use psychoactive substances partly explains why people continue to use them. In effect, people are positively reinforced for using drugs. All drugs seem to affect the reward or pleasure centers of the brain.
   a. The pleasure center is believed to include the **dopaminergic system** and its opiod-releasing neurons that begin in the midbrain ventral tegmental area and then work their way through the nucleus accumbens and on to the frontal cortex.
   b. Amphetamines and cocaine (including nicotine and alcohol) act directly on the dopamine system, whereas other drugs increase the availability of dopamine indirectly. GABA, as a major inhibitory neurotransmitter

system, helps to turn off the continued activity of the reward system. Opiates (e.g., opium, morphine, and heroin) inhibit GABA from doing its job, which in turn stops the GABA neurons from inhibiting dopamine, thus making more dopamine available in the reward center.

2. With several drugs, **negative reinforcement** is related to the drug's anxiolytic effect, particularly alcohol. Such drugs reduce anxiety via the septal/hippocampal system, which includes a large number of GABA sensitive neurons. Such drugs may enhance the activity of GABA in this region, thereby inhibiting the brain's normal reaction (anxiety/fear) to anxiety-producing situations.
    a. Sons of alcoholics appear more able to appreciate the initial highs of drinking and are less sensitive to the lows that come later compared to sons of non-alcoholics.

C. Psychological dimensions

1. **Positive and negative reinforcement** seems involved in drug use behavior. **Positive reinforcement** is the main reason people use drugs (i.e., the pleasurable experience or high). **Negative reinforcement** may be involved as drugs also tend to reduce or eliminate unpleasant feelings, or to escape from unpleasant circumstances in their lives. This phenomena has been explored under several different names, including tension reduction, negative affect, and self-medication.
2. Many view substance abuse as a way that users cope with unpleasant feelings that accompany life circumstances.
    a. Drug use among Vietnam veterans is one example of this phenomenon, where about 42% of these young men reported experimenting with heroin during the war. Interestingly, only 12% of these soldiers continued to use heroin upon return to the U.S.
    b. Children who report more negative affect are more likely to use drugs than children who do not. Moreover, adolescents tend to use drugs as a way to cope with unpleasant feelings. This work suggests that young persons use drugs as a means to escape from unpleasantness, and points to interventions for drug use that are directed at the causes of the unpleasant circumstances to begin with.
3. The **opponent-process theory** has been advanced to explain why people do not cease using drugs after experiencing a crash or other negative side effects. The opponent-process theory integrates positive and negative reinforcement and maintains that positive feelings will be followed by negative feelings and that negative feelings will be followed eventually by positive feelings. This relation is strengthened with repeated drug use and weakened with disuse. Tolerance and more severe withdrawal symptoms create a vicious cycle, and the motivation shifts to alleviating and preventing the next unpleasant crash.
4. Substance abuse may also represent a form of self-medication, though this work is still preliminary.
5. Expectations about a drug's effects can influence one's reactions to the drug. The role of such cognitive factors are known as **expectancy effects**. Such

expectancies may develop prior to actual drug use, and could result from exposure to drug use in others or via the media and advertising. Expectations for positive results from drinking alcohol, for example, tend to increase drinking behavior. Positive expectations have an indirect influence on drug problems, but do increase the likelihood that one will use certain drugs. Expectations may explain relapse.

a. A cognitive phenomenon with respect to alcohol use is **alcohol myopia**, or a condition where immediate experience tends to substantially influence behavior and emotion. Alcohol myopia may help explain why people continue to drink as they may not be able to evaluate properly the risks involved in continued drinking.

D. Social dimensions

1. Exposure to psychoactive substances is a necessary prerequisite for their use and possible abuse. Media advertising may be more influential than peer pressure in determining whether teens smoke. Children appear to learn about alcohol and other drugs from relatives and acquaintances rather than television alone.
    a. Drug addicted parents spend less time monitoring their children than parents without drug problems and this is an important factor in early adolescent substance abuse.
2. **Society** tends to view substance abuse as either a sign of moral weakness or in terms of a disease model of dependence.
    a. The **moral weakness view** maintains that drug use is a failure of self-control in the face of temptation, and that drug users lack the character or moral fiber to resist the lure of drugs (i.e., a psychological view).
    b. The **disease model** stipulates that drug dependence is caused by an underlying disorder, or a disease (i.e., a biological view). Alcoholics Anonymous and similar organizations accept the disease model.
3. A comprehensive view of substance-related disorder includes both psychological and biological influences.

E. Cultural dimensions

1. **Cultural norms** affect the rates of substance abuse and dependence in important ways. For example, in Korea, members are expected to drink alcohol heavily on certain social occasions.
2. Cultural factors also determine how substance-related disorders manifest. Expectancies about the effects of alcohol use differ across cultures, and whether substance use is considered a harmful dysfunction often depends on the cultural group. This work on cultural factors is in its infancy.

IX. An Integrative Model of Substance-Related Disorders

A. Exposure or access to a drug is a necessary but not a sufficient condition for drug use. Drug use will also depend on social and cultural expectations. The path from drug use to abuse is more complicated; here, the presence of major stressors increases the risk of substance abuse and dependence. Genetic influences may also play a key role, with some people inheriting a sensitivity to drug effects and/or inheriting greater tolerance.

B. **Equifinality** refers to the fact that a disorder may arise from multiple and different paths, and seems particularly relevant to substance-related problems. Repeated drug use may lead to biological and cognitive reactions that contribute to dependence. In addition, tolerance and conditioning with pleasurable experiences may increase one's motivation toward continued drug use.

X. Treatment of Substance-Related Disorders

A. **Treatment** of substance-related disorders is difficult and often begins with the person admitting that s/he needs help, that s/he does have a problem with drugs, and that s/he needs the help of others to overcome dependence. The motivation to work on a drug problem appears to be essential in the treatment of substance abuse. Generally, the prognosis for drug dependent persons is not positive.

B. Treatment for substance-related disorders may focus on several of the following areas:

1. Assistance through the withdrawal process, with the ultimate goal being abstinence.
2. Another goal might be to get the person to maintain a certain level of drug use without escalating its intake, and/or preventing exposure to drugs

C. Biological treatments

1. **Agonist substitution** involves providing the person with a safe drug that has a chemical composition similar to the abused drug.
    a. **Methadone** is an opiate agonist used as a heroin substitute. Methadone does not produce the quick high of heroin, but provides that same analgesic and sedative effects. Heroin and methadone are cross-tolerant (i.e., act on the same neurotransmitter receptors). As a result, a person may become addicted to methadone.
    b. Addiction to cigarette smoking is also treated with substitution in the form of nicotine gum or nicotine patch. Both can help persons quit smoking in combination with psychosocial interventions, with the patch being somewhat more effective than gum.
2. **Antagonist treatment** involves drugs that block or counteract the positive effects of psychoactive drugs.
    a. **Naltrexone** is the most commonly prescribed opiate-antagonist. This drug produces immediate and extremely unpleasant withdrawal symptoms in persons addicted to opiates; however, it has limited success in persons who are not also involved in a structured treatment program. Naltrexone may also work for alcohol dependence in combination with other forms of psychotherapy.
    b. **Ondansetron** is a newer drug being studied for people who develop alcoholism at or before their early 20s.

3. **Aversive** treatments involve the use of drugs to make the ingestion of abused substances extremely unpleasant.
    a. A common aversive is **disulfiram** (**Antabuse**), which prevents the breakdown of acetaldehyde following alcohol use. A build-up of acetaldehyde then produces severe illness that is associated with drinking alcohol. The effect of this drug lasts a few days.
    b. Efforts to make smoking aversive have focused on **silver nitrate** in lozenges or gum. This chemical combines with the saliva of a smoker to produce a bad taste in the mouth; however, success has been limited.
4. Several **other biological treatments** are available. For example, medication is often used to address withdrawal symptoms.
    a. **Clonidine**, a drug for hypertension, has been used for persons withdrawing from opiates.
    b. **Sedatives or benzodiazepines** are sometimes used for those withdrawing from alcohol.
    c. The antidepressant drug **desipramine** is also effective in increasing abstinence from cocaine.

D. Psychosocial treatments

1. **Inpatient hospital treatment** is expensive and is often used to assist people through the withdrawal stage of substance abuse and to provide supportive therapy so they such persons can return to the community. Comparative outcome research indicates that there may be no difference in effectiveness between inpatient and outpatient care.
2. **Alcoholics Anonymous (AA)** is a popular 12-step program that views alcoholism as a disease that people are powerless to overcome without help. Social support is also a key element. Total abstinence is required of members. However, opinions are mixed as to the effectiveness of this approach, and systematic research has been made difficult due to anonymity of participants. Those who regularly participate in AA activities and carefully follow its guidelines are more likely to have a positive outcome than those who do not.
3. Teaching people to achieve **controlled use of substances** is extremely controversial. Controlled drinking as a treatment for alcoholism is widely accepted in the United Kingdom. Some evidence supports the idea that controlled drinking is a useful alternative to abstinence. Long-term outcomes are less positive for both controlled use and abstinence-based treatments.
4. Most **comprehensive treatment programs** aimed at helping people with substance abuse and dependence problems include several components.
    a. **Aversion therapy** is a conditioning form of therapy where substance use is paired with something extremely unpleasant, such as shock or nausea. The goal is to counteract the positive associations with substance use and to establish negative associations with the substance and its use.
    b. **Covert sensitization** is a variation of aversion therapy, but done entirely in imagination.

c. **Contingency management** involves setting up a system of goals and rewards for reaching certain goals.
d. **Community reinforcement** approaches address several different facets of the drug problem to help identify and correct aspects of the person's life that might contribute to substance use or interfere with efforts to abstain. Treatment may include family therapy, avoidance of cues for drug use, occupational assistance, and development of recreational alternatives. Preliminary results are encouraging, but more research is needed to address the long-term effectiveness of this approach.
e. **NIAAA Project MATCH** attempted to fit treatment with client characteristics. Though no specific treatment-person matches have been identified, this work suggests that well-run programs can be effective for several types of substance abuse problems.
f. **Relapse prevention** is a treatment model that views relapse as failure to use cognitive and behavioral coping skills. Therapy involves the removal of ambivalence about stopping drug use, examines beliefs about the positive aspects of a drug, confronts negative consequences of its use, and identifies adaptive strategies to cope with high-risk situations. This approach is particularly effective for alcohol problems, marijuana dependence, smoking, and cocaine abuse.

5. **Prevention efforts** have increasingly shifted from education-based approaches to more wide-ranging approaches including changes in the laws regarding drug possession and use and community-based interventions. The widely used DARE (i.e., Drug Abuse Resistance Education) program encourages a "no drug use" message through fear of consequences, rewards for commitments not to use drugs, and strategies for refusing offers of drugs. DARE, however, does not appear particularly effective. The more powerful prevention efforts may come from large-scale social changes, including advertising, stigmatization for use of certain drugs, and so on.

IX. Impulse-Control Disorders

A. DSM-IV-TR includes five **impulse-control disorders** that are not included under other categories: intermittent explosive disorder, kleptomania, pyromania, pathological gambling, and trichotillomania.

1. Persons with **intermittent explosive disorder** have episodes where they act on aggressive impulses that result in very serious assaults or destruction of property. Cognitive-behavioral interventions and approaches modeled after drug treatments appear the most effective for these individuals, although few controlled studies exist.
2. **Kleptomania** involves a recurrent failure to resist urges to steal things that are not needed for personal use or their monetary value. There appears to be a high comorbidity between kleptomania and the mood disorders, and to a lesser extent with substance abuse and dependence.
3. **Pyromania** involves having an irresistible urge to set fires. Very little research has been conducted on this rare disorder.

4. **Pathological gambling** affects an increasing number of people, approximately 3% to 5% of adults. This disorder has some parallels with substance abuse, such as the need to gamble increasing amounts of money over time, and the presence of "withdrawal symptoms" when attempting to stop. There is a growing body of research on the nature and treatment of pathological gambling.
5. **Trichotillomania** is the urge to pull out one's own hair from anywhere on the body, including the scalp, eyebrows, and arms. This disorder can often have severe social consequences, and those affected may go to great lengths to conceal their behavior.

OVERALL SUMMARY

This chapter outlines the major features of substance-related disorders (i.e., use, dependence, abuse, intoxication, withdrawal), including categories regarding depressants (i.e., alcohol, barbiturates, and benzodiazepines), stimulants (i.e., amphetamines, cocaine, nicotine, and caffeine), opiates (i.e., heroin, codeine, morphine), and hallucinogens (i.e., marijuana, and LSD). In addition, patterns of drug use, etiological factors, mechanisms of action, and treatments are discussed within an integrative bio-psycho-social framework. The chapter concludes with a review and discussion of impulse control disorders.

KEY TERMS

Agonist substitution (p. 408)
Alcohol dehydrogenase (p.387)
Alcohol use disorders (p. 385)
Amphetamine use disorders (p. 390)
Antagonist drugs (p. 408)
Barbiturates (p. 389)
Benzodiazepines (p. 389)
Caffeine use disorders (p. 395)
Cocaine use disorders (p. 392)
Controlled drinking (p. 410)
Depressants (p. 385)
Fetal alcohol syndrome (p. 387)
GABA system (p. 386)
Hallucinogen use disorder (p. 398)
Hallucinogens (p. 385)
Impulse-control disorders (p.379)
Intermittent explosive disorder (p.413)
Kleptomania (p.413)
LSD (d-lysergic acid diethylamide) (p. 399)
Marijuana (p. 398)
Nicotine use disorders (p. 393)
Opiates (p. 385)

Opiod use disorders (p. 396)
Pathological gambling (p. 413)
Polysubstance use (p. 379)
Psychoactive substances (p. 380)
Pyromania (p. 413)
Relapse prevention (p. 411)
Stimulants (p. 385)
Substance abuse (p. 381)
Substance dependence (p. 381)
Substance-related disorders (p. 379)
Substance intoxication (p. 381)
Tolerance (p. 381)
Trichotillomania (p. 414)
Withdrawal (p. 381)
Withdrawal delirium (delirium tremens/"DTs")(p. 386)

INFOTRAC KEY TERM EXERCISES

Each exercise is linked to key terms from the Wadsworth InfoTrac on-line searchable database. Key terms must be entered exactly as written.

Exercise 1: **Pulling Your Hair Out: An Impulse Control Problem or Variant of OCD?**
Article: A17716186
Citation: (Childhood trichotillomania: clinical phenomenology, comorbidity, and family genetics.). Robert A. King, Larry Scahill, Lawrence A. Vitulano, Mary Schwab-Stone, Kenneth P. Tercyak, & Mark A. Riddle. Journal of the American Academy of Child and Adolescent Psychiatry, Nov 1995 v34 n11 p1451(9)

According to the DSM-IV-TR, trichotillomania is an impulse control disorder, grouped along with other serious antisocial conditions as kleptomania, pathological gambling, pyromania, and intermittent explosive disorder. In contrast to the current DSM-IV approach, the present article suggests that trichotillomania may resemble obsessive-compulsive disorder (OCD) in its phenomenology, pathophysiology, and reported response to serotonergic agents. You are to review this InfoTrac article and then make a case, backed by appropriate data, for one of the following positions: (a) trichotillomania is an impulse control disorder not a variant of OCD, or (b) trichotillomania is a variant of OCD and belongs with the anxiety disorders. Limit your answer to 3-5 double-spaced pages.

Exercise 2: **Efficacy of Nicotine Nasal Spray as a Treatment for Nicotine Addiction**
Key Term: *Nicotine Nasal Spray*

Nicotine nasal spray represents one of the latest medical treatments for nicotine addiction. Your task here is to review the InfoTrac articles on the efficacy of nicotine nasal spray relative to other medical and psychological treatments for nicotine addition. What do we know about this new form of treatment? And, is there enough evidence to warrant its continued use as a treatment for nicotine addition? Limit your answer to 3-5 double-spaced pages.

Exercise 3: **College Binge Drinking: A Potentially Problematic Facet of College Life**
Key Term: *Binge Drinking*

Alcohol use appears to be a regularly accepted part of college life and many college students appear to binge drink regularly. What constitutes binge drinking?, and when does alcohol use among college students border on abuse? Does college drinking predict later alcoholism and other related problems? Review the InfoTrac articles on college drinking behaviors. In so doing, assume the role of a writer for the New York Times. Assimilate what is known about the prevalence of college drinking, particularly binge drinking, and include information about psychological and other factors that seem related to regular use and abuse of alcohol among college students. In light of the evidence, does you believe that college binge drinking is a problem? Take a position and defend it. Limit your answer to 3-5 double-spaced pages.

Exercise 4 (Future Trend): Addiction by Prescription: A Growing National Problem

A recent 2002 National Survey on Drug Use and Health, sponsored by the Substance Abuse and Mental Health Services Administration (SAMHSA), showed that the second most popular category of drug use after marijuana is the non-medical use of prescription drugs. An estimated 6.2 million people, 2.6 percent of the population aged 12 or older are misusing prescription drugs. Of these, an estimated 4.4 million used narcotic pain relievers, 1.8 million used anti-anxiety medications (also known as tranquilizers), 1.2 million used stimulants and 0.4 million used sedatives. The growing problem of abuse and addiction to prescription medications can be described and illustrated. The following link is to a SAMHSA web site with extensive information on prescription drug abuse, relevant links, including a multi-media video segment that you can show in the classroom.

http://www.recoverymonth.gov/2004/multimedia/w.aspx?ID=245

CLASSROOM ACTIVITIES, DEMONSTRATIONS, AND LECTURE TOPICS

1. **Activity: Survey on Drug Use/Abuse Patterns.** Many students believe that drug use and abuse have declined dramatically over the years, regardless of the drug type or classification (e.g., licit vs. illicit, hallucinogens vs. stimulants, etc.). One way to foster discussion on this topic is to ask students to complete HANDOUT 11.1; a survey developed by Dr. George F. Koob of the University of California, San Diego Department of Psychology before discussing Chapter 3. Dr. Koob has compiled the survey results from his *Drugs, Addiction, and Mental Disorder* classes for more than a decade and shares indications of certain trends in drug use with his students each year. A good follow-up assignment would allow students to research articles addressing the prevalence of drug use among certain populations (e.g. 18-24 yr old male vs. female smoking rates, etc.); do the survey results match what the scientific literature concludes regarding drug use in the U.S.?

2. **Activity: Demonstrate Cigarette Smoking Residue.** This exercise can be used to demonstrate the residue that remains in the body when smoking a cigarette. You will need two cigarettes and a "smoking apparatus" in this exercise. The apparatus can be borrowed

from a local chapter of the American Cancer Society or American Lung Association, or it can be built at home. To build the apparatus, you need the following items:

a. A clean, empty, flexible plastic bottle such as a dishwashing soap container with a top (transparent bottle would be ideal).
b. Plastic tubing about the size of a cigarette; a cigarette must be able to fit snugly within the tubing.
c. A small ball of clay, a cotton ball or loose cotton, a book of matches, and two index cards on which to place cigarette parts and transparent tape.

Make an opening in the bottle cap so the tubing fits snugly. Insert the tubing through the hole, leaving about an inch extending out of the top. Use the clay to form a seal where the tube meets the top. Insert loosely packed cotton into the opposite end of the tubing. Be sure to do this demonstration in a well-ventilated room. The procedure is as follows:

a. Squeeze air out of the bottle and place cigarette firmly into the end of the tubing.
b. Light the cigarette and begin to slowly compress and release the sides of the bottle. Continue until the cigarette is almost completely "smoked."
c. Remove the cigarette, cut off the filter, tape it to the index card, and pass it around. Discuss the residue that remains and the effectiveness of filters.
d. Remove the cotton from the tubing, tape it to the index card, and pass it around. This represents the residue that is introduced into a "smoker's" lungs despite the presence of a filter.

3. **Activity: Should Mandatory Drug Testing Become Part of Campus Life?** Mandatory random drug testing is increasingly routine in large corporations. Yet, whether such drug testing curbs drug abuse is a matter for which there is still considerable debate. Mandatory drug testing raises a host of ethical and constitutional issues about right to privacy. Discuss the issues related to mandatory drug testing and ask students to consider whether colleges and universities should adopt a regular policy of random drug testing among their students. What would be the implications of this move for drug use on college campuses? Would such a policy work to deter drug use? This topic should result in some lively discussion and debate.

4. **Activity: Student Response to Signs of Addiction in Friends and Family.** Ask students to break up in small groups for this exercise and have each group address how they would approach a situation where they strongly suspected that either a family member or close friend was on the road to addiction. Would they be comfortable saying anything to that person about his or her use of drugs? How would they broach the subject? What sorts of reactions might they expect in the other person after they confronted him or her? What steps would they take to help that person? Sample the responses from different groups, tally them on an overhead or the blackboard, and open the discussion up to an analysis of the assets and liabilities of different proposals.

5. **Video Activity: The Case of Tim and the Problem of Alcohol Dependence.** Show the film segment on Part II of the videotape "Abnormal Psychology: Inside/Out, Video 1, Vol 1" that presents an interview with a patient (Tim) who suffers from alcohol

dependence. Ask the students to consider how why it took the negative consequences of alcohol abuse to lead Tim to the realization he had a problem with alcohol. What role did Tim's family play in perpetuating Tim's pattern of addiction and what might have been done to prevent Tim from developing full-blow alcoholism. Finally, what treatment do the students think would be best for Tim (e.g., controlled drinking or complete alcohol abstinence)?

HANDOUT 11.1

Substance Abuse Questionnaire

A. Do not write your name on the questionnaire (responses are anonymous)
B. Please circle the most correct response
C. State both medical and recreational experiences

Age: _____ Sex: M F

1.	Do you smoke cigarettes (tobacco)?		No	Yes
2.	Do you smoke other tobacco products (cigar, pipe, clove)?		No	Yes
3.	Do you chew or snuff tobacco?		No	Yes
4.	Have you ever consumed marijuana or hashish?		No	Yes
5.	Have you consumed marijuana/hashish *within the last 30 days?*		No	Yes
6.	Have you ever tried amphetamines (speed, crystal)?		No	Yes
7.	Have you consumed amphetamines *within the last 30 days?*		No	Yes
8.	Have you ever tried cocaine?		No	Yes
9.	Have you ever tried crack cocaine (smoke freebase)?		No	Yes
10.	Have you consumed cocaine *within the last 30 days?*		No	Yes
11.	Have you ever tried:			
		LSD (acid)?	No	Yes
		Heroin?	No	Yes
		Morphine?	No	Yes
		Barbiturates (e.g., Luminal, Nembutal, etc.)	No	Yes
		PCP (angel dust)?	No	Yes
		Darvon (propoxyphene)?	No	Yes
		Hallucinogenic mushrooms?	No	Yes
		Ecstasy (MDMA)?	No	Yes
		Inhalants (e.g., nitrous oxide, etc.)	No	Yes
12.	Do you drink:			
		Alcoholic beverages?	No	Yes
		Some beer each week?	No	Yes
		Some wine each week?	No	Yes
		Some mixed drinks each week?	No	Yes
13.	*Within the last 30 days* have you used:			
		Prescription sleeping pills?	No	Yes
		Over-the-counter pain relievers?	No	Yes
		Minor tranquilizers (e.g., Xanax, etc.)?	No	Yes
		Diet pills?	No	Yes
14.	Do you *think* you have a problem with substance abuse?		No	Yes
	If yes, which substance(s)______________________________			
15.	If you previously had a problem, are you now problem-free?		No	Yes

SUPPLEMENTARY READING MATERIAL FOR CHAPTER ELEVEN

(🔍 = These sources can be found on *"Infotrac, the online library"* provided by Wadsworth and Brooks/Cole Publishing.)

🔍 Bell, D. C., Montoya, I. D., Richard, A. J., & Dayton, C. A. (1998). The motivation for drug abuse treatment: Testing cognitive and 12-step theories. American Journal of Drug and Alcohol Abuse, 24, 551(1).

Donovan, D. M., & Marlatt, G. A. (Eds.) (1988). Assessment of addictive behaviors. New York: Guilford.

Galanter, M. (1996). Recent developments in alcoholism, Volume 13: Alcohol and violence: Epidemiology, neurobiology, psychology, and family issues. New York: Plenum.

Galanter, M., & Kleber, H. D. (Eds). (1994). Textbook of substance abuse treatment. Washington, DC: American Psychiatric Press.

Goldstein, A. (1994). Addiction from biology to drug policy. New York: Freeman.

Gomberg, E., & Nirenberg, T. D. (Eds.) (1994). Women and substance abuse. Norwood, NJ: Ablex Press.

Gorski, T., & Miller, M. (1986). Staying sober: A guide for relapse prevention. Independence, MO: Independence Press.

Gootenberg, P. (1999). Cocaine: Global histories. New York: Routledge.

Heather, N., Miller, W. R., & Greeley, J. (Eds.) (1994). Self-control and addictive behaviors. New York: Pergamon.

Hester, R., & Miller, W. R. (1989). Handbook of alcoholism treatment approaches. New York: Pergamon.

Marlatt, G. A., & Gordan, J. R. (1985). Relapse prevention: Maintenance strategies in the treatment of addictive behaviors. New York: Guilford.

McCrady, B. S., & Miller, W. R. (Eds.) (1993). Research on Alcoholics Anonymous: Opportunities and alternatives. New Brunswick, NJ: Alcohol Research Documentation.

Meyers, R. J., & Smith, J. D. (1995). Clinical guide to alcohol treatment: The community reinforcement approach. New York: Guilford.

Rotgers, F., Keller, D. S., & Morgenstern, J. (Eds.) (1996). Treating substance abuse: Theory and technique. New York: Guilford.

Stoil, M. J., & Hill, G. (1996). Preventing substance abuse: Interventions that work. New York: Plenum.

Streissguth, A. (1999). Fetal alcohol syndrome: A guide for families and communities. New York: Brooks Cole.

Tucker, J. A., Donovan, D. M., & Marlatt, G. A. (Eds.) (2001). Changing addictive behavior: Bridging clinical and public health strategies. New York: Guilford.

Westermeyer, J., & Boedicker, A. E. (2000). Course, severity, and treatment of substance abuse among women versus men. American Journal of Drug and Alcohol Abuse, 26, 523.

SUPPLEMENTARY 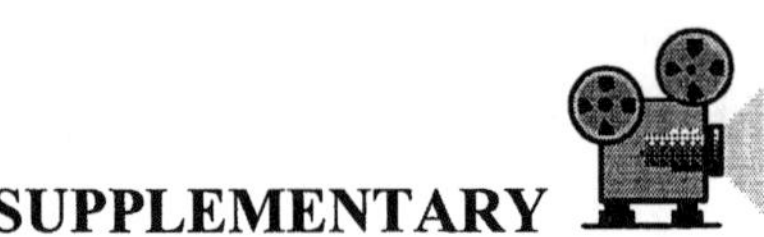 VIDEO RESOURCES FOR CHAPTER ELEVEN

Abnormal psychology inside/out, video 2, vol 1. (*available through your International Thomson Learning representative).* The video presents an interview with Tim; a patient who suffers from alcohol abuse/dependence. Tim describes how he first came to realize he had a problem with alcohol when he was arrested for assaulting others, including family problems and accumulated DWIs. (13 min)

Addictions and mental illness. (Insight Media: 2162 Broadway, New York, NY 10024/ (800)-233-9910). Many mentally ill people are also addicted to drugs and alcohol. Explaining that these are separate problems that require separate treatments, this video discusses the theory of "self-medicating" and addresses the historic failure of the psychiatric and substance-abuse counseling communities to share information. It includes case profiles and discusses current research that might help identify at-risk adolescents before they start to have problems. (28 min)

Clean and sober. (Hollywood Film; Drama). This film provides a nice portrayal of AA, cocaine addiction, and alcoholism.

CNN today: Abnormal psychology, vol. 1. (*available through your International Thomson Learning representative).* This video contains three segments related to substance abuse and its disorders.

The first segment, titled "Substance-Related Disorders: Teen Drug Abuse" discusses how drugs can also be found in the suburbs and presents the cases of teenagers who died of heroin overdoses. (3 min, 8 sec)

The second segment, titled "Fighting Addiction," presents the case of an alcoholic, including an overview of animal research regarding the mechanisms involved in relapse and research efforts to better understand and treat addictions more generally. (2 min, 16 sec)

The third segment, titled "Marijuana Brains," describes the negative consequences of regular marijuana use on brain function, including an overview of associated attention-related problems. (3 min, 21 sec)

Cognitive-behavioral relapse prevention for addictions. (Insight Media: 2162 Broadway, New York, NY 10024/ (800)-233-9910). Presenting G. Alan Marlatt in an unscripted session with an improvisational actor portraying a client, this video offers viewers the opportunity to witness a wholly naturalistic client-therapist interaction. It focuses on the use of cognitive-behavioral techniques to prevent relapse. (40 min)

Drug addiction. (Insight Media: 2162 Broadway, New York, NY 10024/ (800)-233-9910). The first volume of this set discusses the psychological and physical reasons people start and continue to use drugs. The second offers practical guidelines for treatment. It covers physical and psychological treatments, discusses the legal aspects of prescription, addresses the role of drug screening, and reviews relevant public health issues. (2 Volumes/29 min total)

Drug profiles: Physical and mental aspects. (Insight Media: 2162 Broadway, New York, NY 10024/ (800)-233-9910). This video examines the physical symptoms and psychological effects of ten drugs of abuse — cocaine, heroin, methaqualone, alcohol, marijuana, barbiturates, amphetamines, tranquilizers, PCP, and LSD. It explains their chemical nature and details their effects on the central nervous system. (28 min)

Psychology of addiction. (Insight Media: 2162 Broadway, New York, NY 10024/ (800)-233-9910). This video explains how the physical realities of chemical addiction generate psychological results, showing how chemical substances move through the body to the brain, where psychological effects include denial, rationalization, minimization, and projection of internal problems onto others. It also discusses how these distortions can provoke people closest to an addict to behave similarly in an effort to cope. (34 min)

Stages of change for addictions. (Insight Media: 2162 Broadway, New York, NY 10024/ (800)-233-9910). Featuring the commentary of John C. Norcross, this video identifies the stages of addressing and dealing with addiction. It presents Norcross' sessions with a client who is in early recovery from cocaine addiction and is contemplating changing his use of alcohol. (80 min)

Sweet nothing. (Hollywood Film; Drama). This film depicts the nature of crack addiction and is based on a true story.

Trainspotting. (Hollywood Film; Drama/Comedy). This film depicts the heroin scene in Edinburgh and presents accurate depictions of cold turkey heroin withdrawal symptoms.

Under the influence: The science of drug abuse. (Insight Media: 2162 Broadway, New York, NY 10024/ (800)-233-9910). What happens to the human brain when a person is high, intoxicated, or addicted to drugs? This video examines questions of effect, addiction, and the human hunger for mind-altering substances. It discusses the dynamics of drugs, drug abuse, and human behavior, and includes brain scans and interviews with physicians. (25 min)

INTERNET 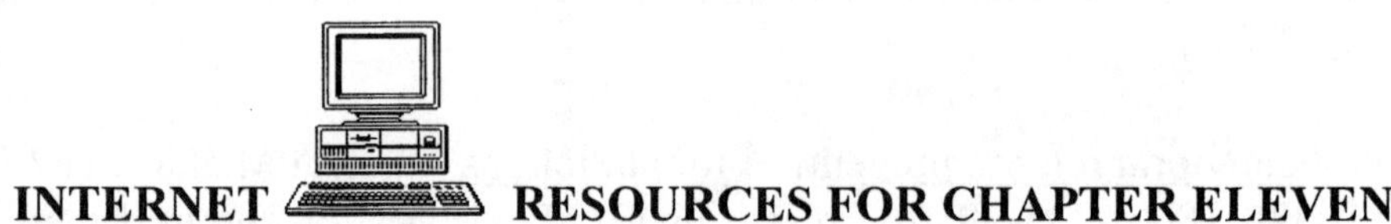 RESOURCES FOR CHAPTER ELEVEN

Alcoholics Anonymous
http://www.alcoholics-anonymous.org/

The official web page for Alcoholics Anonymous; information includes the "Twelve Steps to Recovery".

Center for Education and Drug Abuse Research (CEDAR)
http://cedar.pharmacy.pitt.edu

CEDAR serves to elucidate the factors contributing to the variation in the liability to drug abuse and determine the developmental pathways culminating in drug abuse outcome, normal outcome, and psychiatric/behavioral disorder outcome. CEDAR is a consortium between the University of Pittsburgh and St. Francis Medical Center.

Cocaine Anonymous Home Page
http://www.ca.org/

This group uses the Twelve Steps program to help recovering cocaine addicts. Includes phone numbers for local chapters as well as web links.

King County Department of Community and Human Services, Mental Health, Chemical Abuse, and Dependency Services Division
http://www.metrokc.gov/dchs/mhd/mhlinks.htm

This web site provides links to external web sites that contain reference material on mental health/chemical abuse related subjects.

National Clearinghouse for Alcohol and Drug Information
http://www.health.org/

This web site provides a wealth of information about substance use and abuse provided by the Department of Health and Human Services.

National Council on Problem Gambling
http://www.ncpgambling.org/

This web site is a great resource about issues related to problem gambling and its treatment.

National Institute on Drug Abuse (NIDA)
http://www.nida.nih.gov/

This site provides a wealth of information about drug abuse, drug treatment, and current research, including informative fact sheets about most major drugs of abuse.

Neurobiology of Addition (NIDA)
http://www.nida.nih.gov/Teaching2/Teaching.html

This National Institute of Drug Abuse site is exclusively devoted to the neurobiology of addiction, and includes some excellent free Powerpoint teaching slides. Follow additional NIDA links to other invaluable teaching resources at this site. A must see!!

Web of Addictions
http://www.well.com/user/woa/

This web site provides fact sheets on drugs and abuse, links to other internet resources, and places to get help with addictions.

WARNING SIGNS OF ALCOHOL ABUSE AND DEPENDENCY

- Drinking heavily after a disappointment, a quarrel, or when a boss is difficult
- Drinking more heavily when experiencing difficulties or feeling under pressure
- Ability to "handle" more liquor than when you first started drinking
- Failure to remember events occurring during a previous drinking episode
- Drinking extra amounts of alcohol secretively during social gatherings
- Feeling uncomfortable during occasions when alcohol is not available
- Feeling guilty about drinking
- Feeling irritated when family or friends discuss your drinking
- An increase in the frequency of memory blackouts
- Wishing to continue drinking after others say "enough is enough"
- Having a reason for the occasions when you drink heavily
- Feeling regret while sober for things said or done while drinking
- Attempts to switch brands or to follow different plans to control drinking
- Failure to keep promises about cutting down on drinking
- Failed attempts to control drinking by making a change in jobs or moving
- Avoidance of family or close friends while drinking
- Having an increasing number of financial and work problems
- Feeling as though more people are treating you unfairly without good reason
- Eating very little or irregularly while drinking
- Drinking in the morning to alleviate the shakes
- Noticing that it is difficult to drink as much as previously
- Staying drunk for several days at a time
- Feeling depressed and wondering whether life is worth living
- Hearing or seeing things that aren't there following a period of drinking
- Experiencing extreme fear after heavy drinking

WARNING SIGNS OF ADDICTION (GENERAL)

- Losing time from work due to drinking/drugs
- Drinking/using drugs makes home life unhappy
- Drinking/using drugs because of shyness around other people
- Drinking/using drugs is negatively affecting your reputation
- Feeling remorse after drinking/using drugs
- Experiencing financial difficulties as a result of drinking/drugs
- Decreased ambition since drinking/using drugs
- Craving a drink/drugs at a definite time daily
- Wanting a drink/drugs the next morning
- Experiencing sleeping problems related to drinking/using drugs
- Decreased efficiency since drinking/using drugs
- Drinking/using drugs is jeopardizing one's job or business
- Drinking/using drugs to escape from worries or troubles
- Drinking/using drugs while alone
- Experiencing a complete loss of memory as a result of drinking/using drugs
- Drinking/using drugs to build up self-confidence
- Hospitalization or medical care due to drinking/drug use

WARNING SIGNS OF COMPULSIVE GAMBLING

- Preoccupation with gambling (e.g., thinking of ways to get money to gamble)
- Lost time from work or family due to your gambling
- Neglected responsibilities to yourself or family to gamble
- Pawned or sold personal possessions for gambling money
- Borrowed money under false pretences to gamble
- Need to gamble with increasing amounts of money to achieve excitement
- Repeated unsuccessful efforts to control, cut back, or stop gambling
- Restless or irritable when attempting to cut down or stop gambling
- Gamble as a way of escaping from problems or of relieving negative feelings
- After losing money gambling, do you often return another day to get even?
- Lying to conceal the extent of involvement with gambling
- Committing illegal acts (e.g., forgery, fraud, theft) to finance gambling
- Jeopardizing a significant relationship, job, educational/career opportunity because of gambling
- Relying on others to provide money to relieve a desperate financial situation caused by gambling
- Feeling hopeless, depressed or suicidal due to gambling

DSM-IV-TR Criteria for Substance Abuse

A. A maladaptive pattern of substance use leading to clinically significant impairment or distress, as manifested by one (or more) of the following, occurring within a 12-month period:

1. recurrent substance use resulting in a failure to fulfill major role obligations at work, school, or home (e.g., repeated absences or poor work performance related to substance use; substance-related absences, suspensions, or expulsions from school; neglect of children or household)
2. recurrent substance use in situations in which it is physically hazardous (e.g., driving an automobile or operating a machine when impaired by substance use)
3. recurrent substance-related legal problems (e.g., arrests for substance-related disorderly conduct)
4. continued substance use despite having persistent or recurrent social or interpersonal problems caused or exacerbated by the effects of the substance (e.g., arguments with spouse about consequences of Intoxication, physical fights)

B. The symptoms have never met the criteria for Substance Dependence for this class of substance.

DSM-IV-TR Criteria for Substance Dependence

A maladaptive pattern of substance use, leading to clinically significant impairment or distress, as manifested by three (or more) of the following, occurring at any time in the same 12-month period:

1. tolerance, as defined by either of the following:
    a. a need for markedly increased amounts of the substance to achieve Intoxication or desired effect
    b. markedly diminished effect with continued use of the same amount of the substance
2. Withdrawal, as manifested by either of the following:
    a. the characteristic withdrawal syndrome for the substance (refer to Criteria A and B of the criteria sets for Withdrawal from the specific substances)
    b. the same (or a closely related) substance is taken to relieve or avoid withdrawal symptoms
3. the substance is often taken in larger amounts or over a longer period than was intended
4. there is a persistent desire or unsuccessful efforts to cut down or control substance use
5. a great deal of time is spent in activities necessary to obtain the substance (e.g., visiting multiple doctors or driving long distances), use the substance (e.g., chain-smoking), or recover from its effects
6. important social, occupational, or recreational activities are given up or reduced because of substance use
7. the substance use is continued despite knowledge of having a persistent or recurrent physical or psychological problem that is likely to have been caused or exacerbated by the substance (e.g., current cocaine use despite recognition of cocaine-induced depression, or continued drinking despite recognition that an ulcer was made worse by alcohol consumption)

Specify if:

With Physiological Dependence: evidence of tolerance or withdrawal (i.e., either Item 1 or 2 is present)

Without Physiological Dependence: no evidence of tolerance or withdrawal (i.e., neither Item 1 nor 2 is present)

Course specifiers (see text for definitions):

Early Full Remission **Sustained Partial Remission**
Early Partial Remission **On Agonist Therapy**
Sustained Full Remission In a Controlled Environment

DSM-IV-TR Criteria for Substance Intoxication

A. The development of a reversible substance-specific syndrome due to recent ingestion of (or exposure to) a substance.

Note: Different substances may produce similar or identical syndromes.

B. Clinically significant maladaptive behavioral or psychological changes that are due to the effect of the substance on the central nervous system (e.g., belligerence, mood lability, cognitive impairment, impaired judgment, impaired social or occupational functioning) and develop during or shortly after use of the substance.

C. The symptoms are not due to a general medical condition and are not better accounted for by another mental disorder.

DSM-IV-TR Criteria for Substance Withdrawal

A. The development of a substance-specific syndrome due to the cessation of (or reduction in) substance use that has been heavy and prolonged.

B. The substance-specific syndrome causes clinically significant distress or impairment in social, occupational, or other important areas of functioning.

C. The symptoms are not due to a general medical condition and are not better accounted for by another mental disorder.

DSM-IV-TR Criteria for Alcohol Intoxication

A. Recent ingestion of alcohol.

B. Clinically significant maladaptive behavioral or psychological changes (e.g., inappropriate sexual or aggressive behavior, mood lability, impaired judgment, impaired social or occupational functioning) that developed during, or shortly after, alcohol ingestion.

C. One (or more) of the following signs, developing during, or shortly after, alcohol use:

1. slurred speech
2. incoordination
3. unsteady gait
4. nystagmus
5. impairment in attention or memory
6. stupor or coma

D. The symptoms are not due to a general medical condition and are not better accounted for by another mental disorder.

Transparency 11-6

DSM-IV-TR Criteria for Alcohol Withdrawal

A. Cessation of (or reduction in) alcohol use that has been heavy and prolonged.

B. Two (or more) of the following, developing within several hours to a few days after Criterion A:

1. autonomic hyperactivity (e.g., sweating or pulse rate greater than 100)
2. increased hand tremor
3. insomnia
4. nausea or vomiting
5. transient visual, tactile, or auditory hallucinations or illusions
6. psychomotor agitation
7. anxiety
8. grand mal seizures

C. The symptoms in Criterion B cause clinically significant distress or impairment in social, occupational, or other important areas of functioning.

D. The symptoms are not due to a general medical condition and are not better accounted for by another mental disorder. Specify if: With Perceptual Disturbance

DSM-IV-TR Criteria for Sedative, Hypnotic, or Anxiolytic Intoxication

A. Recent use of a sedative, hypnotic, or anxiolytic.

B. Clinically significant maladaptive behavioral or psychological changes (e.g., inappropriate sexual or aggressive behavior, mood lability, impaired judgment, impaired social or occupational functioning) that developed during, or shortly after, sedative, hypnotic, or anxiolytic use.

C. One (or more) of the following signs, developing during, or shortly after, sedative, hypnotic, or anxiolytic use:

1. slurred speech
2. incoordination
3. unsteady gait
4. nystagmus
5. impairment in attention or memory
6. stupor or coma

D. The symptoms are not due to a general medical condition and are not better accounted for by another mental disorder.

DSM-IV-TR Criteria for Sedative, Hypnotic, or Anxiolytic Withdrawal

A. Cessation of (or reduction in) sedative, hypnotic, or anxiolytic use that has been heavy and prolonged.

B. Two (or more) of the following, developing within several hours to a few days after Criterion A:

1. autonomic hyperactivity (e.g., sweating or pulse rate greater than 100)
2. increased hand tremor
3. Insomnia
4. nausea or vomiting
5. transient visual, tactile, or auditory hallucinations or illusions
6. psychomotor agitation
7. anxiety
8. grand mal seizures

C. The symptoms in Criterion B cause clinically significant distress or impairment in social, occupational, or other important areas of functioning.

D. The symptoms are not due to a general medical condition and are not better accounted for by another mental disorder.

Specify if:

With Perceptual Disturbances

DSM-IV-TR Criteria for Amphetamine Intoxication

A. Recent use of amphetamine or a related substance (e.g., methylphenidate).

B. Clinically significant maladaptive behavioral or psychological changes (e.g., euphoria or affective blunting; changes in sociability; hypervigilance; interpersonal sensitivity; anxiety, tension, or anger; stereotyped behaviors; impaired judgment; or impaired social or occupational functioning) that developed during, or shortly after, use of amphetamine or a related substance.

C. Two (or more) of the following, developing during, or shortly after, use of amphetamine or a related substance:

1. tachycardia or bradycardia
2. pupillary dilation
3. elevated or lowered blood pressure
4. perspiration or chills
5. nausea or vomiting
6. evidence of weight loss
7. psychomotor agitation or retardation
8. muscular weakness, respiratory depression, chest pain, or cardiac arrhythmias
9. confusion, seizures, dyskinesias, dystonias, or coma

D. The symptoms are not due to a general medical condition and are not better accounted for by another mental disorder.

Specify if:

With Perceptual Disturbances

DSM-IV-TR Criteria for Amphetamine Withdrawal

A. Cessation of (or reduction in) amphetamine (or a related substance) use that ha been heavy and prolonged.

B. Dysphoric mood and two (or more) of the following physiological changes, developing within a few hours to several days after Criterion A:

1. fatigue
2. vivid, unpleasant dreams
3. Insomnia or Hypersomnia
4. increased appetite
5. psychomotor retardation or agitation

C. The symptoms in Criterion B cause clinically significant distress or impairmen in social, occupational, or other important areas of functioning.

D. The symptoms are not due to a general medical condition and are not better accounted for by another mental disorder.

DSM-IV-TR Criteria for Cocaine Intoxication

A. Recent use of cocaine.

B. Clinically significant maladaptive behavioral or psychological changes (e.g., euphoria or affective blunting; changes in sociability; hypervigilance; interpersonal sensitivity; anxiety, tension, or anger; stereotyped behaviors; impaired judgment; or impaired social or occupational functioning) that developed during, or shortly after, use of cocaine.

C. Two (or more) of the following, developing during, or shortly after, cocaine use:

1. tachycardia or bradycardia
2. pupillary dilation
3. elevated or lowered blood pressure
4. perspiration or chills
5. nausea or vomiting
6. evidence of weight loss
7. psychomotor agitation or retardation
8. muscular weakness, respiratory depression, chest pain, or cardiac arrhythmias
9. confusion, seizures, dyskinesias, dystonias, or coma

D. The symptoms are not due to a general medical condition and are not better accounted for by another mental disorder.

Specify if:

With Perceptual Disturbances

Transparency 11-12

DSM-IV-TR Criteria for Cocaine Withdrawal

A. Cessation of (or reduction in) cocaine use that has been heavy and prolonged.

B. Dysphoric mood and two (or more) of the following physiological changes, developing within a few hours to several days after Criterion A:

1. fatigue
2. vivid, unpleasant dreams
3. Insomnia or Hypersomnia
4. increased appetite
5. psychomotor agitation or retardation

C. The symptoms in Criterion B cause clinically significant distress or impairmer in social, occupational, or other important areas of functioning.

D. The symptoms are not due to a general medical condition and are not better accounted for by another mental disorder.

DSM-IV-TR Criteria for Nicotine Withdrawal

A. Daily use of nicotine for at least several weeks.

B. Abrupt cessation of nicotine use, or reduction in the amount of nicotine used, followed within 24 hours by four (or more) of the following signs:

1. dysphoric or depressed mood
2. Insomnia
3. irritability, frustration, or anger
4. anxiety
5. difficulty concentrating
6. restlessness
7. decreased heart rate
8. increased appetite or weight gain

C. The symptoms in Criterion B cause clinically significant distress or impairment in social, occupational, or other important areas of functioning.

D. The symptoms are not due to a general medical condition and are not better accounted for by another mental disorder.

DSM-IV-TR Criteria for Caffeine Intoxication

A. Recent consumption of caffeine, usually in excess of 250 mg (e.g., more than 2-3 cups of brewed coffee).

B. Five (or more) of the following signs, developing during, or shortly after, caffeine use:

1. restlessness
2. nervousness
3. excitement
4. Insomnia
5. flushed face
6. diuresis
7. gastrointestinal disturbance
8. muscle twitching
9. rambling flow of thought and speech
10. tachycardia or cardiac arrhythmia
11. periods of inexhaustibility
12. psychomotor agitation

C. The symptoms in Criterion B cause clinically significant distress or impairmen in social, occupational, or other important areas of functioning.

D. The symptoms are not due to a general medical condition and are not better accounted for by another mental disorder (e.g., an Anxiety Disorder).

DSM-IV-TR Criteria for Opiod Intoxication

A. Recent use of an opioid.

B. Clinically significant maladaptive behavioral or psychological changes (e.g., initial euphoria followed by apathy, dysphoria, psychomotor agitation or retardation, impaired judgment, or impaired social or occupational functioning) that developed during, or shortly after, opioid use.

C. Pupillary constriction (or pupillary dilation due to anoxia from severe overdose) and one (or more) of the following signs, developing during, or shortly after, opioid use:

1. drowsiness or coma
2. slurred speech
3. impairment in attention or memory

D. The symptoms are not due to a general medical condition and are not better accounted for by another mental disorder.

Specify if:

With Perceptual Disturbances

Transparency 11-16

DSM-IV-TR Criteria for Opiod Withdrawal

A. Either of the following:
1. cessation of (or reduction in) opioid use that has been heavy and prolonged (several weeks or longer)
2. administration of an opioid antagonist after a period of opioid use

B. Three (or more) of the following, developing within minutes to several days after Criterion A:
1. dysphoric mood
2. nausea or vomiting
3. muscle aches
4. lacrimation or rhinorrhea
5. pupillary dilation, piloerection, or sweating
6. diarrhea
7. yawning
8. fever
9. Insomnia

C. The symptoms in Criterion B cause clinically significant distress or impairmer in social, occupational, or other important areas of functioning.

D. The symptoms are not due to a general medical condition and are not better accounted for by another mental disorder.

DSM-IV-TR Criteria for Hallucinogen Intoxication

A. Recent use of a hallucinogen.

B. Clinically significant maladaptive behavioral or psychological changes (e.g., marked anxiety or depression, ideas of reference, fear of losing one's mind, paranoid ideation, impaired judgment, or impaired social or occupational functioning) that developed during, or shortly after, hallucinogen use.

C. Perceptual changes occurring in a state of full wakefulness and alertness (e.g., subjective intensification of perceptions, depersonalization, derealization, illusions, hallucinations, synesthesias) that developed during, or shortly after, hallucinogen use.

D. Two (or more) of the following signs, developing during, or shortly after, hallucinogen use:

1. pupillary dilation
2. tachycardia
3. sweating
4. palpitations
5. blurring of vision
6. tremors
7. incoordination

E. The symptoms are not due to a general medical condition and are not better accounted for by another mental disorder.

DSM-IV-TR Criteria for Hallucinogen Persisting Perception Disorder (Flashbacks)

A. The reexperiencing, following cessation of use of a hallucinogen, of one or more of the perceptual symptoms that were experienced while intoxicated with the hallucinogen (e.g., geometric hallucinations, false perceptions of movement in the peripheral visual fields, flashes of color, intensified colors, trails of images of moving objects, positive afterimages, halos around objects, macropsia, and micropsia).

B. The symptoms in Criterion A cause clinically significant distress or impairment in social, occupational, or other important areas of functioning.

C. The symptoms are not due to a general medical condition (e.g., anatomical lesions and infections of the brain, visual epilepsies) and are not better accounted for by another mental disorder (e.g., Delirium, Dementia, Schizophrenia) or hypnopompic hallucinations.

DSM-IV-TR Criteria for Inhalant Intoxication

A. Recent intentional use or short-term, high-dose exposure to volatile inhalants (excluding anesthetic gases and short-acting vasodilators).

B. Clinically significant maladaptive behavioral or psychological changes (e.g., belligerence, assaultiveness, apathy, impaired judgment, impaired social or occupational functioning) that developed during, or shortly after, use of or exposure to volatile inhalants.

C. Two (or more) of the following signs, developing during, or shortly after, inhalant use or exposure:

1. dizziness
2. nystagmus
3. incoordination
4. slurred speech
5. unsteady gait
6. lethargy
7. depressed reflexes
8. psychomotor retardation
9. tremor
10. generalized muscle weakness
11. blurred vision or diplopia
12. stupor or coma
13. euphoria

D. The symptoms are not due to a general medical condition and are not better accounted for by another mental disorder.

DSM-IV-TR Criteria for Phencyclidine Intoxication

A. Recent use of phencyclidine (or a related substance).

B. Clinically significant maladaptive behavioral changes (e.g., belligerence, assaultiveness, impulsiveness, unpredictability, psychomotor agitation, impaired judgment, or impaired social or occupational functioning) that developed during, or shortly after, phencyclidine use.

C. Within an hour (less when smoked, "snorted," or used intravenously), two (or more) of the following signs:

1. vertical or horizontal nystagmus
2. hypertension or tachycardia
3. numbness or diminished responsiveness to pain
4. ataxia
5. dysarthria
6. muscle rigidity
7. seizures or coma
8. hyperacusis

D. The symptoms are not due to a general medical condition and are not better accounted for by another mental disorder.

Specify if:

With Perceptual Disturbances

DSM-IV-TR Criteria for Intermittent Explosive Disorder

A. Several discrete episodes of failure to resist aggressive impulses that result in serious assaultive acts or destruction of property.

B. The degree of aggressiveness expressed during the episodes is grossly out of proportion to any precipitating psychosocial stressors.

C. The aggressive episodes are not better accounted for by another mental disorder (e.g., Antisocial Personality Disorder, Borderline Personality Disorder, a Psychotic Disorder, a Manic Episode, Conduct Disorder, or Attention-Deficit/Hyperactivity Disorder) and are not due to the direct physiological effects of a substance (e.g., a drug of abuse, a medication) or a general medical condition (e.g., head trauma, Alzheimer's disease).

Transparency 11-22

DSM-IV-TR Criteria for Kleptomania

A. Recurrent failure to resist impulses to steal objects that are not needed for personal use or for their monetary value.

B. Increasing sense of tension immediately before committing the theft.

C. Pleasure, gratification, or relief at the time of committing the theft.

D. The stealing is not committed to express anger or vengeance and is not in response to a delusion or a hallucination.

E. The stealing is not better accounted for by Conduct Disorder, a Manic Episode or Antisocial Personality Disorder.

DSM-IV-TR Criteria for Pathological Gambling

A. Persistent and recurrent maladaptive gambling behavior as indicated by five (or more) of the following:

1. is preoccupied with gambling (e.g., preoccupied with reliving past gambling experiences, handicapping or planning the next venture, or thinking of ways to get money with which to gamble)
2. needs to gamble with increasing amounts of money in order to achieve the desired excitement
3. has repeated unsuccessful efforts to control, cut back, or stop gambling
4. is restless or irritable when attempting to cut down or stop gambling
5. gambles as a way of escaping from problems or of relieving a dysphoric mood (e.g., feelings of helplessness, guilt, anxiety, depression)
6. after losing money gambling, often returns another day to get even ("chasing" one's losses)
7. lies to family members, therapist, or others to conceal the extent of involvement with gambling
8. has committed illegal acts such as forgery, fraud, theft, or embezzlement to finance gambling
9. has jeopardized or lost a significant relationship, job, or educational or career opportunity because of gambling
10. relies on others to provide money to relieve a desperate financial situation caused by gambling

B. The gambling behavior is not better accounted for by a Manic Episode.

DSM-IV-TR Criteria for Pyromania

A. Deliberate and purposeful fire setting on more than one occasion.

B. Tension or affective arousal before the act.

C. Fascination with, interest in, curiosity about, or attraction to fire and its situational contexts (e.g., paraphernalia, uses, consequences).

D. Pleasure, gratification, or relief when setting fires, or when witnessing or participating in their aftermath.

E. The fire setting is not done for monetary gain, as an expression of sociopolitic ideology, to conceal criminal activity, to express anger or vengeance, to improve one's living circumstances, in response to a delusion or a hallucination, or as a result of impaired judgment (e.g., in Dementia, Mental Retardation, Substance Intoxication).

F. The fire setting is not better accounted for by Conduct Disorder, a Manic Episode, or Antisocial Personality Disorder.

DSM-IV-TR Criteria for Trichotillomania

A. Recurrent pulling out of one's hair resulting in noticeable hair loss.

B. An increasing sense of tension immediately before pulling out the hair or when attempting to resist the behavior.

C. Pleasure, gratification, or relief when pulling out the hair.

D. The disturbance is not better accounted for by another mental disorder and is not due to a general medical condition (e.g., a dermatological condition).

E. The disturbance causes clinically significant distress or impairment in social, occupational, or other important areas of functioning.

CHAPTER TWELVE

PERSONALITY DISORDERS

LEARNING OBJECTIVES

1. Describe the essential features of personality disorders according to DSM-IV-TR and why they are listed on Axis II.
2. Describe controversies over the reliability and validity of personality disorder diagnoses in the context of categorical vs. dimensional approaches.
3. Describe the essential characteristics of each of the Cluster A (odd/eccentric) personality disorders, including information pertaining to etiology and treatment.
4. Describe the essential characteristics of each of the Cluster B (dramatic/erratic) personality disorders, including information pertaining to etiology and treatment.
5. Understand the distinction and overlap between psychopathy and antisocial personality disorder, including the relation between antisocial personality, violence, criminality, neurobiological influences, and socialization.
6. Describe the essential characteristics of each of the Cluster C (anxious/fearful) personality disorders, including information pertaining to etiology and treatment.
7. Understand problems related to estimating prevalence of personality disorders, including issues related to gender bias, comorbidity, and difficulties in treatment.

OUTLINE

I. An Overview of Personality Disorders
   A. According to DSM-IV-TR, personality disorders are defined as:
      1. "Enduring patterns of perceiving, relating to, and thinking about the environment and oneself that are exhibited in a wide range of social and personal contexts."
      2. Such patterns are also "inflexible and maladaptive, and cause either significant functional impairment or subjective distress."

   B. Personality is a more general term that is used to describe characteristic ways that people think and behave.

   C. Overview of personality disorders
      1. In DSM-IV-TR, personality disorders are coded on **Axis II**, indicating that the problems are chronic and long-term in nature.
      2. The DSM-IV-TR lists 10 specific personality disorders.
      3. Such disorders originate in childhood and continue throughout adulthood, and most are associated with high rates of comorbidity with other Axis I and II conditions. Such problems pervade every aspect of a person's life.
      4. According to the DSM-IV-TR, a person with the personality disorder may or may not be distressed by it. Other persons are often distressed by persons with personality disorders.

D. **Categorical versus dimensional models** reflects the debate over whether personality disorders are extreme versions of normal personality variations (i.e., dimensions) or fundamentally different ways of relating (i.e., categories) as compared to psychologically healthy behaviors.

1. **Categorical models** like the DSM-IV-TR are designed to differentiate syndromes according to separate kinds, and not as problems of degree. Yet, most persons in the field view personality disorders as extremes on one or more personality dimensions.
2. **Dimensional classification models** view personality disorders on a continuum of normal personality and behavior. For example, within a DSM categorical system, one either has or does not have borderline personality disorder; under a more flexible dimensional approach, different characteristics of borderline personality disorder would be viewed along a profile of traits and/or severity.
    a. Advocates of dimensional classification models would like to see DSM categories for personality disorders be supplemented by additional personality dimensions.
    b. The **five factor model** that includes extraversion, agreeableness, conscientiousness, emotional stability, and openness to experience has been proposed for consideration.
    c. Westen and Shedler (1999) proposed **12 personality dimensions** as illustrated in the textbook (i.e., psychological health, psychopathy, hostility, narcissism, emotional dysregulation, dysphoria, schizoid orientation, obsessionality, thought disorder, oedipal conflict, dissociated consciousness, and sexual conflict). This newer system has yet to receive extensive research attention.

E. Personality disorders are organized within the DSM-IV-TR in terms of three groups or **clusters** based on shared resemblance.

1. **Cluster A** is the *odd or eccentric cluster* and includes paranoid, schizoid, and schizotypal personality disorders.
2. **Cluster B** is the *dramatic, emotional, or erratic cluster* and includes antisocial, borderline, histrionic, and narcissistic personality disorders.
3. **Cluster C** is the *anxious or fearful cluster* and includes avoidant, dependant, and obsessive-compulsive personality disorders.

F. Statistics and development

1. Personality disorders are found in 0.5% to 2.5% of the general population, with higher rates in inpatient and outpatient settings.
2. Personality disorders are thought to originate in childhood and continue into the adult years; though relatively little is known about the developmental course of the personality disorders.
3. Significant comorbidity marks this population, with about half of those diagnosed with a personality disorders also meeting diagnostic criteria for another personality disorder.

G. Diagnoses of personality disorders suggest possible gender biases.
   1. For example, borderline personality disorder is diagnosed much more frequently in females, who make up 75% of the identified cases.
   2. Knowledge of whether a client is male or female appears to significantly influence whether s/he receives one personality disorder diagnosis or another.
   3. For example, antisocial personality disorder is assigned more often when the patient is male, whereas a similar description of antisocial personality features with a fictitious female client is more likely to be labeled histrionic personality disorder. Many features of histrionic personality disorder are characteristic of the stereotypical Western female.
   4. **Gender bias** is extremely controversial and may reflect one of the following:
      a. The criteria for a disorder may be biased (i.e., **criterion gender bias**).
      b. The measures and how they are used to assess disorders may be biased (i.e., **assessment gender bias**).

II. Cluster A Personality Disorders
A. Persons with **paranoid personality disorder (PPD)** are excessively mistrustful and suspicious of others, without any justification, and assume that others are out to harm or trick them.
   1. Clinical description of PDD
      a. The defining characteristic of PPD is a pervasive and unjustified distrust and suspiciousness.
      b. Behavioral manifestations of PPD may include being argumentative, voicing frequent complaints, utter silence, ongoing doubt about the reliability and faithfulness of others, reluctance to confide in others, reading hidden, destructive meanings into the innocuous behaviors of others, bearing grudges, and consistent perception of threats from others
      c. Feelings of hostility toward other people are common, and such individuals are very sensitive to criticism and have an excessive need for autonomy.
   2. The textbook illustrates paranoid personality disorder with the case of Jake.
   4. Evidence for a **biological contribution** to PPD is limited, and evidence for a **psychological contribution** is more unclear. The most salient psychological feature is a pervasive negative view of the world and the motives of others; a view that may originate in early childhood.
   5. **Cultural factors** have also been implicated in PPD, particularly in certain groups of people such as prisoners, refugees, people with hearing impairments, and the elderly.
   5. **Treatment for PPD** is made difficult by the fact that few persons with this disorder seek professional help, and when they do, difficulties in developing trusting relationships make establishing a therapeutic relationship with a therapist more difficult.
      a. Treatment focuses on development of trust and may include cognitive therapy to counter the person's mistaken assumptions about others.
      b. There are no good studies showing that treatment is effective for PPD.

B. Persons with **schizoid personality disorder (SZPD)** show a pervasive pattern of detachment from social relationships and a very limited range of emotions in interpersonal situations. The textbook illustrates the features of schizoid personality disorder with the case of Mr. Z.

1. Primary characteristics of SZPD include lack of desire for either close or sexual relationships, preference for solitary activities and few friends, little pleasure in most activities, and indifference or aloofness to the behaviors of others.
   a. The DSM-IV-TR recognizes that at least some people with SZPD are sensitive to the opinions of others but are unwilling or unable to express this emotion. For this group, social isolation may be painful.
   b. Homelessness is quite prevalent in persons with SZPD.
2. The **etiology** of SZPD is unclear. Interestingly, the preference for social isolation resembles aspects of autism; though a link between autism and SZPD has not been established.
3. **Treatment** for SZPD focuses on the value of social relationships, including learning empathy skills, social skills training.
   a. Role playing is used to help the person learn to establish and maintain social relationships.
   b. Treatment prognosis is poor for people with SZPD, and most rarely seek treatment, except in response to a crisis.

C. Persons with **schizotypal personality disorder (STPD)** are typically socially isolated like those with schizoid personality disorder. In addition, those with STPD think and behave in odd and unusual ways, and tend to be highly suspicious and hold odd beliefs. The textbook illustrates schizotypal personality disorder with the case of Mr. S.

1. Such persons show **ideas of reference** (i.e., they think insignificant events relate directly to them), engaging in **magical thinking** (e.g., believing they are clairvoyant or telepathic), and report unusual perceptual experiences such as **illusions** (e.g., feeling the presence of another person when they are alone).
2. Such persons tend not to improve on their own over time, and there is some increased risk that many may go on to develop more severe characteristics of schizophrenia.
3. Several factors are thought to cause STPD and include:
   a. STPD is viewed by some as a phenotype of a schizophrenia genotype and genetic research seems to support such a relationship. Family, twin, and adoption studies have shown an increased prevalence of STPD among relatives of people with schizophrenia who do not have schizophrenia themselves.
   b. Exposure to influenza during pregnancy may increase risk of STPD in the unborn fetus.
   c. Cognitive factors include mild-to-moderate deficits in memory and learning, suggesting damage to the left hemisphere of the brain,

whereas MRI studies suggest more generalized brain abnormalities in STPD individuals.

4. Few controlled treatment studies for STPD exist.
    a. The main treatment focus tends to be on developing social skills.
    b. Given that as many as 30% to 50% of persons with STPD who seek treatment meet criteria for major depressive disorder, therapy also tends to focus on alleviating depressed mood.
    c. Medical treatment tends to follow that for people with schizophrenia.
    d. The prognosis for persons with STPD is not good.

III. Cluster B Personality Disorders

A. Persons with **antisocial personality disorder (ASPD)** tend to have long histories of failing to comply with social norms, violating the rights of others, and engaging in behavior that most persons would find unacceptable (e.g., stealing from friends or family). The textbook illustrates antisocial personality disorder with the case of Ryan.

1. **Clinical Description**: Persons with ASPD tend to be irresponsible, impulsive, and deceitful, lack a conscience and empathy, and selfishly take what they want and do as they please without guilt, regret, or remorse.
    a. Substance abuse occurs in about 83% of persons with antisocial personality disorder.
    b. Long-term outcome of persons with ASPD is poor, regardless of gender.
5. **Psychopathy** was an older term used to characterize what is now ASPD, and included 16 major characteristics; characteristics that are referred to as the Cleckley Criteria after the name of the psychiatrist, Hervey Cleckley, who proposed them.
    a. Examples of **Cleckley criteria** for psychopathy include superficial charm and good intelligence, absence of delusions and other signs of irrational thinking, absence of nervousness, unreliability, untruthfulness and insincerity, lack of remorse or shame, to name few.
    b. **Robert Hare** has done extensive research on the nature of psychopathy and developed a 20-item **Revised Psychopathy Checklist-PCL-R** to assess the following six main criteria: glibness/superficial charm, grandiose sense of self-worth, proneness to boredom/need for stimulation, pathological lying, conning/manipulative, and lack of remorse. Persons scoring high of the PCL-R are less likely to benefit from treatment and are more likely to repeat criminal offenses.
    a. The DSM-IV-TR criteria for ASPD focuses almost entirely on **observable behaviors**, whereas the **Cleckley/Hare** criteria focus primarily on **underlying personality traits**. Some psychopaths are not criminals, nor do they display the DSM-IV-TR criteria of aggressiveness that is part of the criterion for ASPD.
    d. **Dyssocial psychopathy** (i.e., antisocial behavior that is thought to originate in a person's allegiance to a culturally deviant group, such as

a gang) may be included with ASPD, but not psychopathy. Dyssocial psychopaths are presumed to have the capacity for guilt and loyalty.

   e. Psychopathy and ASPD are not synonymous with legal problems. Those that get into legal problems seem to have lower IQs.

3. The diagnosis of **conduct disorder** is reserved for children who engage in behaviors that violate cultural norms.
   a. Many with this disorder become juvenile offenders and tend to become involved with drugs. Many adults with ASPD or psychopathy had conduct disorder as children.
   b. Lack of remorse is not part of the DSM-IV-TR criteria for conduct disorder, but is present for ASPD.
4. Genetic influences
   a. **Family, twin, and adoption studies** all suggest a genetic influence on ASPD and criminality.
   b. A gene-environment interaction appears involved, suggesting that genetic vulnerability interacts with environmental factors such as deficits in early, high quality contact with parents or parent-surrogates.
   c. The average concordance rate for criminality among monozygotic twins is 55%, whereas with dizygotic twins the rate drops to about 13%.
5. Research suggests that **general brain damage** does not explain why people become psychopaths or criminals. Two theories have attracted a great deal of attention: the underarousal hypothesis and the Fearlessness hypothesis.
   a. According to the **underarousal hypothesis**, psychopaths have abnormally low levels or cortical arousal. The Yerkes-Dodson curve suggests that people with either very high or very low levels of arousal tend to experience negative affect and perform poorly in many situations, whereas persons with moderate levels of arousal tend to be relatively content and perform satisfactorily across situations. Low cortical arousal is used to explain antisocial risk taking behavior as such behavior is thought to boost low cortical arousal to acceptable levels. Future criminal behavior is predicted by low skin conductance activity, lower heart rate during rest, and slow brain wave activity.
   b. The **cortical immaturity hypothesis** suggests that the cerebral cortex of psychopaths is at a primitive stage of development and may explain why the behavior of psychopaths is often childlike and impulsive.
   c. According to the **fearlessness hypothesis**, psychopaths show higher thresholds for experiencing fear than most persons. Research suggests that psychopaths have difficulty associating cues with impending punishment or danger.
6. **Jeffrey Gray's model of brain functioning** has also been applied to psychopathy.
   a. The **behavioral inhibition system (BIS)** is responsible for behavior control in response to impending punishment, nonreward, or novel situations that lead to anxiety or frustration. The BIS is thought to be

located in the septohippocampal system and involves noradrenergic and serotonergic neurotransmitter systems.
   b. The **reward system (REW)** is responsible for approach behavior, particularly positive rewards.
   c. An imbalance between the BIS and REW may make the fear and anxiety produced by the BIS less apparent, and positive feelings associated with the REW more prominent which may explain why psychopaths are not concerned about committing antisocial acts.
7. **Psychological and social dimensions** of psychopathy and ASPD include the following:
   a. Psychopaths and persons with ASPD are less likely to be deterred from reaching a goal, despite not being able to attain it.
   b. Family and social factors may also contribute to psychopathy and ASPD, particularly inconsistent parental discipline, trust and solidarity in the family and community neighborhood.
8. **An integrative model of ASPD** includes a genetic vulnerability for antisocial behaviors and related personality traits, perhaps resulting from underarousal or fearlessness, or a propensity for a weak BIS system and an overactive REW system. Family stress and family interaction styles may activate the biological vulnerability, and the resulting antisocial behavior, including problems at school, may further alienate other children that may serve as good role models.
9. **Treatment for ASPD** is complicated by the fact the few persons with such problems see any need for treatment. Antisocial behavior is generally predictive of poor prognosis, even in childhood. Therapists agree that incarceration is often the best alternative.
   a. Most common intervention for children is parent training, where parents are taught to recognize behavior problems early and how to use praise and privileges to reduce problem behavior and to encourage prosocial behaviors.
   b. Juvenile offenders are often treated with a combination of behavioral and family interventions.
10. **Prevention** programs may be the best alternative in the long run, given the ineffectiveness of treatment for adults.

B. Persons with **borderline personality disorder (BPD)** lead tumultuous lives, characterized by patterns of unstable moods and relationships, impulsivity, fear of abandonment, coupled with a very poor self-image and lack of control over their emotions. The textbook illustrates borderline personality disorder with the case of Claire.
1. Clinical description of BPD
   a. Persons with BPD engage in suicidal and/or self-mutilative behaviors, and are often perceived as very intense, moving from anger to deep depression in a short time.
   b. BPD is one of the most common personality disorders in psychiatric settings, and accounts for 50% of patients with personality disorders.

c. BPD often co-occurs with mood disorders, including eating disorders (i.e., particularly bulimia), and many improve without treatment between the ages of 30 and 50.

2. Causes of BPD
   a. BPD **runs in families** and is somehow linked to mood disorders.
   b. **Early trauma** in the development of BPD has received a great deal of attention, specifically sexual and physical abuse. BPD is associated with greater reports of early abuse than other psychiatric conditions.
   c. This connection may help explain why women are more likely to develop BPD than men, particularly as girls are 2 to 3 times more likely to be sexually abused than boys. However, 20% to 40% of persons with BPD do not have a clear history of early abuse.
   d. Some argue that BPD is really a case of PTSD in women.
3. Few studies exist evaluating **treatment for BPD**.
   a. **Medications**, such as tricyclic antidepressants and lithium seem to have some efficacy.
   b. **Psychosocial treatment** research is limited. The most promising approach is **dialectical behavior therapy (DBT)**.
   c. DBT involves helping persons with BPD cope with stressors that seem to trigger suicidal behaviors, including teaching the patient how to identify and regulate their emotions. Problem solving is also emphasized in DBT, and other treatment components resemble those used for PTSD, particularly trauma reexperiencing. DBT seems efficacious in reducing suicide attempts, dropouts from treatment, and hospitalizations.

C. Persons with **histrionic personality disorder (HPD)** tend to be overly dramatic and often appear as if they are acting. The textbook illustrates histrionic personality disorder with the case of Pat.

1. Clinical description of HPD
   a. Persons with HPD tend to express their emotions in an exaggerated fashion, are vain and self-centered, and are uncomfortable when not the center of attention.
   b. Many dress and behave seductively, are often overly concerned about their appearance, and tend to seek reassurance and approval constantly.
   c. Many are also impulsive and have difficulty in delaying gratification.
   d. Such persons tend to view situations in very global, or black and white terms; speech is often vague, lacking in detail, and characterized by hyperbole.
   e. HPD is more commonly diagnosed in females.
2. Causes of HPD
   a. The etiology of HPD is largely unknown; though some have speculated a relation between HPD and antisocial personality disorder.

b. Roughly 66% of persons with HPD also meet criteria for ASPD, leading some to suggest that HPD and ASPD may represent sex-typed alternative expressions of the same unidentified underlying condition.

3. **Treatment** for persons with HPD has not been extensively studied.
    a. Therapists usually target attention-getting behavior, problematic interpersonal relationships (e.g., manipulation of others through emotional crises, using charm, sex, or seductiveness to attain desired ends).
    b. Efforts are made to show persons with HPD that the short-terms gains they derive from their behavior have long-term costs, to teach them more appropriate ways of meeting their needs.

D. Persons with **narcissistic personality disorder (NPD)** show an exaggerated and unreasonable sense of self-importance and preoccupation with receiving attention to such an extent that they lack sensitivity and compassion for other people. The feelings and fantasies of greatness (i.e., grandiosity) create a number of negative attributes, such as demanding special attention, exploitation of others for their own interests, and showing little empathy. Such persons also tend to be envious and arrogant, and many are also depressed. The textbook illustrates narcissistic personality disorder with the case of David.

1. The **etiology of NPD** has been linked to an early failure in childhood to learn how to show empathy. The result is a child who remains fixated in a self-centered, grandiose stage of development.
2. **The sociological view** argues that NPD results from large-scale social changes in Westernized society, particularly an emphasis on hedonism, individualism, competitiveness, and success (i.e., the me generation).
4. **Treatment research for NPD** is extremely limited. Therapy often focuses on grandiosity, hypersensitivity to evaluation, lack of empathy for others, unrealistic thinking, and coping strategies to reduce sensitivity to criticism. Treatment also addresses depression.

IV. Cluster C Personality Disorders

A. Persons with **avoidant personality disorder (APD)** are extremely sensitive to the opinions of others and therefore avoid most relationships. Their low self-esteem, coupled with fear of rejection, causes such persons to have limited friendships and to show a high degree of dependence on those they feel comfortable with. The textbook illustrates avoidant personality disorder with the case of Jane.

1. Primary characteristics of APD include avoidance of interpersonal contact in occupational or other settings, unwillingness to participate in intimate relationships or take risks, preoccupation with being criticized, and a belief that one is socially inept.
2. Unlike persons with schizoid personality disorder, those with APD are asocial because they are interpersonally anxious and fearful of rejection.
3. Persons with APD feel chronically rejected by others and pessimistic about their future.
4. **Etiological factors** involved in APD are numerous and include the following:

a. **Millon** suggested that APD individuals are born with a difficult temperament or personality characteristics, and that these features lead their parents to reject them. The result is low self-esteem and social alienation. Many persons with APD report childhood experiences of isolation, rejection, and conflict with others.

5. There are several well-controlled **treatment studies for APD**.
   a. Behavioral interventions for anxiety and social problems are successful and resemble those used for social phobia and may include **systematic desensitization** and **behavioral rehearsal**.

B. Persons with **dependent personality disorder (DPD)** tend to rely on others to make ordinary and important life decisions, resulting in an unreasonable fear of abandonment. The textbook illustrates dependent personality disorder with the case of Karen.

1. Clinical Description of DPD
   a. Persons with DPD tend to agree with others to avoid rejection, and may show submissiveness, timidity, and passivity.
   b. Persons with DPD are like those with APD in that they are prone to similar feelings of inadequacy, are sensitive to criticism, and need reassurance. Unlike persons with APD who respond by avoiding relationships, persons with DPD respond to such feelings by clinging to relationships.
2. The **etiology of DPD** has been linked to disruptions in the normal early process of moving from dependence to independence. This view originates in the work on child attachment (i.e., how children learn to bond with their parents and other important people in their lives). If such bonding is interrupted, persons may end up being constantly anxious that they will lose people close to them.
3. The **treatment** literature for DPD is mostly descriptive. Therapy typically progresses gradually and attempts to help the patient foster a sense of independence in making important life decisions.

C. Persons with **obsessive-compulsive personality disorder (OCPD)** show a fixation on things being done the right way to such an extent that it prevents them from actually completing much of anything. The textbook illustrates obsessive-compulsive personality disorder with the case of Daniel.

1. Clinical Description of OCPD
   a. Persons with OCPD tend to be work-oriented, spend little time pursuing enjoyable non-work activities, and tend to have poor interpersonal relationships because of their rigidity.
   b. Persons with OCPD do not tend to have the obsessive thoughts and compulsive behaviors characteristic of obsessive-compulsive disorder. OCPD is common among gifted children.
2. The etiology of OCPD is weakly related to genetics, and little is known about other etiologic contributing factors that may be involved.
4. **Treatment** outcome data for OCPD are limited. Therapy often targets the fears that underlie the need for orderliness, fears of inadequacy, and

procrastination and rumination about important issues and minor details, and may include relaxation procedures and distraction techniques.

OVERALL SUMMARY

This chapter outlines the nature of personality and the clinical characteristics, epidemiology, etiology, and treatment for the DSM-IV-TR personality disorders. Cluster A, B, and C disorders are described as well as personality disorders under study for future consideration in the DSM. In addition, specific issues regarding the classification of personality disorders are covered; namely, the debate over categorical vs. dimensional models of taxonomy, the diagnostic validity of personality disorders, and gender bias with respect to diagnosis.

KEY TERMS

Antisocial personality disorder (p. 432)
Avoidant personality disorder (p. 446)
Borderline personality disorder (p. 440)
Dependent personality disorder (p. 447)
Histrionic personality disorder (p. 443)
Narcissistic personality disorder (p. 444)
Obsessive-compulsive personality disorder (p. 448)
Paranoid personality disorder (p. 427)
Personality disorders (p. 421)
Psychopathy (p. 434)
Schizoid personality disorder (p. 429)
Schizotypal personality disorder (p. 430)

INFOTRAC KEY TERM EXERCISES

Each exercise is linked to key terms from the Wadsworth InfoTrac on-line searchable database. Key terms must be entered exactly as written.

Exercise 1: **Borderline Personality or PTSD?: You Decide**
Article: A110526680
Citation: (Borderline personality disorder and posttraumatic stress disorder: Time for integration?). Shannon Hodges.
Journal of Counseling and Development, Fall 2003 v81 i4 p409(9)

Borderline personality disorder is one of several diagnoses that has been the subject of some criticism, particularly in the context of gender bias favoring females. This InfoTrac article addresses whether PTSD is a more appropriate label than BPD and places such issues in a broader developmental context. The author argues that the pejorative view of the BPD category has resulted from a "caste system" of diagnosis and treatment that fails to adequately serve women labeled with BPD. What does the author have to say about the following issues: (a) labeling women as "borderline", (b) the subjectivity of BPD criteria, (c) the overlapping comorbidity with BPD and PTSD, and (d) the difficulties created by attempting to fit BPD into the category of trauma disorders. In your answer, make a case for or against the view that BPD should be dropped and replaced with the label PTSD. Limit your answer to 3-5 double-spaced pages.

Exercise 2: Antisocial Personality by Proxy: A Critical Evaluation
Key Term: *Antisocial Personality Disorder*

Antisocial personality disorder by proxy is defined by a proposed set of diagnostic criteria and a general description of proxy and perpetrator characteristics. The main feature of an antisocial personality disorder by proxy is the expression of antisocial impulses by eliciting or inciting antisocial behavior in another individual, the "proxy." Though this condition does not appear anywhere in the DSM-IV, it does raise a host of issues related to the nature of antisocial personality disorder, diagnosis, and personality more generally. Review the InfoTrac article on this topic, and critically evaluate whether there is enough evidence to warrant antisocial personality disorder by proxy as a disorder warranting further study in the DSM-IV. In your answer, be sure to address why the diagnosis of antisocial personality disorder is insufficient for the proxy him or herself. Limit your answer to 3-5 double-spaced pages.

Exercise 3: Borderline Personality Disorder In Children: What are the Tell Tale Signs?
Key Term: *Borderline Personality Disorder in Children*

Most personality disorders are thought to originate early in development and borderline personality disorder is no exception. Your task here is to review the InfoTrac article on neuropsychological and behavioral risk factors associated with borderline personality disorder in children, and then to propose a basic prevention program that might help reduce the risk for developing borderline personality disorder. Be creative in your answer and try to create a prevention program in line with the material you read about in the personality disorders chapter in the textbook. Limit your answer to 3-5 double-spaced pages.

Exercise 4 (Future Trend): Other Personality Disorders Under Study

The DSM-IV-TR includes 10 personality disorders, and several others are under study (e.g., passive-aggressive, depressive). One such disorder resembles depression and is termed "depressive personality disorder." A link to the criteria for this disorder appears below. You may review these criteria and ask students to differentiate depression as a personality trait vs. depression as a mood disorder. How are they the same and where do they differ. You may take this discussion in any number of directions. For instance, can students come up with other types of personality problems other than those described in the DSM-IV-TR?

http://www.enter.net/~planetearth/depress.htm
http://www.geocities.com/ptypes/overviews.html

CLASSROOM ACTIVITIES, DEMONSTRATIONS, AND LECTURE TOPICS

1. **Activity: Identifying Personality Disorders.** It is often difficult to discriminate between normal and abnormal behavior, especially where personality disorders are concerned. In fact, many students will identify their own behavior in various personality disorders. To illustrate concretely the difficulty in drawing diagnostic lines, make a list of behaviors and

have your students judge and justify whether the behavior is normal or abnormal. Some examples of these behaviors may include:

a. A woman who is careful to lock her car and house immediately after entering them because she fears intruders. Would you consider this behavior paranoid? Why or why not? When would it become paranoid?
b. A car salesman who lies to people to manipulate them into buying a car, and feels no guilt about making an unethical sale. Would you consider this behavior antisocial?
c. A woman who does not socialize with other people. She communicates with people at her job, but outside of work she has no social contact with others. Would you consider this behavior schizoid?
d. A man who becomes upset when his wife rearranges his shirt drawer, does not have dinner ready on schedule, or in any way interferes with his rigidly planned work schedule. Would you consider this behavior obsessive-compulsive?

2. **Activity: Gender Bias and "Normal" Behavior.** With respect to the discussion on gender bias, it is useful to have students experience this bias themselves. Pass out the vignette depicted in HANDOUT 12.1 to half of your students. Give the remaining students in your class HANDOUT 12.2 that depicts identical vignettes, but with the gender of the pronounces changed. Do not tell your students there are alternate versions of the vignettes. Ask each student to write down their "clinical" opinion about the person's behavior in the scenarios. Ask them to judge if the behavior is "normal" or not. Furthermore, ask them to assign adjectives to the person in the vignette that would portray an accurate description of their personality. Collect and record the opinions on the blackboard. Ask your students if any noticeable differences exist between students based on the gender of the subject. This can lead to a discussion on the potential impact gender biases can have on the diagnostic process.

3. **Activity: Diagnose A Film Character With a Personality Disorder.** Have students watch Fatal Attraction and/or Misery, or show clips from both films in class. Then, ask students to arrive at a diagnosis of the lead characters in each film. In Fatal Attraction, Glenn Close depicts what many believe is a classic case of borderline personality disorder, whereas Kathy Bates in the film Misery depicts features of either paranoid or schizoid personality disorder.

4. **Activity: Student Identification With Personality Disorder Features.** Students will often report that they see portions of themselves in the chapter descriptions of the features of some of the personality disorders. An exercise that may be useful to spark discussion about the relation between normal and disordered personality would be to have students identify one personality disorder that they feel shares much in common with aspects of their own personality. Obviously you are not asking students to self-diagnose, but to select the disorder that descriptively comes closest to their own personality features. Have students write down the name of the disorder that is closest to them, including whether they are male and female, and then collect the response anonymously. Tally up the class information and put it up on the board or overhead. Use this exercise to talk about personality generally and what makes personality a disorder. You should find

some interesting gender differences in the labels students most identity with. As an aside, to add humor to this exercise, you can tell the students that the label that best fits you as an instructor is narcissistic.

5. **Video Activity: The Case of George and His Antisocial Personality.** Show your class the segment from Abnormal Psychology: Inside /Out depicting an interview with a patient named George who describes his history of criminality and antisocial behavior. Ask the students whether they can identity either etiological or diagnostic criteria from George's recounting of his history that would warrant a diagnosis of antisocial personality disorder. The answer is that George does meet DSM-IV-TR criteria for antisocial personality disorder.

HANDOUT 12.1

The Case of Robert and Karen

1. Robert is 10 years old. He attends school, but is often in trouble because he is inattentive or rebellious towards the teacher. He has friends in class, but frequently gets into physical fights with them and on one occasion hurt a classmate. He teases his younger brother at home, and prefers to be outside playing baseball with friends rather than completing homework or chores.

2. Karen is a 35-year-old single woman. She is depressed because she wants to have children but has not found a suitable partner. Karen has recently quit her job and spends most of her time talking with friends on the telephone. She has no immediate plans to return to work, and will look to her family to provide for her during this difficult time.

HANDOUT 12.2

The Case of Karen and Robert

1. Karen is 10 years old. She attends school, but is often in trouble because she is inattentive or rebellious towards the teacher. She has friends in class, but frequently gets into physical fights with them and on one occasion hurt a classmate. She teases her younger brother at home, and prefers to be outside playing baseball with friends rather than completing homework or chores.

2. Robert is a 35-year-old single man. He is depressed because he wants to have children but has not found a suitable partner. Robert has recently quit his job and spends most of his time talking with friends on the telephone. He has no immediate plans to return to work, and will look to his family to provide for him during this difficult time.

SUPPLEMENTARY READING MATERIAL FOR CHAPTER TWELVE

(= These sources can be found on "*Infotrac, the online library*" provided by Wadsworth and Brooks/Cole Publishing.)

Clarkin, J. F., & Lenzenweger, M. F. (1996). Major theories of personality disorder. New York: Guilford.

Clarkin, J. F., Marziali, E., & Munroe-Blum, H. (1992). Borderline personality disorder: Clinical and empirical perspectives. New York: Guilford.

Cooper, A. M., Frances, A. J., & Sacks, M. H. (1991). The personality disorders and neuroses. New York: Basic.

Funder, D. C. (2001). Personality. Annual Review of Psychology, 197.

Linehan, M. M. (1993). Cognitive-behavioral treatment of borderline personality disorder. New York: Guilford.

Livesley, W. J. (1995). The DSM-IV-TR personality disorders. New York: Guilford.

Millon, T. (1990). Toward a new personology: An evolutionary model. New York: Wiley.

Millon, T., & Davis, R. D. (1995). Disorders of personality: DSM-IV-TR and beyond. New York: Wiley.

Mischel, W., & Shoda, Y. (1998). Reconciling processing dynamics and personality dispositions. Annual Review of Psychology, 49, 229(30).

Oldham, J. M. (Ed.). (1991). Personality disorders: New perspectives on diagnostic validity. Washington, DC: American Psychiatric Press.

Stone, M. H. (1993). Abnormalities of personality: Within and beyond the realm of treatment. New York: Norton.

Tyrer, P. (1988). Personality disorders: Diagnosis, management, and course. Boston: Wright.

SUPPLEMENTARY 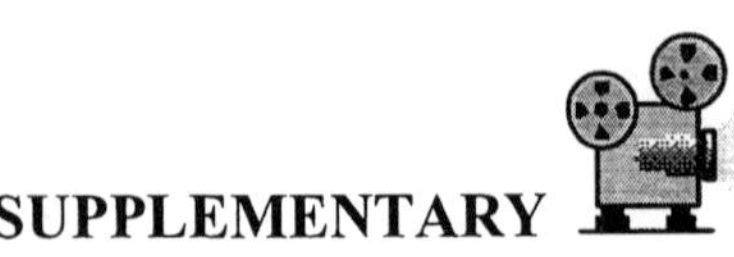 VIDEO RESOURCES FOR CHAPTER TWELVE

Abnormal psychology inside/out, video 2, vol 1. (*available through your International Thomson Learning representative).* An interview with a patient named George is presented where he describes his antisocial personality, including selling drugs, holding a gun to his father's head, and lack of empathy and caring toward other people and himself. This segment nicely illustrates how personality disorders often develop early. (15 min)

A streetcar named desire. (Hollywood Film; Drama). This film provides a nice depiction of histrionic personality.

Borderline syndrome: Personality disorder of our time. (Insight Media: 2162 Broadway, New York, NY 10024/ (800)-233-9910). Using rare footage of conversations with patients, this video explores borderline personality disorder and the clinical issues it raises. (74 min)

Born to be bad. (Insight Media: 2162 Broadway, New York, NY 10024/ (800)-233-9910). Presenting the research and commentary of scientists who believe a person's genetic makeup, brain chemistry, and brain function may put them at risk for committing impulsive crimes, this video investigates how new technologies may help detect those at risk. (25 min)

Fatal attraction. (Hollywood Film; Thriller/Romance). Glenn close displays classic characteristics of borderline personality disorder.

Girl interrupted. (Hollywood Film; Drama). This film, set in the 1960s, illustrates a compelling true story of a woman who attempted suicide and subsequently self-committed to a mental institution. The range of psychopathology of the characters, including the depiction of treatment and life in a mental institution during the 1960s, is outstanding. This film nicely illustrates depression, suicide, but it is particularly useful as an illustration of borderline personality disorder.

La cage aux folles. (Hollywood Film; Comedy). This film provides a nice example of histrionic personality disorder.

Personality disorders. (Insight Media: 2162 Broadway, New York, NY 10024/ (800)-233-9910). Intended for students and practitioners in the mental-health field, this video examines the characteristic features and phenomenology of personality disorders. It presents a doctor's interviews with patients and discusses the rudiments of performing a differential diagnosis. (45 min)

Silence of the lambs. (Hollywood Film; Drama). Sir Anthony Hopkins depicts a serial killer named Hannibal Lector. The film nicely illustrates severe antisocial personality disorder.

Taxi driver. (Hollywood Film; Drama). This film nicely illustrates delusional, paranoid thinking and particularly features of schizotypal personality disorder.

The conversation. (Hollywood Film; Drama). This film stars Gene Hackman who plays a surveillance expert with a paranoid personality.

The odd couple. (Hollywood Film; Comedy). This film depicts Jack Lemmon as the obsessive-compulsive Felix Unger.

The psychopath: Mad or bad? (Insight Media: 2162 Broadway, New York, NY 10024/ (800)-233-9910). This program describes the psychopath as an individual suffering from a type of personality disorder characterized by a lack of such normal feelings as guilt, love, stress, and concern. It discusses such traits as being asocial, highly impulsive, and aggressive, and explains that the psychopath is unable to feel — but can cleverly mimic human personalities, thus frequently coming off as rational and even charming. The video also explores possible causes of psychopathy, linking it with retarded maturation and discussing such factors as the lack of a role model or parental rejection. (60 min)

Understanding borderline personality disorder. (Insight Media: 2162 Broadway, New York, NY 10024/ (800)-233-9910). This video presents clinical features of borderline personality disorder (BPD) and shows strategies for counseling BPD clients. Marsha Linehan describes causes of the disorder, emphasizing biosocial factors, and traces the development of her Dialectical Behavior Therapy. (35 min)

INTERNET 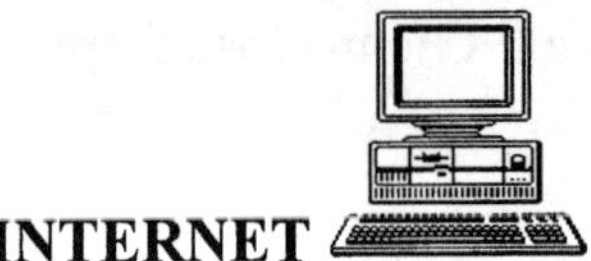 RESOURCES FOR CHAPTER TWELVE

Antisocial Personality Disorder
http://www.mentalhealth.com/dis/p20-pe04.html
This web site (part of internet mental health) is devoted to information pertaining to the diagnosis, etiology, and treatment of antisocial personality disorder.

Avoidant Personality Disorder
http://www.mentalhealth.com/p20-grp.html
This web site (part of internet mental health) is devoted to information pertaining to the diagnosis, etiology, and treatment of avoidant personality disorder.

Borderline Personality Disorder
http://www.mentalhealth.com/p20-grp.html
This web site (part of internet mental health) is devoted to information pertaining to the diagnosis, etiology, and treatment of borderline personality disorder.

BPD Central
http://www.BPDCentral.com/
A web site devoted to furthering the understanding of borderline disorder, written with those who live with a BPD patient in mind.

Histrionic Personality Disorder
http://www.mentalhealth.com/p20-grp.html
This web site (part of internet mental health) is devoted to information pertaining to the diagnosis, etiology, and treatment of histrionic personality disorder.

Narcissistic Personality Disorder
http://www.mentalhealth.com/p20-grp.html

This web site (part of internet mental health) is devoted to information pertaining to the diagnosis, etiology, and treatment of narcissistic personality disorder.

Obsessive Compulsive Personality Disorder
http://www.mentalhealth.com/p20-grp.html

This web site (part of internet mental health) is devoted to information pertaining to the diagnosis, etiology, and treatment of obsessive-compulsive personality disorder.

Paranoid Personality Disorder
http://www.mentalhealth.com/p20-grp.html

This web site (part of internet mental health) is devoted to information pertaining to the diagnosis, etiology, and treatment of paranoid personality disorder.

Schizoid Personality Disorder
http://www.mentalhealth.com/p20-grp.html

This web site (part of internet mental health) is devoted to information pertaining to the diagnosis, etiology, and treatment of schizoid personality disorder.

Schizotypal Personality Disorder
http://www.mentalhealth.com/p20-grp.html

This web site (part of internet mental health) is devoted to information pertaining to the diagnosis, etiology, and treatment of schizotypal personality disorder.

WARNING SIGNS OF PARANOID PERSONALITY DISORDER

- An unmistakable sign of paranoia is continual mistrust
- Feel as though one needs to be constantly on their guard
- Tendency to view the world as a threatening place
- Expect trickery and doubt the loyalty of others
- Being hyperalert for signs of threat
- Vigilance for any slight against them
- Show a tendency to be defensive and antagonistic
- Inability to accept blame and mild criticism
- Tendency to be highly critical of others
- Often argumentative and uncompromising
- Appear cold and aloof socially
- Often avoid intimacy with other people

WARNING SIGNS OF SCHIZOID PERSONALITY DISORDER

- No desire for social relationships
- Lack ability to form close social relationships
- Often single and unmarried, with little interest in sex or intimacy
- Preference for solitary activities
- Limited range of emotions, particularly in social settings (e.g., coldness, detachment, or flatness)
- Often appear indifferent to compliments and criticisms
- Find little or no joy in activities or in life

WARNING SIGNS OF SCHIZOTYPAL PERSONALITY DISORDER

- Behavior or appearance that is odd, eccentric, or peculiar
- Ideas of reference (excluding delusions of reference)
- Few close relationships
- Odd beliefs or magical thinking (e.g., superstitiousness, belief in clairvoyance, telepathy, or "sixth sense"; in children and adolescents, bizarr fantasies or preoccupations)
- Unusual perceptual experiences, including bodily illusions
- Suspiciousness or paranoid ideation
- Inappropriate or constricted affect
- Lack of close friends or confidants other than immediate family members
- Excessive social anxiety that does not diminish with familiarity and tends tc be associated with paranoid fears rather than negative judgments about self

WARNING SIGNS OF ANTISOCIAL PERSONALITY DISORDER

- Defiance and disregard for social norms or the rights of other people
- Regularly performing illegal acts that are grounds for arrest
- Show little empathy for others
- Lack remorse for persons they have hurt
- Tendency to be self-absorbed (i.e., concerned with themselves)
- Often appear superficial
- Show difficulties in fulfilling responsibilities and commitments (e.g., work or financial obligations)
- Habitually lying or being manipulative
- Use of aliases and conning people for personal profit or pleasure
- Frequent physical aggression and conflict with other people
- Having had serious behavioral problems in childhood and teenage years
- Blaming others or offering rationalizations for antisocial behavior
- Being impulsive
- May be accompanied with unusually early age of drug and/or alcohol abuse
- Problems with the legal system

WARNING SIGNS OF BORDERLINE PERSONALITY DISORDER

- Frantic efforts to avoid real or imagined abandonment
- A pattern of unstable and intense interpersonal relationships characterized b alternating between extremes of idealization and devaluation
- Identity disturbances (e.g., unstable self-image or sense of self)
- Impulsivity in areas that are potentially self-damaging (e.g., spending, sex, substance abuse, reckless driving, binge eating)
- Affective (emotional) instability due to a marked reactivity of mood (e.g., intense episodic dysphoria, irritability, or anxiety usually lasting a few hou and only rarely more than a few days)
- Chronic feelings of emptiness
- Inappropriate, intense anger or difficulty controlling anger(e.g., frequent displays of temper, constant anger, recurrent physical fights)
- Transient (brief) stress-related paranoid ideation or severe dissociative symptoms

WARNING SIGNS OF HISTRIONIC PERSONALITY DISORDER

- Acting more emotional than a situation warrants
- Constantly seeking praise & approval from others
- Consistently seeking to be the center of attention
- Self-centered and demand to be the center of attention
- Inappropriately seductive or sexual
- Excessively concerned with appearance
- Tendency to dramatize situations
- Theatrical speech, dress, and mannerism
- Overly trusting and gullible and overly adjustable
- Verbal communication is expressive but lacks detail
- Easily alter emotions
- Trapped in the present and caring little for the future or future plans
- Often accompanied with an underlying feeling of low self-esteem
- Very social and extroverted however, self-absorbed
- May be accompanied with impotence in men and inability to orgasm in women

WARNING SIGNS OF NARCISSISTIC PERSONALITY DISORDER

- Physical posture implying and exuding an air of superiority
- Amused indifference
- Lack of eye and bodily contact
- Speaks from the standpoint of condescension
- Assumes a social posture as an "observer," and is otherwise asocial
- Demanding "special treatment" of some kind (e.g., not waiting for a turn)
- Either idealizes or devalues others
- Tendency to try and "belong," while maintaining a stance as an outsider
- Seeking constant admiration
- A preference for showing off, but lacking substance
- A tendency to be shallow (i.e., a pond pretending to be an ocean)
- Inability to admit ignorance about something
- Speech containing frequent usage of "I," "my," "myself," and "mine"
- Show a grandiose sense of self-importance (e.g., if a scientist – s/he is on th very brink of a discovery with cosmic and global consequences)
- Tendency to be easily hurt and/or insulted

WARNING SIGNS OF AVOIDANT PERSONALITY DISORDER

- Avoids occupational activities that involve significant interpersonal contact, because of fears of criticism, disapproval, or rejection
- Is unwilling to get involved with people unless certain of being liked
- Shows restraint within intimate relationships because of the fear of being shamed or ridiculed
- Is preoccupied with being criticized or rejected in social situations
- Is inhibited in new interpersonal situations because of feelings of inadequacy
- Views self as socially inept (not fitting in), personally unappealing, or inferior to others
- Is unusually reluctant to take personal risks or to engage in any new activities because they may prove embarrassing

WARNING SIGNS OF DEPENDENT PERSONALITY DISORDER

- Need for others to control their lives
- Difficulty in making decisions or initiating new projects on their own
- Lack self-confidence and trust in their own abilities
- Often belittle themselves (e.g., saying "I'm dumb," or "I'm stupid)
- Tendency to be submissive and clingy in social relationships
- Avoidance of conflict
- Feel a strong need to be taken care of
- Fear of separation and abandonment

WARNING SIGNS OF OBSESSIVE-COMPULSIVE PERSONALITY DISORDER

- A tendency toward perfectionism
- Hold inflexible ethical and behavioral standards
- Tendency to be highly organized and rigidly disciplined
- Pay excessive attention to details, rules, lists, schedules
- Difficulties in expressing warm feelings or emotions
- Premium is placed on mental and emotional control

Transparency 12-1

DSM-IV-TR General Criteria for Personality Disorder

A. An enduring pattern of inner experience and behavior that deviates markedly from the expectations of the individual's culture. This pattern is manifested in two (or more) of the following areas:

1. cognition (i.e., ways of perceiving and interpreting self, other people, and events)
2. affectivity (i.e., the range, intensity, lability, and appropriateness of emotional response)
3. interpersonal functioning
4. impulse control

B. The enduring pattern is inflexible and pervasive across a broad range of personal and social situations.

C. The enduring pattern leads to clinically significant distress or impairment in social, occupational, or other important areas of functioning.

D. The pattern is stable and of long duration and its onset can be traced back at least to adolescence or early adulthood.

E. The enduring pattern is not better accounted for as a manifestation or consequence of another mental disorder.

F. The enduring pattern is not due to the direct physiological effects of a substance (e.g., a drug of abuse, a medication) or a general medical condition (e.g., head trauma).

DSM-IV-TR Criteria for Paranoid Personality Disorder

A. A pervasive distrust and suspiciousness of others such that their motives are interpreted as malevolent, beginning by early adulthood and present in a variety of contexts, as indicated by four (or more) of the following:

1. suspects, without sufficient basis, that others are exploiting, harming, or deceiving him or her
2. is preoccupied with unjustified doubts about the loyalty or trustworthiness of friends or associates
3. is reluctant to confide in others because of unwarranted fear that the information will be used maliciously against him or her
4. reads hidden demeaning or threatening meanings into benign remarks or events
5. persistently bears grudges, i.e., is unforgiving of insults, injuries, or slights
6. perceives attacks on his or her character or reputation that are not apparent to others and is quick to react angrily or to counterattack
7. has recurrent suspicions, without justification, regarding fidelity of spouse or sexual partner

B. Does not occur exclusively during the course of Schizophrenia, a Mood Disorder With Psychotic Features, or another Psychotic Disorder and is not due to the direct physiological effects of a general medical condition.
Note: If criteria are met prior to the onset of Schizophrenia, add "Premorbid," e.g., "Paranoid Personality Disorder (Premorbid)."

Transparency 12-3

DSM-IV-TR Criteria for Schizoid Personality Disorder

A. A pervasive pattern of detachment from social relationships and a restricted range of expression of emotions in interpersonal settings, beginning by early adulthood and present in a variety of contexts, as indicated by four (or more) of the following:

1. neither desires nor enjoys close relationships, including being part of a family
2. almost always chooses solitary activities
3. has little, if any, interest in having sexual experiences with another person
4. takes pleasure in few, if any, activities
5. lacks close friends or confidants other than first-degree relatives
6. appears indifferent to the praise or criticism of others
7. shows emotional coldness, detachment, or flattened affectivity

B. Does not occur exclusively during the course of Schizophrenia, a Mood Disorder With Psychotic Features, another Psychotic Disorder, or a Pervasive Developmental Disorder and is not due to the direct physiological effects of a general medical condition.

Note: If criteria are met prior to the onset of Schizophrenia, add "Premorbid," e.g., "Schizoid Personality Disorder (Premorbid)."

DSM-IV-TR Criteria for Schizotypal Personality Disorder

A. A pervasive pattern of social and interpersonal deficits marked by acute discomfort with, and reduced capacity for, close relationships as well as by cognitive
or perceptual distortions and eccentricities of behavior, beginning by early adulthood and present in a variety of contexts, as indicated by five (or more) of the following:

1. ideas of reference (excluding delusions of reference)
2. odd beliefs or magical thinking that influences behavior and is inconsistent with subcultural norms (e.g., superstitiousness, belief in clairvoyance, telepathy, or "sixth sense"; in children and adolescents, bizarre fantasies or preoccupations)
3. unusual perceptual experiences, including bodily illusions
4. odd thinking and speech (e.g., vague, circumstantial, metaphorical, overelaborate, or stereotyped)
5. suspiciousness or paranoid ideation
6. inappropriate or constricted affect
7. behavior or appearance that is odd, eccentric, or peculiar
8. lack of close friends or confidants other than first-degree relatives
9. excessive social anxiety that does not diminish with familiarity and tends to be associated with paranoid fears rather than negative judgments about self

B. Does not occur exclusively during the course of Schizophrenia, a Mood Disorder With Psychotic Features, another Psychotic Disorder, or a Pervasive Developmental Disorder.

Note: If criteria are met prior to the onset of Schizophrenia, add "Premorbid," e.g., "Schizotypal Personality Disorder (Premorbid)."

DSM-IV-TR Criteria for Antisocial Personality Disorder

A. There is a pervasive pattern of disregard for and violation of the rights of others occurring since age 15 years, as indicated by three (or more) of the following:

1. failure to conform to social norms with respect to lawful behaviors as indicated by repeatedly performing acts that are grounds for arrest
2. deceitfulness, as indicated by repeated lying, use of aliases, or conning others for personal profit or pleasure
3. impulsivity or failure to plan ahead
4. irritability and aggressiveness, as indicated by repeated physical fights or assaults
5. reckless disregard for safety of self or others
6. consistent irresponsibility, as indicated by repeated failure to sustain consistent work behavior or honor financial obligations
7. lack of remorse, as indicated by being indifferent to or rationalizing having hurt, mistreated, or stolen from another

B. The individual is at least age 18 years.

C. There is evidence of Conduct Disorder with onset before age 15 years.

D. The occurrence of antisocial behavior is not exclusively during the course of Schizophrenia or a Manic Episode.

DSM-IV-TR Criteria for Borderline Personality Disorder

A pervasive pattern of instability of interpersonal relationships, self-image, and affects, and marked impulsivity beginning by early adulthood and present in a variety of contexts, as indicated by five (or more) of the following:

1. frantic efforts to avoid real or imagined abandonment. Note: Do not include suicidal or self-mutilating behavior covered in Criterion 5.
2. a pattern of unstable and intense interpersonal relationships characterized by alternating between extremes of idealization and devaluation
3. identity disturbance: markedly and persistently unstable self-image or sense of self
4. impulsivity in at least two areas that are potentially self-damaging (e.g., spending, sex, Substance Abuse, reckless driving, binge eating). Note: Do not include suicidal or self-mutilating behavior covered in Criterion 5.
5. recurrent suicidal behavior, gestures, or threats, or self-mutilating behavior
6. affective instability due to a marked reactivity of mood (e.g., intense episodic dysphoria, irritability, or anxiety usually lasting a few hours and only rarely more than a few days)
7. chronic feelings of emptiness
8. inappropriate, intense anger or difficulty controlling anger (e.g., frequent displays of temper, constant anger, recurrent physical fights)
9. transient, stress-related paranoid ideation or severe dissociative symptoms

DSM-IV-TR Criteria for Histrionic Personality Disorder

A pervasive pattern of excessive emotionality and attention seeking, beginning by early adulthood and present in a variety of contexts, as indicated by five (or more) of the following:

1. is uncomfortable in situations in which he or she is not the center of attention
2. interaction with others is often characterized by inappropriate sexually seductive or provocative behavior
3. displays rapidly shifting and shallow expression of emotions
4. consistently uses physical appearance to draw attention to self
5. has a style of speech that is excessively impressionistic and lacking in detail
6. shows self-dramatization, theatricality, and exaggerated expression of emotion
7. is suggestible, i.e., easily influenced by others or circumstances
8. considers relationships to be more intimate than they actually are

DSM-IV-TR Criteria for Narcissistic Personality Disorder

A pervasive pattern of grandiosity (in fantasy or behavior), need for admiration, and lack of empathy, beginning by early adulthood and present in a variety of contexts, as indicated by five (or more) of the following:

1. has a grandiose sense of self-importance (e.g., exaggerates achievements and talents, expects to be recognized as superior without commensurate achievements)
2. is preoccupied with fantasies of unlimited success, power, brilliance, beauty, or ideal love
3. believes that he or she is "special" and unique and can only be understood by, or should associate with, other special or high-status people (or institutions)
4. requires excessive admiration
5. has a sense of entitlement, i.e., unreasonable expectations of especially favorable treatment or automatic compliance with his or her expectations
6. is interpersonally exploitative, i.e., takes advantage of others to achieve his or her own ends
7. lacks empathy: is unwilling to recognize or identify with the feelings and needs of others
8. is often envious of others or believes that others are envious of him or her
9. shows arrogant, haughty behaviors or attitudes

Transparency 12-9

DSM-IV-TR Criteria for Avoidant Personality Disorder

A pervasive pattern of social inhibition, feelings of inadequacy, and hypersensitivity to negative evaluation, beginning by early adulthood and present in a variety of contexts, as indicated by four (or more) of the following:

1. avoids occupational activities that involve significant interpersonal contact, because of fears of criticism, disapproval, or rejection
2. is unwilling to get involved with people unless certain of being liked
3. shows restraint within intimate relationships because of the fear of being shamed or ridiculed
4. is preoccupied with being criticized or rejected in social situations
5. is inhibited in new interpersonal situations because of feelings of inadequac
6. views self as socially inept, personally unappealing, or inferior to others
7. is unusually reluctant to take personal risks or to engage in any new activities because they may prove embarrassing

DSM-IV-TR Criteria for Dependent Personality Disorder

A pervasive and excessive need to be taken care of that leads to submissive and clinging behavior and fears of separation, beginning by early adulthood and present in a variety of contexts, as indicated by five (or more) of the following:

1. has difficulty making everyday decisions without an excessive amount of advice and reassurance from others
2. needs others to assume responsibility for most major areas of his or her life
3. has difficulty expressing disagreement with others because of fear of loss of support or approval. Note: Do not include realistic fears of retribution.
4. has difficulty initiating projects or doing things on his or her own (because of a lack of self-confidence in judgment or abilities rather than a lack of motivation or energy)
5. goes to excessive lengths to obtain nurturance and support from others, to the point of volunteering to do things that are unpleasant
6. feels uncomfortable or helpless when alone because of exaggerated fears of being unable to care for himself or herself
7. urgently seeks another relationship as a source of care and support when a close relationship ends
8. is unrealistically preoccupied with fears of being left to take care of himself or herself

DSM-IV-TR Criteria for Obsessive-Compulsive Personality Disorder

A pervasive pattern of preoccupation with orderliness, perfectionism, and mental and interpersonal control, at the expense of flexibility, openness, and efficiency, beginning by early adulthood and present in a variety of contexts, as indicated by four (or more) of the following:

1. is preoccupied with details, rules, lists, order, organization, or schedules to the extent that the major point of the activity is lost
2. shows perfectionism that interferes with task completion (e.g., is unable to complete a project because his or her own overly strict standards are not met)
3. is excessively devoted to work and productivity to the exclusion of leisure activities and friendships (not accounted for by obvious economic necessity)
4. is overconscientious, scrupulous, and inflexible about matters of morality, ethics, or values (not accounted for by cultural or religious identification)
5. is unable to discard worn-out or worthless objects even when they have no sentimental value
6. is reluctant to delegate tasks or to work with others unless they submit to exactly his or her way of doing things
7. adopts a miserly spending style toward both self and others; money is viewed as something to be hoarded for future catastrophes
8. shows rigidity and stubbornness

CHAPTER THIRTEEN

SCHIZOPHRENIA AND OTHER PSYCHOTIC DISORDERS

LEARNING OBJECTIVES

1. Define schizophrenia and explain the difference between schizophrenia and psychosis.
2. Trace the history of schizophrenia, including contributions of Kraepelin and Bleuler.
3. Distinguish between positive, negative, and disorganized symptoms of schizophrenia.
4. Describe the clinical characteristics and major subtypes of schizophrenia: paranoid, catatonic, disorganized, undifferentiated, and residual.
5. Describe diagnostic and clinical features of other psychotic disorders in the textbook.
6. Describe the prevalence of schizophrenia, including the potential genetic, neurobiological, developmental, and psychosocial contributions and risk factors.
7. Describe what is known about abnormalities in neurocognitive and biological functioning and their relation to the symptom clusters of schizophrenia.
8. Distinguish among the different classification schemes used to describe the onset and course of schizophrenia (e.g., process vs. reactive, poor vs. good premorbid, Type I vs. Type II) and explain why they are important.
9. Describe the role of expressed emotion in the course of schizophrenia, particularly with regard to risk of relapse.
10. Describe biological and psychosocial treatments for schizophrenia, including the short and long-term side-effects of neuroleptic medications, and the general goals of therapy.

OUTLINE

I. Perspectives on Schizophrenia
   A. **Schizophrenia** is characterized by a broad spectrum of cognitive and emotional dysfunctions that include hallucinations and delusions, disorganized speech and behavior, and inappropriate emotions.
      1. Schizophrenia affects about 1 out of 100 persons at some point in their lives.
      2. Despite advances in treatment, complete recovery from schizophrenia is rare.
      3. In 1991, the cost of schizophrenia in the U.S. was estimated to be $65 billion.

   B. The **history of schizophrenia** includes the early writings of **John Haslam** in 1809 and those of **Philippe Pinel** in France at about the same time. Some 50 years later another physician, **Benedict Morel**, used the French term **demence** (loss of mind) **precoce** (early, premature) because the onset of the disorder is often during adolescence.

1. **Emil Kraepelin** built on the work of Haslam, Pinel, and Morel to provide the most enduring description of schizophrenia. Two of Kraepelin's accomplishments stand out:
    a. First, he combined **catatonia** (i.e., alternating immobility and excited agitation), **hebephrenia** (i.e., silly and immature emotionality), and **paranoia** (i.e., delusions of grandeur and persecution) and labeled them as falling under the heading **dementia praecox**.
    b. Second, Kraepelin distinguished dementia praecox from manic-depressive illness by emphasizing onset and outcome.
2. **Eugen Bleuler**, a Swiss psychiatrist, was the first to introduce the term schizophrenia; a term derived from the Greek words for **split** (skhizen) and **mind** (phren). Unlike Kraepelin, Bleuler believed that the core of schizophrenia rests in an **associative splitting** of basic personality functions. This concept emphasized the following:
    a. "Breaking of associative threads," or the breakdown of forces that connect one function to the next.
    b. Bleuler also believed that an inability to keep a constant train of thought was characteristic of all persons with schizophrenia.
3. Schizophrenic symptoms are **heterogeneous**, meaning that this disorder includes a number of symptoms and behaviors that are not shared by all persons with the diagnosis. Both Kraepelin and Bleuler emphasized that schizophrenia was a heterogeneous condition.

II. Clinical Description, Symptoms, and Subtypes

A. The term **psychotic** is often used to characterize unusual behaviors, but it really refers to either delusions or hallucinations. The textbook illustrates the symptom clusters associated with schizophrenia with the cases of David and Arthur

B. **Positive symptoms** of schizophrenia refer to active manifestations of abnormal behavior or an excess or distortion of normal behavior. Examples include delusions, hallucinations, and disorganized speech.

1. **Delusions** refer to a belief that would be seen by most members of society as a misrepresentation of reality; often referred to as a disorder of thought content. Delusions are often called the basic characteristic of madness. Some research suggests that delusions give some patients a sense of meaning and purpose in life and result in less depression. Thus, delusions may serve an adaptive function. Types of delusions include:
    a. **Delusions of grandeur**, or the belief that one is particularly famous or important.
    b. **Delusions of persecution** refer to a common belief that other people are out to get or harm the person.
    c. More unusual delusions include **Capgras syndrome,** or the belief that someone a person knows has been replaced by a double, and **Cotard's syndrome**, where the person believes that a part of the body (e.g., brain) has changed in some impossible way.

2. **Hallucinations** refer to the experience of sensory events without any input from the surrounding environment. Hallucinations can involve any of the senses; though auditory hallucinations (i.e., hearing things that are not there) are most common in persons with schizophrenia.
   a. **Single photon emission tomography (SPECT)** has been used to study cerebral blood flow in schizophrenic patients during their auditory hallucinations. The part of the brain most active during auditory hallucinations is **Broca's area** (i.e., the area involved in speech production), *not* **Wernicke's area** (i.e., the area involved in understanding and language comprehension). This research supports the idea that auditory hallucinations do not involve hearing voices of others, but rather patients listening to their own thoughts or their own voices, and a failure to recognize the difference.

C. **Negative symptoms** of schizophrenia indicate the absence or insufficiency of normal behavior and include emotional or social withdrawal, apathy, and poverty of thought or speech.
1. **Avolition** or apathy refers to the inability to initiate and persist in activities. Persons with this feature show little interest in performing even the most basic daily functions, such as personal hygiene
2. **Alogia** refers to the relative absence of speech. This feature may manifest as brief replies to questions with little content, delayed comments or slowed responses to questions, or as disinterest in conversation. This feature is thought to reflect a negative thought disorder, not inadequate communication skills.
3. **Anhedonia** refers to a lack of pleasure, or indifference to activities that would normally be considered pleasurable, including eating, social interactions, and sexual relations.
4. **Affective flattening**, or flat affect, occurs in about two-thirds of persons with schizophrenia, and refers to an absence of normally expected emotional responses. Persons with flat affect show little change in facial expression, but not the experience of appropriate emotions. This work suggests that flat affect in schizophrenia may represent difficulty in expressing emotion, not an inability to feel emotion. Lack of expressed affect may be important in the development of schizophrenia. For example, children who later develop schizophrenia show less positive and more negative affect than normal siblings.

D. **Disorganized symptoms** of schizophrenia include rambling speech, erratic behavior, and inappropriate affect.
1. **Disorganized speech** refers to several often frustrating forms of communication problems in persons with schizophrenia. Examples include:
   a. **Cognitive slippage** often manifests as illogical and incoherent speech where the person jumps from one topic to the next.
   b. **Tangentiality** manifests as "going off on a tangent" rather than answering a question directly.

c. **Loose associations** or **derailment** refers to changing a conversational topic in unrelated areas.

2. Persons with schizophrenia often show **inappropriate affect** (e.g., laughing or crying at improper times) and **disorganized behavior** (e.g., boarding objects or acting in unusual ways in public). Such problems include the following:
   a. **Catatonia**, which involves motor dysfunctions that range from wild agitation to immobility. At one end of the spectrum, the person may pace restlessly or move their arms and fingers in stereotyped ways, whereas at the other end the person may hold unusual postures for hours on end (i.e., (**catatonic immobility**) and/or **waxy flexibility** (i.e., the tendency to keep limbs in a position that they were placed in by someone else).

E. DSM-IV-TR **subtypes of schizophrenia** include catatonic, disorganized, and paranoid.

1. Persons with the **paranoid type** of schizophrenia stand out because of their hallucinations and delusions. Such persons have relatively intact cognitive skills and affect and do not generally show disorganized speech or flat affect. The paranoid type is associated with the best prognosis.
   a. Delusions and hallucinations usually have a theme of grandeur or persecution.
   b. DSM-IV-TR criteria specify a preoccupation with one or more delusions or auditory hallucinations but without marked display of disorganized speech, disorganized or catatonic behavior, or flat or inappropriate affect.
2. Persons with the **disorganized type** (**hebephrenia**) show marked disruptions in their speech and behavior, including flat or inappropriate affect, self-absorption. If hallucinations or delusions are present, they tend to be organized around a theme, but are more fragmented. Such persons with this subtype show problems early and their problems tend to be chronic, lacking periods of remissions that characterize other forms of this disorder.
3. Persons with the **catatonic type** show unusual motor responses and odd mannerisms. In addition, such persons often show **echolalia** (i.e., repeating or mimicking the words of others) and **echopraxia** (i.e., imitating the movements of others). This subtype is relatively rare.
4. Persons with the **undifferentiated type** do not neatly fit into any of the other subtypes and include people with major symptoms of schizophrenia but who do not meet criteria for paranoid, disorganized, or catatonic types.
5. Persons with the **residual type** have had at least one episode of schizophrenia but are no longer displaying major symptoms. Such persons often display residual symptoms, such as negative beliefs, unusual or bizarre ideas, social withdrawal, inactivity, or flat affect.

F. Other psychotic disorders

1. Persons with **schizophreniform disorder** have experienced symptoms of schizophrenia for a few months only and usually resume normal lives. There are few studies of this disorder, with a lifetime prevalence of 0.2%.
    a. DSM-IV-TR criteria for schizophreniform disorder include onset of psychotic symptoms within 4 weeks of the first noticeable change in usual behavior, confusion at the height of the psychotic episode, good premorbid social and occupational functioning, and the absence of blunted affect.
2. Persons with **schizoaffective disorder** suffer from symptoms of schizophrenia and a mood disorder. The prognosis is similar as for people with schizophrenia and such persons do not tend to get better on their own.
    a. DSM-IV-TR criteria for schizoaffective disorder require the presence of a mood disorder and delusions or hallucinations for at least 2 weeks in the absence of prominent mood disorder symptoms.
3. Persons with **delusional disorder** display a persistent belief that is contrary to reality in the absence of other schizophrenia symptoms. Such persons tend not to have flat affect, anhedonia, or other negative symptoms of schizophrenia. They may, however, become socially isolated as a function of their delusions that tend to be long-standing. The DSM-IV-TR recognizes the several delusional subtypes:
    a. The **erotomanic type** is a delusion reflecting the irrational belief that one is loved by another person, usually of higher status (e.g., celebrity stalkers).
    b. The **grandiose type** of delusion involves believing in one's inflated worth, power, knowledge, identity, or special relationship to a deity or famous person.
    c. Persons with a **jealous type** of delusion believes that a sexual partner is unfaithful.
    d. The **persecutory type** involves believing oneself (or someone close) is being malevolently treated in some way.
    e. The **somatic type** of delusion involves events that could be happening but are not (e.g., believing that one is being followed), whereas in schizophrenia such events are not even possible.
    f. Delusional disorder is rare, affecting 24-30 people out of every 100,000. Average age of onset is in middle adulthood, and the disorder is slightly more common in females than males. Prognosis is better than schizophrenia, and features of delusional disorder may have a genetic component.
4. Persons with **brief psychotic disorder** experience one or more positive symptoms of schizophrenia (e.g., delusions, hallucinations, or disorganized speech or behavior) within one month. This disorder is often precipitated by an extremely stressful situation and commonly dissipates on its own.
5. Persons with **shared psychotic disorder** (folie a deux) develop delusions as a result of a close relationship with someone else who has delusions. Content of delusions span the spectrum and little is known about this condition.

6. **Schizotypal personality disorder** (Chapter 12) is related to psychotic disorders. The characteristics of this personality disorder are similar to schizophrenia, but less severe.

III. Prevalence and Causes of Schizophrenia

A. Schizophrenia is generally chronic and most persons with the disorder have difficulty functioning in society, particularly social relationships. The prevalence of schizophrenia worldwide is 0.2% to 1.5%, meaning that it will affect about 1% of the population at some point. Life expectancy in persons with schizophrenia is slightly less than average. Although there is some disagreement about sex differences in diagnosis of schizophrenia, women appear to have more favorable outcomes than men. Onset of schizophrenia is greatest in early adulthood and declines with age for males, whereas the reverse is true for females.

B. Several **classification systems** exist that emphasize onset of schizophrenia; namely process vs. reactive, poor vs. good premorbid, Type I vs. Type II.

1. **Process schizophrenia** is similar to Kraepelin's dementia praecox and was thought to develop slowly, without an obvious stress trigger, to be physiologically based and associated with poor prognosis, leaving the person withdrawn and apparently emotionless. **Reactive schizophrenia** was thought to be a response to extreme stress, with a sudden onset and good prognosis, and accompanied by highly social, volatile, and intense behavior.
    a. Process-reactive categories do not apply neatly to many people. Moreover, some people with reactive schizophrenia eventually show characteristics of process schizophrenia.
    b. The process-reactive distinction is no longer widely accepted.
2. **Poor** versus **good premorbid** is another related classification scheme referring to social functioning before major symptoms of schizophrenia emerge. The poor-good premorbid scheme is no longer considered useful.
3. A more widely accepted classification system, introduced in the mid-1970s, emphasizes positive, negative, and more recently disorganized symptoms. Accordingly, schizophrenia can be dichotomized into **Type I and Type II** based on several characteristics, including symptoms, response to medication, outcome, and presence of intellectual impairment.
    a. **Type I** is associated with positive symptoms, a good response to medication, an optimistic prognosis, and absence of intellectual impairment.
    b. **Type II** includes people with negative symptoms (i.e., flat affect, poverty of speech), poor response to medication, a pessimistic prognosis, and intellectual impairments.

C. **Developmental research** suggests that children who eventually develop schizophrenia tend to show early abnormal signs such as more negative affect and less positive affect. It may be that **brain damage** early in development causes schizophrenia. Research suggests that people with schizophrenia who demonstrate early signs of abnormality at birth and during early childhood tend to do better in the long run than those that do not. This finding is explained, in part, by appeal to **brain plasticity**. That is, early onset schizophrenia allows the brain to compensate for such deficits over time, whereas this is more difficult in a fully developed brain later in life. Other research suggests that older adults display fewer positive symptoms and more negative symptoms, suggesting that schizophrenia may improve over time. Most persons with schizophrenia fluctuate between severe and moderate levels of impairment throughout their lives, and relapse is common.

D. Schizophrenia appears to be a universal **world-wide phenomenon**; however, the course and outcome of schizophrenia varies from culture to culture. In the U.S., more African-Americans are diagnosed with schizophrenia than whites, and may reflect misdiagnosis due to bias against some minority groups.

E. **Genetic influences** are responsible for making some individuals vulnerable to schizophrenia.

1. **Family studies** have shown that the more severe the parent's schizophrenia, the more likely the children were to develop it also. All forms of schizophrenia were also seen within families, meaning that we do not inherit a specific type of schizophrenia, but a general predisposition for schizophrenia that may differ from the parent or close relatives. Family members of a person with schizophrenia are also at increased risk not just for schizophrenia, but a spectrum of psychotic disorders.
    a. Risk for schizophrenia is associated with degree of genetic relatedness to the person with schizophrenia. Having any family member with schizophrenia increases the risk of schizophrenia in other family members above what is expected in the general population.
2. **Twin studies** indicate a confluence of genetic and environmental factors. The risk of schizophrenia in monozygotic twins is 48%. The risk drops to 17% for fraternal (dizygotic) twins. This effect is also represented by the Genain quadruplets who shared identical genes and were raised in the same household, but differed in terms of the onset of schizophrenia, the symptoms, diagnoses, course of the disorder, and outcomes. Genain comes from the Greek meaning "dreadful gene." This case reveals the concept of unshared environments, which may lead to different outcomes of the same disorder even within the same household.
3. **Adoption studies** allow one to differentiate between the role of environment and genetics in the development of schizophrenia. The **adoptees' study method** examines rates of schizophrenia in mothers who gave up their child for adoption. This research suggests that children of parents with schizophrenia (i.e., the mothers in this case) have a much higher chance of developing schizophrenia themselves, even when raised away from their biological parents.

4. Research on the **children of twins with schizophrenia** helps to address whether a genetic link in necessary for one to develop schizophrenia. Such research may identify identical and fraternal twin pairs with a history of

schizophrenia and their children. Then, risk for schizophrenia is assessed in relation to the parent and the parent's related twin in terms of whether either has schizophrenia.

   a. This research suggests that a child has a 17% chance of developing schizophrenia when either the identical twin parent has schizophrenia or if their parent's twin is unaffected.
   b. If the parent is a fraternal twin with schizophrenia, then their children have about a 17% chance of developing schizophrenia. If the fraternal twin parent does not have schizophrenia but their fraternal twin does, the risk in the children drops to about 2%.
   c. The only way to explain such findings is through genetics. This research suggests that genes predispose people to developing schizophrenia, and that one may not show the disorder and yet still pass the genes on to children.

5. **Linkage and association studies** initially focused on a gene located on the fifth chromosome; a finding that has since been refuted. Several sites for genes responsible for schizophrenia have been explored subsequently. Regions of chromosomes 1, 6, 8, 10, 13, 18 and 22 have been implicated in schizophrenia, and a particular gentic deficit (**22q11 deletion syndrome**) is also being explored as a cause of a subtype of schizophrenia. Because dopamine is involved in schizophrenia, researchers have been looking for genes related to dopamine function; however, linkage studies attempted to establish a relation between dopamine sites (D1, D2, D3, and D4 loci) and the presence of schizophrenia genes have not produced strong supportive evidcnce.
6. Several potential markers for schizophrenia have been studied. **Smooth-pursuit eye movement or eye-tracking** refers to a procedure involving keeping one's head still while tracking a moving pendulum back and forth with one's eyes. This tracking ability is deficient in many persons with schizophrenia, including relatives of schizophrenia persons. This work suggests that eye-tracking may be a marker for schizophrenia.
7. Schizophrenia is likely associated with more than one gene; a phenomenon referred to as **quantitative trait loci (QTL)**.

F. **Neurobiological influences** in schizophrenia with regard to brain functioning goes back as far as Emil Kraepelin and several hypotheses have been proposed since then.

1. Schizophrenia may be the result of an **excess of dopamine** in the brain. This hypothesis was propelled by several of the following findings showing that when drugs are administered that are known to increase dopamine (agonists), schizophrenic behavior increases, whereas with drugs that are known to decrease dopamine activity (antagonists), schizophrenia symptoms tend to diminish:
   a. Antipsychotic neuroleptic drugs (i.e., dopamine antagonists) are effective in treating schizophrenia. Such drugs work primarily by blocking the D_2 dopamine receptors

b. The negative side effects are similar to those seen in persons with **Parkinson's disease**; a disorder known to be due to insufficient dopamine.
c. The drug **L-dopa** (i.e., a dopamine agonist) that is used to treat people with Parkinson's disease, and can produce schizophrenia-like symptoms.
d. **Amphetamines** (i.e., drugs that activate dopamine) can make psychotic symptoms worse in people with schizophrenia.
e. Such observations led to the view that schizophrenia was due to excessive dopamine activity.

2. **Arguments against the dopamine theory** include the following:
    a. Many persons with schizophrenia are not helped with dopamine antagonists.
    b. Neuroleptics work to block dopamine quickly, but the relevant symptoms remit long after.
    c. Neuroleptics do little to help the negative symptoms.
    d. The drug **clozapine** is effective for many persons not helped by traditional neuroleptic medication, and yet it is one of the weakest dopamine antagonists.
3. Three specific neurochemical anomalies may be involved in the development of schizophrenia:
    a. The most effective antipsychotic drugs all help block the stimulation of D_2 receptors. This effect leads us to believe that schizophrenia may be the result of **excessive stimulation of striatal dopamine (DA) D_2 receptors**.
    b. Recent work focused on schizophrenia has found that persons with schizophrenia have a **deficiency in the stimulation of prefrontal DA D_2 receptors**.
    c. Two recreational drugs, "PCP" and ketamine produce psychotic-like behavior in persons without schizophrenia. These drugs are NMDA antagonists, meaning that they interact with glutamate receptors. As a result of these findings, it is currently thought that the blocking of NMDA receptors, or **alterations in prefrontal activity involving glutamate transmission**, may be involved in the production of schizophrenic symptoms.
4. Evidence for **neurological damage** in persons with schizophrenia is partially derived from the fact that children at risk for the disorder often show abnormal reflexes and attention problems. Such problems tend to persist into adulthood.
    a. Positive symptoms of schizophrenia may be related to excessive dopamine activity, but negative symptoms may be related to structural brain abnormalities such as **enlarged lateral ventricles**. However, many people without schizophrenia have such abnormalities.
    b. The **frontal lobes** of people with schizophrenia tend to be less active than in people without the disorder; a phenomenon known as **hypofrontality,** or they tend to be too active, termed **hyperfrontality**.

These deficits appear in a dorsolateral prefrontal cortex of the frontal lobes, and are associated with the negative symptoms of schizophrenia. This prefrontal area is also one site of a major dopamine pathway in the brain.

5. Some have hypothesized that schizophrenia is a recent phenomenon historically, appearing during the past 200 years, and may involve some recently introduced **virus**. There is evidence that a virus-like disease may account for some cases of schizophrenia, particularly prenatal exposure to influenza. For example, a higher prevalence of schizophrenia is seen among urban males, implying exposure to infectious agents.
    a. Evidence for developmental problems during the second trimester of fetal development has led to an interest in **fingertip dermal cells** that migrate to the cortex of the brain and produce fingerprint ridges. Migration of such cells would be disrupted if a virus occurred during this critical period of development. The number of fingertip ridges in twins without schizophrenia differs little, but substantial differences are seen in one-third of twins discordant for the disorder. This work suggests that fingertip ridge count may be a marker of potential brain damage.

G. Psychological and social influences

1. Research on **stress** and schizophrenia suggests that extreme stress can produce psychotic-like symptoms in otherwise normal persons. Stress appears related to activation of a schizophrenia predisposition and risk for relapse.
2. **Family interactions** and their effect on schizophrenia has been the focus of a great deal of research. The term **schizophrenogenic** was used for a time to describe a mother whose cold, dominant, and rejecting nature was thought to cause schizophrenia in her children. The term **double-bind** was also used to portray a type of communication that produced conflicting messages, resulting in schizophrenia. Both terms are no longer widely used. Recent work has focused on how family interactions contribute to relapse from schizophrenia, not in the onset of schizophrenia.
    a. **Expressed emotion** is a term describing a particular family communication style that is related to schizophrenic relapse. High expressed emotion, characterized by criticism, hostility, and emotional over-involvement, is strongly related to risk of relapse. Persons with schizophrenia living in a family with high expressed emotion are 3.7 times more likely to relapse than if they lived in a family low in expressed emotion.

IV. Treatment of Schizophrenia

A. Historically the treatment of schizophrenia was highly medicalized. For instance, primitive brain surgeries were used as early as the 1500s, and similar, albeit more sophisticated, procedures were used in the 1950s (e.g., **prefrontal lobotomies**). Modern Westernized treatment of schizophrenia usually begin with **neuroleptic drugs** in combination with psychosocial treatments aimed at reducing relapse, compensating for skills deficits, and to improve compliance with medication regimens.

B. Biological interventions

1. During the 1930s, persons with schizophrenia may have undergone one of several biological interventions, including:
    a. **Insulin coma therapy** involved injections of massive doses of insulin to induce a coma in persons suffering from schizophrenia. Though many thought this procedure was helpful, serious illness and death often occurred.
    b. **Psychosurgery**, including prefrontal lobotomies was also introduced in the 1930s. **Prefrontal lobotomies** involved severing the frontal lobes from the lower portion of the brain, resulting in calmed behavior but severe cognitive and emotional deficits. Such procedures are still used in some primitive cultures.
    c. In the late 1930s, **electroconvulsive therapy (ECT)** was advanced as a treatment for schizophrenia, but was found to be of little help.
2. During the 1950s, several **neuroleptic drugs** were introduced to relieve the symptoms of schizophrenia. Such drugs affect the positive symptoms of schizophrenia (i.e., reduce or eliminate hallucinations and delusions), and help persons think more clearly. Such drugs are not equally effective for all persons and often involve a trial and error process to find a medication that works best. Many persons with schizophrenia stop taking their medications from time to time, mostly because of the negative side effects of such drugs.
    a. The earliest neuroleptic drugs, called **conventional antipsychotics**, work in about 60% of persons who try them, but include several unpleasant side effects.
    b. **Newer medications**, such as clozapine, risperidone, and olanzapine, have fewer serious side effects than conventional antipsychotics.
3. Factors affecting **noncompliance** with medications include a negative patient-doctor relationship, cost of medication, poor social support, and unwanted negative side effects. Side effects of neuroleptics may include **extrapyramidal** or **Parkinsonian symptoms**.
    a. One such symptom is **akinesia**, which is characterized by an expressionless face, slowed motor activity, and monotonous speech.
    b. Another extrapyramidal symptom is **tardive dyskinesia**, which involves involuntary movements of the tongue, face, mouth, or jaw and can include protrusions of the tongue, puffing of the cheeks, puckering of the mouth, and chewing movements. Tardive dyskinesia results from high doses of antipsychotic medications over long time periods and often is irreversible.
4. A newer and not-as-yet validated procedure for the treatment of hallucinations involves exposing the individual to magnetic fields. This procedure, called **transcranial magnetic stimulation**, uses wire coils to repeatedly generate magnetic fields that pass through the skull to the brain. Recent research has

demonstrated reductions in hallucinations following this procedure; however, further research is needed to assess the effectiveness of this treatment.

C. Psychosocial interventions

1. Today, few believe that psychological factors cause schizophrenia or that traditional psychotherapeutic approaches will cure them; however, psychosocial approaches have an important role in treatment.
2. **Behavioral approaches** for inpatients are designed to encourage and foster appropriate socialization, participation in group sessions, and self-care, while discouraging violent outbursts. Such interventions rely on **token economy** systems, in which residents earn access to meals and small luxuries by behaving appropriately. Patients in such programs do better than those who are not part of them.
3. Clinicians also reduce the routine institutionalization of persons with schizophrenia by implementing **community care programs**.
4. The more insidious negative effects of schizophrenia are on **social behavior**, or the person's ability to relate with other people. Treatments here target and attempt to re-teach social skills such as how to have a basic conversation, assertiveness, and relationship building. Modeling, role-play, feedback, and practice are emphasized. Maintenance of these skills may be problematic, however.
5. **Independent living skills programs** focus on teaching a range of skills that persons with schizophrenia can use to adapt to their disorder and still live in the community. Such programs are multidisciplinary and help prevent relapse.
6. **Behavioral family therapy** has been used as a means to teach families of persons with schizophrenia to be more supportive, particularly families high in expressed emotion. Such procedures provide education about schizophrenia, teach communication skills, address more constructive ways of expressing negative feelings, and emphasize problem solving. This type of therapy seems to require ongoing work, as its effectiveness diminishes after 1 year.
7. **Vocational rehabilitation** is used to help persons with schizophrenia gain and maintain employment, and may include hands-on job coaches.

D. Treatment across cultures

1. **Cultural factors** seem to play a role in the treatment of schizophrenia. For example, Hispanics are less likely to seek help in institutional settings and rely instead on family support. In China, the preferred treatment for schizophrenia is antipsychotic medication and most are treated outside of hospitals. In Africa, persons with schizophrenia are kept in prisons.

E. Prevention efforts

1. **Prevention** of schizophrenia focuses on identifying and treating children who may be at risk for the disorder later in life. Instability of early family rearing environment seems related to subsequent risk of developing schizophrenia in

at risk children. Preventive efforts may focus on birth complications and early illnesses, particularly among those who are genetically predisposed.

OVERALL SUMMARY

This chapter outlines the primary features of schizophrenia and related psychotic disorders. Positive and negative symptoms as well as subtypes of schizophrenia are described. Related problems include schizophreniform, schizoaffective, delusional, brief psychotic, and shared psychotic disorder. Etiological factors, relapse, and treatment are discussed.

KEY TERMS

Alogia (p. 461)
Anhedonia (p. 461)
Associative splitting (p. 456)
Avolition (p. 461)
Brief psychotic disorder (p. 466)
Catatonia (p. 455)
Catatonic immobility (p. 462)
Catatonic type of schizophrenia (p. 464)
Delusional disorder (p. 465)
Delusion (p. 458)
Dementia praecox (p. 456)
Disorganized speech (p. 462)
Disorganized type of schizophrenia (p. 463)
Double bind (p. 477)
Expressed emotion (p. 477)
Flat affect (p. 461)
Good premorbid (p. 468)
Hallucination (p. 460)
Hebephrenia (p. 455)
Inappropriate affect (p. 462)
Negative symptoms (p. 468)
Paranoia (p. 456)
Paranoid type of schizophrenia (p. 463)
Poor premorbid (p. 468)
Positive symptoms (p. 468)
Process schizophrenia (p. 467)
Psychotic (p. 458)
Reactive schizophrenia (p. 468)
Residual type of schizophrenia (p. 464)
Schizoaffective disorder (p. 464)
Schizophrenia (p. 455)
Schizophreniform disorder (p. 464)
Schizophrenogenic (p. 477)

Schizotypal personality disorder (p. 466)
Shared psychotic disorder (folie à deux) (p. 466)
Token economy (p. 480)
Undifferentiated type of schizophrenia (p. 464)

INFOTRAC KEY TERM EXERCISES

Each exercise is linked to key terms from the Wadsworth InfoTrac on-line searchable database. Key terms must be entered exactly as written.

Exercise 1: **Reducing Violent Behavior in Persons Suffering From Schizophrenia**
Article: A80485496
Citation: (Reducing violence in severe mental illness: Randomised controlled trial of intensive case management compared with standard care). Elizabeth Walsh; Catherine Gilvarry; Chiara Samele; Kate Harvey; Catherine Manley; Peter Tyrer; Francis Creed; Robin Murray; Thomas Fahy.
British Medical Journal, Nov 10, 2001 v323 i7321 p1093(4)

Violent acts are rare events in persons with mental illness, including severe forms of mental illness such as schizophrenia. Nonetheless, schizophrenic individuals do, on occasion, commit violent acts. Usually such acts make there way into the media and create the false impression that violence and mental illness go hand in hand. This InfoTrac article describes a Randomized Clinical Trial comparing the efficacy of intensive case management vs. standard case management in reducing violence in patients with psychosis. Read the article and answer the following questions: (a) what is the relation between violence and mental illness?, (b) describe what the authors of this study were testing, including the interventions, the participants, and dependent variables, (c) briefly summarize the main findings of the study, and (d) based on the findings, what intervention appears to offer the best hope in reducing violent acts by persons suffering from schizophrenia and other severe forms of mental illness? Limit your answer to 3-5 double-spaced pages.

Exercise 2: **What do We Know About the Brains of Children With Schizophrenia**
Key Term: *Schizophrenia, Development and Progression*

The neurobiological connection in schizophrenia seems clear and linked, in some respect, to early changes in brain function. Yet, surprisingly little is known about neurobiological markers for schizophrenia in children. What are the childhood neurobiological markers (if any), and what do we know about the brains of schizophrenic children? Review the InfoTrac article on this topic, and draw parallels between recent neurobiological markers in children with schizophrenia and what is known about similar neurobiological markers in adults with schizophrenia (see your textbook). Limit your answer to 3-5 double-spaced pages.

Exercise 3: **Expressed Emotion: A Concept Stretching Beyond Schizophrenia's Borders**
Key Term: *Expressed Emotion*

Relapse in schizophrenia has been linked to the construct of high expressed emotion, particularly in family members of persons suffering from schizophrenia. Yet, the expressed emotional concept is finding its way into other areas of psychopathology as a toxic risk factor for psychopathology more generally. What psychological problems show a relation with expressed emotion, and what is so toxic about this particularly style of family communication. Review the InfoTrac article on this topic and summarize current research on the expressed emotion concept in relation to schizophrenia and other forms of psychopathology. Is expressed emotion a general risk factor for some forms of psychopathology, or is it specific to schizophrenia? Limit your answer to 3-5 double-spaced pages.

Exercise 4 (Future Trend): Recent Developments in Atypical Antipsychotic Medications

Atypical antipsychotic medications have fewer negative side effects than earlier conventional neuroleptic medications and are considered a first line treatment for most forms of schizophrenia. Such drugs are being developed at a rapid clip. The links below provide detailed information about these newer drugs, how they work, side effect profiles, and related resources. You may use this activity as an opportunity to describe these newer medications in more detail, including information about what can be done to help individuals suffering from schizophrenia.

http://www.healthyplace.com/Communities/Thought_Disorders/schizo/medications/index.htm

http://www.healthyplace.com/Communities/Thought_Disorders/schizo/news/index.htm

http://www.abpi.org.uk/publications/publication_details/targetSchizophrenia-2003/section5.asp

http://www.schizophrenia-help.com/

CLASSROOM ACTIVITIES, DEMONSTRATIONS, AND LECTURE TOPICS

1. **Demonstration: Symptoms of Schizophrenia.** Osberg (1992) developed a monologue which simulates the thought disorders and disorganized language typical of schizophrenia. Osberg recommends displaying the monologue on an overhead projector and asking students to identify examples of specific schizophrenic symptoms.

   Source Information. Osberg, T. M. (1992) The disordered monologue: A classroom demonstration of the symptoms of schizophrenia. Teaching of Psychology, 19, 47-48.

   National public radio also has an excellent on-line multimedia segment illustrating auditory and visual hallucinations of a person going to a pharmacy for medications. This is perhaps the best segment I have seen showing what positive symptoms (mostly paranoid) are like. The link to the web site is:
   http://www.npr.org/programs/atc/features/2002/aug/schizophrenia/

2. **Activity: The Social Anhedonia Scale.** Students will have a better idea of one of the most common symptoms of schizophrenia after completing this scale (which is also an appropriate way to elaborate on one of the symptoms of major depression). This scale is a true-false questionnaire which can be completed within class time.

   Source Information. Leak, G. K. (1991). An examination of the construct validity of the Social Anhedonia scale. Journal of Personality Assessment, 56, 84-95.

3. **Activity: Name that Symptom!** To test students' understanding of the different symptoms of schizophrenia, divide the class into several teams. Prepare clinical examples of the various symptom categories. Take turns reading an example to each team, who then has a chance to determine what symptom is being described. If the first team does not get the answer correct, then the next team can try to answer. Examples of the clinical symptoms include:

   a. *Disorder of thought content or delusion:* The flicker of candles communicates secret messages about me to aliens.
   b. *Delusion of grandeur:* I am Queen of Eastern Europe.
   c. *Delusion of persecution:* The CIA is tracking me and planning on assassinating me in my sleep.
   d. *Auditory hallucination:* Voices tell me to jump out of windows.
   e. *Visual hallucination:* I can see large spiders crawling up my walls.
   f. *Olfactory hallucination:* I smell my family's pets around me.
   g. *Tactile hallucination:* I feel little bugs crawling under my skin.
   h. *Tangentiality:* Oh, you want to know where I was, well, my brother called me to come over and he works on cars at a shop in town that has money problems.
   i. *Loose association:* I went to the store but the violin was fixed so I could return to church and pray.
   j. *Waxy flexibility and catatonic immobility:* (Demonstrate).
   k. *Alogia:* (Ask a student to question you and then respond in monosyllables).

   These represent one example per symptom, but you can provide additional examples. Keep score so you can determine the team that wins the most points. You may want to reward the winning team with extra credit points to get students invested in learning the material.

4. **Activity: Lecture on Hallucinations in "Normal" Individuals.** Hallucinations can occur in people *without* schizophrenia. In fact, one study conducted by Chapman, Edell, and Chapman (1980) found that 15% of normal subjects have experienced psychotic-like symptoms involving auditory hallucinations. Certain conditions like fatigue, hunger, drugs, stress, and religious fervor can cause psychotic-like symptoms in normal people. For example, Kendall and Hammen (1984) noted the following in their *Abnormal Psychology* text: "Have you ever been so tired while driving at night that the bright lights of an oncoming car became a huge orange rolling down the road? Or have you ever ingested a drug that caused you to "hear" colors or made you think that you could see inside people's heads? Or maybe in your place of worship you felt that God spoke through you in a language that you couldn't understand" (p. 297). Have students discuss any hallucinatory experiences they may have had and explore what the experience was like for them. This exercise serves to enhance student empathy and help reduce the fear that is often elicited by people who have schizophrenia.

   You may also want to administer to the class the Perceptual Aberration Scale (1980) that measures unusual experiences. This scale is referenced in the following article:

Source Information. Chapman, L. J., Edell, W. S., & Chapman, J. P. (1980). Physical anhedonia, perceptual aberration, and psychosis proneness. Schizophrenia Bulletin, 6, 639-653.

5. **Video Activity: Schizophrenia.** Show the film segment from *Abnormal psychology inside/out, vol 1, Video 2* that presents an interview with a patient named Edna, who displays disordered thoughts and delusions. This segment nicely demonstrates positive and negative symptoms, disorganized thoughts, and delusions associated with schizophrenia. During the interview, Edna also displays extrapyramidal symptoms. Ask you students to try and identify and classify the symptoms she displays during the interview and to attempt to diagnose her type of schizophrenia.

SUPPLEMENTARY READING MATERIAL FOR CHAPTER THIRTEEN

(I = These sources can be found on "*Infotrac, the online library*" provided by Wadsworth and Brooks/Cole Publishing.)

Birchwood, M. J. (1989). Schizophrenia: An integrated approach to research and treatment. New York: New York University Press.

I Bower, B. (1998). DNA links reported for schizophrenia. Science News, 154, 151(1).

Brown, M. J., & Roberts, D. P. (2000). Growing up with a schizophrenic mother. Jefferson, NC: McFarland.

Cromwell, R. L., & Snyder, C. R. (Eds.) (1993). Schizophrenia: Origins, processes, treatment, and outcome. New York: Oxford University Press.

Farber, S. (Ed.) (1993). Madness, heresy, and the rumor of angels: The revolt against the mental health system. Chicago: Open Court.

Green, M. F. (2001). Schizophrenia revealed: From neurons to social interactions. New York: W. W. Norton.

Hatfield, A. B., & Lefley, H. P. (1993). Surviving mental illness: Stress, coping and adaptation. New York: Guildford.

Heinrichs, R. W. (2001). In search of madness: Schizophrenia and neuroscience. New York: Oxford University Press.

Johnstone, E. C., Humphreys, M. S., Lang, F. H., Lawrie, S. M., & Sandler, R. (1999). Schizophrenia: Concepts and clinical management. New York: Cambridge University Press.

Leudar, I., & Thomas, P. (2000). Voices of reason, voices of insanity: Studies of verbal hallucinations. Florence, KY: Taylor and Francis/Routledge.

Lidz, T. (1985). Schizophrenia and the family. New York: International Universities Press.

Malone, J. A. (1992). Schizophrenia: Handbook for clinical care. Thorofare, NJ: SLACK Inc.

Schiller, L., & Bennett, A. (1996). The quiet room: A journey out of the torment of madness. New York: Harper.

Straube, E. R., & Hahlweg, K. (Eds.) (1990). Schizophrenia: Concepts, vulnerability, and intervention. New York: Springer-Verlag.

Torrey, E. F. (1995). Surviving schizophrenia: A manual for families, consumers, and providers. New York: Harper.

Warner, R. (2000). The environment of schizophrenia: Innovations in practice, policy and communications. Philadelphia, PA: Brunner-Routledge.

Weiden, P. J., Diamond, R. J., Scheifler, P. L., Flynn, L., Diamond, R. I., & Ross, R. (Eds.) (1999). Breakthroughs in antipsychotic medications: A guide for consumers, families, and clinicians. New York: W.W. Norton.

SUPPLEMENTARY VIDEO RESOURCES FOR CHAPTER THIRTEEN

A Beautiful Mind. (Hollywood Film; Drama). This film presents the life of John Nash, a Nobel Prize winning mathematician, and his experience with schizophrenia.

Abnormal psychology inside/out, vol 1, video 2. (*available through your International Thomson Learning representative).* Presents the case of a patient named Edna, who displays disordered thoughts and delusions. This segment nicely demonstrates positive and negative symptoms, disorganized thoughts, and delusions associated with schizophrenia. During the interview, Edna also displays extrapyramidal symptoms. (15 min)

Antipsychotic agents. (Insight Media: 2162 Broadway, New York, NY 10024/ (800)-233-9910). Examining the medications used to alleviate psychotic symptoms, this video features reenactments that illustrate positive and negative symptoms as well as such features as cognitive dysfunction and dysphonic mood. It presents commonly prescribed agents used in the treatment of acute psychotic symptoms; addresses precautions, side effects, and drug interactions; and includes interviews in which professionals and patients discuss the impact of antipsychotic agents on patients with psychotic symptoms. (23 min)

Birdy. (Hollywood; Drama/War). This film depicts a catatonic inpatient in a military hospital who is also a Vietnam veteran.

CNN today: Abnormal psychology, vol. 1. (*available through your International Thomson Learning representative).* The segment titled, "Schizophrenic and Other Psychotic Disorders: Schizophrenia Drug" presents the case of a man with schizophrenia who is on clozapine and how this drug has changed his life and made him able to function in society. Discusses the success clozapine has had on patients who did not respond to any other therapies. Also talks about the side-effects of this medication (e.g., damage to bone marrow). (2 min, 35 sec)

Dark side of the moon. (Fanlight Productions, 1-800-937-4113). This film documents the struggles and successes of three formerly homeless men with mental illnesses. (25 min)

Deficits of mind and brain. (*available through your International Thomson Learning representative).* The second module begins with an overview of schizophrenia. Diagnostic criteria and examples of patients in therapy (showing thought insertion, thought withdrawal, and paranoid delusions) are provided. In the second portion of this module, four patients suffering from schizophrenia are presented. The third portion of this module uses the Wisconsin Card Sorting Task to demonstrate how lesion location has differential effects on task completion. The fourth portion of this module introduces PET imaging techniques for isolating patterns in cerebral processing across brain structures. The fifth portion of this module describes cognitive deficits, the sixth portion covers cognitive neuroscience and schizophrenia, and the last portion covers genetics and schizophrenia.

First break. (Fanlight Productions, 1-800-937-4113). This film documents the impact of the "first break" of mental illness on three young people in their teens and early twenties, as well as the effects on their families. (51 min)

I'm still here: The truth about schizophrenia. (Insight Media: 2162 Broadway, New York, NY 10024/ (800)-233-9910). In this video, medical professionals debunk myths of schizophrenia to provide an accurate and comprehensive picture of this complex disease. It profiles individuals who, though afflicted by this illness, lead lives of extraordinary accomplishment, and it depicts the heartbreak and hope experienced by their families. (67 min)

I never promised you a rose garden. (Hollywood Film; Drama). The patient depicted in this film has command hallucinations that tell her to kill herself. The film provides a sympathetic portrayal of psychiatry and treatment.

One flew over the cukoo's nest. (Hollywood Film; Drama). This is a classic film staring Jack Nicholson as a patient in a psychiatric hospital. The film provides a nice depicting of life on an inpatient ward, including controversial treatments such as ECT and frontal lobotomies.

Repulsion. (Hollywood Film; Horror). This is an intense film about sexual repression and psychotic decompensation, providing good examples of hallucinations.

The shattered mind. (Insight Media: 2162 Broadway, New York, NY 10024/ (800)-233-9910). This video explores the debate over mandatory treatment for schizophrenia, discussed by experts from Bellevue Hospital who detail available options and their dangers. It considers a family whose schizophrenic son refused medication, and profiles a schizophrenic artist whose medication enables her near-normal life. It also dissects a schizophrenic brain. (50 min)

The snake pit. (Hollywood Film; Drama). This is one of the first films to document the treatment of patients in mental hospitals.

Trouble in mind. (Insight Media: 2162 Broadway, New York, NY 10024/ (800)-233-9910). Each of the 13 videos in this set focuses on one common mental disorder, showing typical behavior and symptoms and providing vital information on how to spot and interpret symptoms. The disorders include Alzheimer's disease, anti-social personality disorder, ADHD, bipolar disorder, delirium, depression, eating disorder, obsessive-compulsive disorder, panic disorder, PTSD, postpartum depression, psychosomatic disorder, and schizophrenia. (13 Volumes/30 min each)

INTERNET 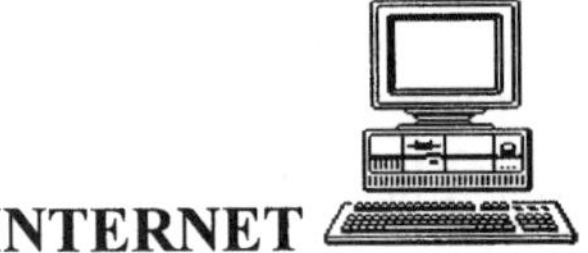 RESOURCES FOR CHAPTER THIRTEEN

About.Com Schizophrenia
http://mentalhealth.about.com/cs/schizophrenia/
A mega site with links and information about schizophrenia and its treatment.

Medical Treatment of Schizophrenia
http://www.psychlaws.org/MedicalResources/index.htm
This site provides information about medical management of schizophrenia.

Mental Health Net Schizophrenia
http://www.mentalhealth.com/dis/p20-ps01.html
This page provides an outstanding starting point for up-to-date information about the diagnosis, etiology, and treatment of schizophrenia, including numerous links to patient and scholarly web sites.

National Alliance of the Mentally Ill
http://www.nami.org/index.html
This site is a useful resource for information related to the treatment of severe mental illness, including legal issues and national health policy guidelines.

NIMH Schizophrenia: Questions and Answers
http://www.nimh.nih.gov/publicat/pubListing.cfm?dID=11
Questions and answers regarding schizophrenia provided by the National Institutes of Health.

Psych Central -- Schizophrenia
http://psychcentral.com/library/meds_schizo.htm
Nice site with lots of information about schizophrenia and available treatment options.

Schizophrenia: A Handbook for Families
http://www.mentalhealth.com/book/p40-sc01.html
This site provides a very detailed description of schizophrenia, including information relevant for families of persons with this disorder, information about causes and medical and psychosocial treatment alternatives.

Schizophrenia.Com Home Page
http://www.schizophrenia.com/
Provides links to other web pages devoted to schizophrenia (this is a good starting place for finding information on schizophrenia on the internet)

WARNING SIGNS OF SCHIZOPHRENIA

- Hearing or seeing something that isn't there
- A constant feeling of being watched
- Peculiar or nonsensical way of speaking or writing
- Strange body positioning
- Feeling indifferent to very important situations
- Deterioration of academic or work performance
- A change in personal hygiene and appearance
- A change in personality
- Increasing withdrawal from social situations
- Irrational, angry or fearful response to loved ones
- Inability to sleep or concentrate
- Inappropriate or bizarre behavior
- Increased withdrawal from social situations
- Extreme preoccupation with religion or the occult

DSM-IV-TR Criteria for Schizophrenia
Criteria A, B, and C

A. Characteristic symptoms: Two (or more) of the following, each present for a significant portion of time during a 1-month period (or less if successfully treated):

1. delusions
2. hallucinations
3. disorganized speech (e.g., frequent derailment or incoherence)
4. grossly disorganized or catatonic behavior
5. negative symptoms, i.e., affective flattening, alogia, or avolition

Note: Only one Criterion A symptom is required if delusions are bizarre or hallucinations consist of a voice keeping up a running commentary on the person's behavior or thoughts, or two or more voices conversing with each other.

B. Social/occupational dysfunction: For a significant portion of the time since the onset of the disturbance, one or more major areas of functioning such as work, interpersonal relations, or self-care are markedly below the level achieved prior to the onset (or when the onset is in childhood or adolescence, failure to achieve expected level of interpersonal, academic, or occupational achievement).

C. Duration: Continuous signs of the disturbance persist for at least 6 months. This 6-month period must include at least 1 month of symptoms (or less if successfully treated) that meet Criterion A (i.e., active-phase symptoms) and may include periods of prodromal or residual symptoms. During these prodromal or residual periods, the signs of the disturbance may be manifested by only negative symptoms or two or more symptoms listed in Criterion A present in an attenuated form (e.g., odd beliefs, unusual perceptual experiences).

DSM-IV-TR Criteria for Schizophrenia
Criteria D, E, F, and Course

D. Schizoaffective and Mood Disorder exclusion: Schizoaffective Disorder and Mood Disorder With Psychotic Features have been ruled out because either (1) no Major Depressive, Manic, or Mixed Episodes have occurred concurrently with the active-phase symptoms; or (2) if mood episodes have occurred during active-phase symptoms, their total duration has been brief relative to the duration of the active and residual periods.

E. Substance/general medical condition exclusion: The disturbance is not due to the direct physiological effects of a substance (e.g., a drug of abuse, a medication) or a general medical condition.

F. Relationship to a Pervasive Developmental Disorder: If there is a history of Autistic Disorder or another Pervasive Developmental Disorder, the additional diagnosis of Schizophrenia is made only if prominent delusions or hallucinations are also present for at least a month (or less if successfully treated).

Classification of longitudinal course (can be applied only after at least 1 year has elapsed since the initial onset of active-phase symptoms):

Episodic With Interepisode Residual Symptoms (episodes are defined by the reemergence of prominent psychotic symptoms); also specify if: With Prominent Negative Symptoms
Episodic With No Interepisode Residual Symptoms
Continuous (prominent psychotic symptoms are present throughout the period of observation); also specify if: With Prominent Negative Symptoms
Single Episode In Partial Remission; also specify if: With Prominent Negative Symptoms
Single Episode In Full Remission
Other or Unspecified Pattern

DSM-IV-TR Criteria for Paranoid Schizophrenia

A type of Schizophrenia in which the following criteria are met:

A. Preoccupation with one or more delusions or frequent auditory hallucinations.

B. None of the following is prominent: disorganized speech, disorganized or catatonic behavior, or flat or inappropriate affect.

Transparency 13-4

DSM-IV-TR Criteria for Disorganized Schizophrenia

A type of Schizophrenia in which the following criteria are met:

A. All of the following are prominent:
   1. disorganized speech
   2. disorganized behavior
   3. flat or inappropriate affect

B. The criteria are not met for Catatonic Type.

DSM-IV-TR Criteria for Catatonic Schizophrenia

A type of Schizophrenia in which the clinical picture is dominated by at least two of the following:

1. motoric immobility as evidenced by catalepsy (including waxy flexibility) or stupor
2. excessive motor activity (that is apparently purposeless and not influenced by external stimuli)
3. extreme negativism (an apparently motiveless resistance to all instructions or maintenance of a rigid posture against attempts to be moved) or mutism
4. peculiarities of voluntary movement as evidenced by posturing (voluntary assumption of inappropriate or bizarre postures), stereotyped movements, prominent mannerisms, or prominent grimacing
5. echolalia or echopraxia

Transparency 13-6

DSM-IV-TR Criteria for Undifferentiated Schizophrenia

A type of Schizophrenia in which symptoms that meet Criterion A are present, but the criteria are not met for the Paranoid, Disorganized, or Catatonic Type.

DSM-IV-TR Criteria for Residual Schizophrenia

A type of Schizophrenia in which the following criteria are met:

A. Absence of prominent delusions, hallucinations, disorganized speech, and grossly disorganized or catatonic behavior.

B. There is continuing evidence of the disturbance, as indicated by the presence of negative symptoms or two or more symptoms listed in Criterion A for Schizophrenia, present in an attenuated form (e.g., odd beliefs, unusual perceptual experiences).

DSM-IV-TR Criteria for Schizophreniform Disorder

A. Criteria A, D, and E of Schizophrenia are met.

B. An episode of the disorder (including prodromal, active, and residual phases) lasts at least 1 month but less than 6 months. (When the diagnosis must be made without waiting for recovery, it should be qualified as "Provisional.")

Specify if:

Without Good Prognostic Features

With Good Prognostic Features: as evidenced by two (or more) of the following:

1. onset of prominent psychotic symptoms within 4 weeks of the first noticeable change in usual behavior or functioning
2. confusion or perplexity at the height of the psychotic episode
3. good premorbid social and occupational functioning
4. absence of blunted or flat affect

DSM-IV-TR Criteria for Schizoaffective Disorder

A. An uninterrupted period of illness during which, at some time, there is either a Major Depressive Episode, a Manic Episode, or a Mixed Episode concurrent with symptoms that meet Criterion A for Schizophrenia.

Note: The Major Depressive Episode must include Criterion A1: depressed mood.

B. During the same period of illness, there have been delusions or hallucinations for at least 2 weeks in the absence of prominent mood symptoms.

C. Symptoms that meet criteria for a mood episode are present for a substantial portion of the total duration of the active and residual periods of the illness.

D. The disturbance is not due to the direct physiological effects of a substance (e.g., a drug of abuse, a medication) or a general medical condition.

Specify type:

Bipolar Type: if the disturbance includes a Manic or a Mixed Episode (or a Manic or a Mixed Episode and Major Depressive Episodes)

Depressive Type: if the disturbance only includes Major Depressive Episodes

DSM-IV-TR Criteria for Delusional Disorder

A. Nonbizarre delusions (i.e., involving situations that occur in real life, such as being followed, poisoned, infected, loved at a distance, or deceived by spouse or lover, or having a disease) of at least 1 month's duration.

B. Criterion A for Schizophrenia has never been met. Note: Tactile and olfactory hallucinations may be present in Delusional Disorder if they are related to the delusional theme.

C. Apart from the impact of the delusion(s) or its ramifications, functioning is not markedly impaired and behavior is not obviously odd or bizarre.

D. If mood episodes have occurred concurrently with delusions, their total duration has been brief relative to the duration of the delusional periods.

E. The disturbance is not due to the direct physiological effects of a substance (e.g., a drug of abuse, a medication) or a general medical condition.

Specify type (the following types are assigned based on the predominant delusiona theme):

Erotomanic Type: delusions that another person, usually of higher status, i in love with the individual

Grandiose Type: delusions of inflated worth, power, knowledge, identity, or special relationship to a deity or famous person

Jealous Type: delusions that the individual's sexual partner is unfaithful

Persecutory Type: delusions that the person (or someone to whom the person is close) is being malevolently treated in some way

Somatic Type: delusions that the person has some physical defect or genera medical condition

Mixed Type: delusions characteristic of more than one of the above types but no one theme predominates

Unspecified Type

DSM-IV-TR Criteria for Brief Psychotic Disorder

A. Presence of one (or more) of the following symptoms:

1. delusions
2. hallucinations
3. disorganized speech (e.g., frequent derailment or incoherence)
4. grossly disorganized or catatonic behavior

Note: Do not include a symptom if it is a culturally sanctioned response pattern.

B. Duration of an episode of the disturbance is at least 1 day but less than 1 month, with eventual full return to premorbid level of functioning.

C. The disturbance is not better accounted for by a Mood Disorder With Psychotic Features, Schizoaffective Disorder, or Schizophrenia and is not due to the direct physiological effects of a substance (e.g., a drug of abuse, a medication) or a general medical condition.

Specify if:

With Marked Stressor(s) (brief reactive psychosis): if symptoms occur shortly after and apparently in response to events that, singly or together, would be markedly stressful to almost anyone in similar circumstances in the person's culture

Without Marked Stressor(s): if psychotic symptoms do not occur shortly after, or are not apparently in response to events that, singly or together, would be markedly stressful to almost anyone in similar circumstances in the person's culture

With Postpartum Onset: if onset within 4 weeks postpartum

Transparency 13-12

DSM-IV-TR Criteria for Shared Psychotic Disorder

A. A delusion develops in an individual in the context of a close relationship wit another person(s), who has an already-established delusion.

B. The delusion is similar in content to that of the person who already has the established delusion.

C. The disturbance is not better accounted for by another Psychotic Disorder (e.g Schizophrenia) or a Mood Disorder With Psychotic Features and is not due to the direct physiological effects of a substance (e.g., a drug of abuse, a medication) or general medical condition.

CHAPTER FOURTEEN

DEVELOPMENTAL DISORDERS

LEARNING OBJECTIVES

1. Define developmental psychopathology.
2. Describe the central defining features of attention deficit/hyperactivity disorder (ADHD), including information about prevalence, known causes, and available treatments.
3. Define the main features and types of learning disorders, including information about their prevalence, course, and how they are typically treated in therapy.
4. Define pervasive developmental disorders and give examples.
5. Describe the three main symptom clusters of autistic disorder, including information about prevalence, course, and information about the kinds of available treatments and their efficacy.
6. Describe the main diagnostic features of Asperger's disorder and distinguish it from autism at the level of symptom presentation, course, and in terms of the kinds of interventions used.
7. Define mental retardation, including the main DSM-IV-TR categories used to classify persons with mental retardation.
8. Describe the four levels of mental retardation based on IQ score and problems associated with using IQ alone to define mental retardation.
9. Describe the American Association of Mental Retardation (AAMR) definition of mental retardation, and outline the three AAMR levels used to classify this problem.
10. Describe the incidence and prevalence of mental retardation.
11. Describe the characteristics of Down and Fragile X syndrome, including what is known about the genetic vs. environmental contribution to mental retardation in general.
12. Discuss available treatment options for persons with mental retardation, including the typical targets of treatment and the efficacy of medications.
13. Briefly outline the nature of prevention programs for developmental disorders.

OUTLINE

I. What is Normal? What is Abnormal?
   A. **Developmental psychopathology** is the study of how disorders arise and change with time. In general, childhood is associated with significant developmental changes that follow a specific pattern. As a result, any disruption in the development of early skills will likely disrupt the development of later skills.

   B. The disorders covered in this chapter are usually diagnosed first in infancy, childhood, or adolescence and include: attention deficit/hyperactivity disorder (ADHD), learning disorders, autism, and lastly mental retardation.

II. Attention Deficit/Hyperactivity Disorder

A. The primary characteristics of persons with **attention deficit/hyperactivity disorder (ADHD)** are inattention, overactivity, and impulsivity. Such persons start many tasks but rarely finish them, have trouble concentrating, and do not seem to pay attention when others speak. These symptoms may lead to other problems such as poor academic performance and peer difficulties. Indeed, children with ADHD are often described as fidgety in school, unable to sit still for more than a few minutes. The textbook illustrates ADHD with the case of Danny.

B. For ADHD, the DSM-IV-TR differentiates two clusters of symptoms.

1. The first cluster includes problems of **inattention**.
2. The second cluster includes symptoms of **hyperactivity and impulsivity**.
3. Either the first (inattention) or the second (hyperactivity and impulsivity) cluster must be present for someone to be diagnosed with ADHD.

C. Inattention, hyperactivity, and impulsivity often result in other problems that are secondary to ADHD. Examples include poor academic performance, unpopularity and peer rejection, and low self-esteem resulting from frequent negative feedback by parents and teachers.

D. ADHD is estimated to occur in 6% of school-aged children, with boys outnumbering girls 4 to 1. The reason for this large gender difference is unknown. \

1. Children with ADHD are first identified as different from their peers around age 3 or 4, and the symptoms of inattention, impulsivity, and hyperactivity become increasingly obvious during the school years.
2. 68% of children with ADHD continue to have problems as adults, mostly inattention.
3. Children are more likely to be labeled ADHD in the United States than anywhere else.

E. The **causes of ADHD** have centered on genetics, brain damage, toxins and food additives, and maternal smoking.

1. With regard to **genetics**, it has been known for some time that ADHD is more common in families with one person having the disorder, and such families display an increase in psychopathology in general, including conduct disorder, mood disorders, anxiety disorders, and substance abuse. More than one gene appears responsible for ADHD, and many are considering possible subtypes of ADHD.
    a. Most of the attention to date focuses on genes associated with the neurochemical dopamine, although norepinepherine, serotonin, and GABA are also implicated in the cause of ADHD.
    b. Families with several individuals with ADHD seem to have a very specific deficit in the region of **chromosome number 20**.

   c. The gene for the D4 receptor, the dopamine transporter gene, and the dopamine D5 receptor gene appear to be associated with ADHD.
2. **Brain damage** has been implicated as a cause of ADHD for several decades as reflected in use of labels such as "minimal brain damage" or "minimal brain dysfunction."
   a. Smaller size of the frontal cortex, the basal ganglia, and the cerebellar vermis have been recently associated with ADHD.
   b. This smaller volume seems to occur early in brain development.
   c. Research has yet to unearth precise neurological mechanisms underlying the basic symptoms of ADHD.
3. **Toxins**, such as allergens and food additives have been considered as possible causes of ADHD, though there is little evidence for this link. Yet, many families continue to put their children on fad diets (e.g., the Feingold Diet), despite the absence of evidence that such diets help.
4. Maternal smoking during pregnancy increases the likelihood of having a child with ADHD threefold.
5. Psychological and social factors of ADHD also influence the disorder itself. Examples include negative responses by parents, teachers, and peers to the affected child's impulsivity and hyperactivity. Such factors may foster a low-self image in ADHD children.

F. **Treatment of ADHD** has proceeded on two fronts: biological and psychosocial interventions.
1. The goal of **biological treatments** is to reduce impulsivity and hyperactivity and to improve attention.
   a. Hundreds of studies have documented the effectiveness of **stimulant medication** in reducing the core symptoms of ADHD. Such medications include methylphenidate (Ritalin), d-amphetamine (Dexedrine), and pemoline (Cylert), which are effective in 70% of cases. Cylert is discouraged from use on a regular basis due to the greater likelihood of negative side effects. The use of stimulant medications causes some concerns, including the potential for abuse. Most common side effects include insomnia, drowsiness, or irritability.
   b. Other drugs such as antidepressants (imipramine) and a drug used to treat high blood pressure (clonidine) have also produced some benefit.
   c. All of these drugs seem to improve compliance and decrease negative behaviors in many children, but they do not affect learning and academic performance. The beneficial effects do not last in the long term once the drug is discontinued.
   d. The paradoxical effects of stimulant medication are the same in children and adults with and without ADHD. Stimulant medications reinforce the brain's ability to focus attention during problem-solving tasks. The theory that these medications produce a paradoxical effect is not supported.

2. **Behavioral interventions** for ADHD involve reinforcement programs to increase appropriate sitting, work, and play. Other programs incorporate parent training.
3. Most clinicians recommend a **combination of biological and psychological approaches** to treat short-term management issues and long-term concerns such as improving social skills and preventing and reversing academic decline.
    a. A recent NIMH sponsored study, titled the "*Multimodal Treatment of Attention-Deficit Hyperactivity Disorder (MTA) Study*," evaluated whether single or combined treatment approaches are most effective.
    b. Initial reports suggest that a combination of behavioral treatments and medication and medication alone were superior to behavioral treatment alone and community care interventions for ADHD symptoms.
    c. Combined treatment seems somewhat better for social skills, parent-child relations, oppositional behavior, and anxiety and depression than single treatments.

III. Learning Disorders

A. **Learning disorders** cover problems related to academic performance in reading, mathematics, and writing that is substantially below what would be expected given the person's age, IQ, and education. The textbook illustrates a reading disorder with the case of Alice.

1. DSM-IV-TR defines a **reading disorder** as a significant discrepancy between a person's reading achievement and what would be expected for someone of the same age.
    a. DSM criteria require that a person read at a level significantly below that of a typical person of the same age, cognitive ability (as measured with an IQ test), and educational background.
    b. The reading problem cannot be caused by a sensory deficit such a trouble with sight or hearing.
2. Similarly, the DSM-IV-TR defines a **mathematics disorder** as achievement below expected performance in mathematics.
3. The DSM-IV-TR **disorder of written expression** represents achievement below expected performance in writing.

B. Definitions of learning disorders vary greatly, making estimates of their incidence and prevalence difficult.

1. There is a 5% to 10% prevalence of learning disorders in the United States, with increased frequency in wealthier regions of the U.S.
2. There appear to be racial differences in the diagnosis of learning disorders, with approximately 1% of white and 2.6% of black children receiving services.
3. Reading difficulties are the most common of the learning disorders and occur in 5% to 15% of the general population, whereas mathematics disorder appears in 6% of the population. Girls and boys are equally likely to have reading disorder.

4. About 32% of students with learning disabilities drop out of school, and employment rates for this group tend to be quite low.
5. Most adults with learning disabilities report that their school experiences were generally negative, with such effects lasting beyond graduation.

C. **Etiological theories** of learning disorders include genetic, neurobiological, and environmental factors.

1. Regarding genetics, reading disorders tend to run in families, and the concordance rate of reading disorders in identical twins is 100%.
    a. Reading disorder may be linked to genetic material on chromosomes 2, 3, 6 and 15, but is likely influenced by several biological and psychosocial factors.
2. Subtle forms of brain damage may be related to learning disabilities; though findings are somewhat mixed.

D. **Treatment** for learning disorders requires intense educational intervention. Biological treatment is typically restricted to those individuals who may also have ADHD.

1. **Educational** interventions focus on the following:
    a. Remediation of the underlying basic **processing** problems (e.g., teaching students visual and auditory perception skills).
    b. Improvement in **cognitive skills** through general instruction in listening, comprehension, and memory.
    c. Targeting **behavioral skills** needed to compensate for specific problems in reading, math, or written expression.
2. Considerable research supports the usefulness of teaching behavioral skills as a means to improve academic skills.

IV. Pervasive Developmental Disorders

A. All persons with **pervasive developmental disorders** have problems with language, socialization, and cognition. **Pervasive** means that the problems affect persons throughout their lives, and includes **autistic disorder**, **Asperger's syndrome, Rett's disorder**, **childhood disintegrative disorder**, and **pervasive developmental disorder – not otherwise specified**. The textbook focuses on autistic disorder and Asperger's disorder.

B. **Autistic disorder**, or autism, is a childhood disorder characterized by significant impairment in social interactions and communication and by restricted patterns of behavior, interest, and activities. The textbook illustrates autism with the case of Amy.

1. The DSM-IV-TR notes **three major characteristics of autism**: impairment in social interactions, impairment in communication, and restricted behavior, interests, and activities.
    a. Persons with autism do not develop the types of **social relationships** expected of their age. Such problems are often more qualitative than quantitative. Such persons are not totally unaware of others, but they

do not seem to enjoy meaningful relationships with others or have the ability to develop them.

   b. Persons with autism have severe problems with **communication**, with about 50% never acquiring useful speech. Some with speech engage in **echolalia**, and others are unable or unwilling to carry on conversations with others.
   c. **Restricted patterns of behavior, interests, and activities** are the most striking aspects of autism. Many prefer that things remain the same; a phenomenon referred to as **maintenance of sameness**. Such persons may also spend countless hours engaging in **stereotyped and ritualistic behaviors** (e.g., spinning around in circles, biting their hands).

2. Autism was once thought to be rare. More recent estimates show an increase in prevalence from 2 to 20 per 10,000 people, to 1 in every 500 births.
   a. Autism is more prevalent in females and for people with IQs under 35, where in the higher IQ range it is more prevalent in males. The reason for this sex difference is unknown.
   b. Autism occurs worldwide and most develop the symptoms before the age of 36 months.
   c. About 50% of persons with autism have IQs in the severe-to-profound range of mental retardation (i.e., IQ less than 50), about 25% test in the mild-to-moderate IQ range (i.e., IQ of 50 to 70), and the remaining people display abilities in the borderline-to-average range (i.e., IQ greater than 70). Better language skills and IQ test performance predicts better lifetime prognosis.
3. Historically, **numerous etiologic theories** have been proposed to explain autism.
   a. In the past, autism was viewed as the result of **bad parenting**. Such parents were thought to be perfectionistic, cold, and aloof. Later research has contradicted this view.
   b. Other theories focused on **unusual speech patterns**; namely the tendency to avoid first-person pronouns such as "I" and "me" and to use he and she instead. This led to the view that autism may reflect a lack of self-awareness. Later research shows that some people with autism do have self-awareness and this follows a developmental progression.
   c. The characteristic idiot savant is not a usual feature of autism.
   d. The phenomenon of **echolalia** (i.e., repeating a word or phrase spoken by another person) was believed to be an unusual characteristic of this disorder; however, this feature is also part of normal development.
   e. The primary characteristic that clearly distinguishes persons with autism from others is social deficiencies.
4. **Biological dimensions** of autism include the following:
   a. **Medical conditions** such as congenital rubella (i.e. German measles), tuberous sclerosis, and difficulties during labor. Such conditions are not always associated with autism.

b. Autism has a **genetic** component. Families with one autistic child have a 3% to 5% risk of having another child with the disorder. The exact genetic contribution is unknown.
c. **Neurobiological** evidence of brain damage is derived from the observation that 3 of 4 people with autism have some level of mental retardation, and 30% to 75% display neurological abnormalities such as clumsiness or abnormal posture or gait.
d. CAT and MRI scans show **abnormalities of the cerebellum,** including reduced size, among people with autism. This appears to be one of the most reliable findings of brain involvement in autism to date.

C. Persons with **Asperger's disorder** suffer from a significant impairment in the ability to engage in meaningful social interaction. Such persons also show restricted and repetitive stereotyped behaviors, but do not show severe delays in language and other cognitive skills characteristic of persons with autism. Examples include following airline schedules or memorizing ZIP codes. Such persons are often quite verbal, but tend to be obsessed with arcane facts and display a pedantic style of speech. Such features led to the name "*Little Professor Syndrome*" to characterize this disorder. Such persons are also often clumsy and exhibit poor coordination. The textbook illustrates Asperger's syndrome with the case of Jim.

1. Many persons with Asperger's disorder probably go undiagnosed, with estimates of prevalence at between 1 and 36 per 10,000.

D. **Treatment** for pervasive developmental disorders relies on a similar approach. The textbook largely focuses on the treatment of autism.

1. **Psychosocial treatments** for autism include behavioral approaches that focus on skill building and treatment of problem behaviors. The behavioral approach is based on the early work of Charles Ferster and Ivar Lovaas. The basic premise is that people with autism can learn and they can be taught some of the skills they lack. Targets for treatment include the following:
    a. **Communication problems** and problems with language are defining characteristics of autism. The basic procedure involves shaping and discrimination training to teach nonspeaking autistic children to imitate others verbally. Alternative methods might include nonverbal gestures and signs.
    b. **Socialization deficits** are profound in persons with autism, and yet limited progress has been achieved toward developing interventions that teach subtle social skills that are important for interactions with peers and others.
    c. Data suggest that early intervention is promising for children with autism. Children placed in regular classrooms tend to do better than those placed in special education classes.
2. No **biological or medical treatment** exists to cure autism. In fact, medical intervention has had little success.

3. **Integrated treatments**, combining several approaches, are the preferred treatment of choice for people with pervasive developmental disorders.
    a. In children, such treatment involves school education combined with special psychological supports for problems with communication and socialization.
    b. Parents likewise need support.
    c. As children with autism grow older, intervention focuses on efforts to integrate them into their communities.

V. Mental Retardation

A. **Mental retardation (MR)** is a disorder of childhood that involves below-average intellectual and adaptive functioning. Historically, persons with mental retardation have been devalued by societies and their treatment has been shameful. Manifestations of mental retardation are varied, with some individuals able to function well in society. Persons with mild-to-moderate impairments (i.e., the majority of persons with MR) can, with proper preparation, carry out most daily activities, whereas those with severe impairments need help to carry out basic living tasks and may, with proper training, achieve a degree of independence. Persons with MR experience impairments that affect most areas of functioning, with language and communication skills being the most obvious problem areas. The textbook illustrates mental retardation with the case of James.

B. The DSM-IV-TR codes MR on **Axis II**, indicating that it is a chronic condition and less amenable to treatment. DSM-IV-TR criteria for MR are arranged in three groups.
1. First a person must have **significantly subaverage intellectual functioning** as determined by one of several IQ tests with a somewhat arbitrary cutoff score set by the DSM-IV-TR at 70 or below. About 2% to 3% of the population score at or below this cutoff.
2. Second, **concurrent deficits or impairments in adaptive functioning** must be evident in at least two of the following areas: communication, self-care, home living, social and interpersonal skills, use of community resources, self-direction, functional academic skills, work, leisure, health, and/or safety.
3. The third criterion is **age of onset**. MR must be evident before the person is 18 years of age. This age criterion rules out the diagnosis of MR for adults who suffer brain trauma or forms of dementia.

C. MR is largely defined by society and most classification systems (including the DSM-IV-TR) identify **four levels of MR**.
1. **Mild MR** includes persons with an IQ score between 50 or 55 and 70.
2. **Moderate MR** includes persons in the IQ range of 35-40 to 50-55.
3. **Severe MR** includes people with IQs ranging from 20-25 up to 35-40.
4. **Profound MR** covers people with IQ scores below 20-25.

D. The most controversial change in the American Association of Mental Retardation (AAMR) definition of MR is its description of different levels of this disorder, based on the level of assistance people need (i.e., intermittent, limited, extensive, or pervasive assistance). The AAMR system identified the role of needed supports in determining level of functioning, whereas the DSM-IV-TR implies that the ability of a person is the sole determining factor.

E. An additional classification method used in education systems to identify abilities of persons with MR relies on three categories. Built into this system is the negative assumption that certain individuals cannot benefit from certain types of training. This system, and the potential stigma of the DSM, led to the AAMR categorization of needed supports.

1. **Educable** mental retardation (i.e., IQ of 50 to approximately 70-75).
2. **Trainable** mental retardation (i.e., IQ of 30 to 50).
3. **Severe** mental retardation (i.e., IQ below 30).

F. About 90% of persons with MR get the label mild mental retardation, and persons with any form of MR represent about 1% to 3% of the general population. The course of MR is chronic; however, prognosis varies greatly. MR occurs more often in males, with a male-to-female ratio of about 6:1; that is, at least in case of mild MR.

G. Etiologic research has identified hundreds of known causes of MR, including **environmental** (e.g., abuse, deprivation), **prenatal** (e.g., exposure to disease, drugs, poor nutrition), **perinatal** (e.g., difficulties during labor and delivery) and **postnatal** (e.g., infections, head injury). Despite the range of known causes, nearly 75% of cases cannot be attributed to any known cause or are thought to be the result of social and environmental influences.

1. **Genetic research** suggests that multiple gene influences are involved in MR. A portion of people with severe MR have identifiable single-gene disorders, involving dominant, recessive, or X-linked genes. Only a few dominant genes result in MR, but can produce conditions related to MR (e.g., tuberous sclerosis, phenylketonuria). **Lesch-Nyhan syndrome** is an X-linked disorder found only in males characterized by MR, signs of cerebral palsy (i.e., spasticity or tightening of the muscles), and self-injurious behavior.
2. Several chromosomal aberrations resulting in MR have been identified.
    a. For example, **Down syndrome** is caused by an extra 21st chromosome and is sometimes referred to as **trisomy 21**. This condition is caused by the failure of cell division (i.e., **nondisjunction**) on chromosome 21, resulting in one cell with one copy that dies and one cell with three copies that divide to create a person with Down syndrome. Down syndrome is associated with characteristic facial features, congenital heart malformations, and dementia of the Alzheimer's type in all adults with Down syndrome past the age of 40. Incidence of Down syndrome increases with the maternal age and risk of this condition can be detected via **amniocentesis**.

b. **Fragile X syndrome** is a second common chromosomally related cause of MR, related to an abnormality on the X chromosome. This condition primarily affects males because they do not have a second X chromosome with a normal gene to balance out the mutation. Female carriers of fragile X syndrome commonly display mild-to-severe learning disabilities. Males with fragile X show moderate-to-severe levels of MR, higher rates of hyperactivity, short attention spans, gaze avoidance, and perseverative speech. Physical characteristics include large ears, testicles, and head circumference. About 1 of every 2,000 males is born with fragile X syndrome.

3. **Psychological and social factors** that are thought to contribute to MR include the following:
    a. **Cultural-familial retardation** is believed to cause about 75% of MR cases and is the least understood. Persons with this form of MR tend to score in the mild MR range on IQ tests and have good adaptive skills. Their MR is thought to result from a combination of psychosocial and biological influences, such as abuse, neglect, and social deprivation. According to the **difference view**, persons with cultural-familiar retardation have a limited subset of deficits (e.g., attentional or memory problems) of those with severe forms of MR and are, therefore, more like persons with severe MR but different from people without MR. The **developmental view** sees the mild MR of people with cultural-familial retardation as a difference in the rate and ultimate ceiling of an otherwise normal developmental sequence. This later view suggests that such children proceed through normal development, but at a slower pace. Support for both views is mixed.

H. **Treatment of MR** parallels treatment of persons with pervasive developmental disorders and attempts to teach such persons skills they need to become more productive and independent. Biological treatment for MR is not a viable option.
1. For mild MR, interventions are similar to learning disorders, and include identification of learning deficits, and assistance with reading and writing. Community support is also included.
2. For severe MR, the goals are generally the same; however, the level of support and community assistance is greatly increased.
3. Persons with MR can acquire skills thorough behavioral interventions, including self-care. Skills are often broken down into component parts via a **task analysis** and the person is taught each skill component in succession until the whole skill can be performed.
4. **Communication training** is also part of treatment. For severe MR, communication training can be challenging, and may include use communication systems such as sign language, picture books, hand gestures, and commuter assisted devices.
5. **Community support** is also critical, and may include supportive employment involving helping the person find, and satisfactorily participate in, a competitive job. Such interventions have been shown to be cost-effective.

VI. Prevention of Developmental Disorders

A. **Prevention** efforts are in the early stages of development. As described previously, early intervention appears promising for some children, and may be helpful for children at risk for cultural-familial mental retardation.

1. The national Head Start program is an early intervention effort that combines educational, medical, and social supports for children and their families.
2. **Prenatal gene therapy** may hold promise for correcting genetic deficits before birth.
3. Prevention efforts also target biological risk factors for development disorders such as malnutrition, exposure to toxins (e.g., lead and alcohol).
4. Behavioral prevention may also include safety training, substance abuse treatment and prevention, and behavioral medicine.

OVERALL SUMMARY

This chapter outlines the primary features of developmental disorders, with a particular emphasis on attention deficit hyperactivity disorder, learning disorders, pervasive developmental disorder (i.e., autistic disorder, Asperger's disorder), and mental retardation. Major features of each of these disorders are outlined within a developmental framework, including integrative coverage of biological, psychological, and sociocultural variables that cause and/or maintain them. Available biological and psychosocial treatments for the developmental disorders are described, including efforts underway to prevent such problems.

KEY TERMS

Amniocentesis (p. 512)
Asperger's disorder (p. 499)
Attention deficit/hyperactivity disorder (ADHD) (p. 490)
Autistic disorder (p. 499)
Childhood disintegrative disorder (p. 499)
Cultural-familial retardation (p. 512)
Disorder of written expression (p. 495)
Down syndrome (p. 511)
Expressive language disorder (p. 497)
Fragile X syndrome (p. 512)
Learning disorders (p. 495)
Mathematics disorder (p. 495)
Mental retardation (p. 507)
Pervasive developmental disorder (p. 499)
Reading disorder (p. 495)
Rett's disorder (p. 499)
Selective mutism (p. 497)
Stuttering (p. 497)
Tic disorder (p. 497)

INFOTRAC KEY TERM EXERCISES

Each exercise is linked to key terms from the Wadsworth InfoTrac on-line searchable database. Key terms must be entered exactly as written.

Exercise 1: The Nature of Intelligence

Article: A13858763

Citation: (On what intelligence is). Robert W. Howard. British Journal of Psychology, Feb 1993 v84 n1 p27(11)

Stupid? Smart? Dumb? We have all heard these socially loaded labels and are in some sense guided by them. At the core, these labels reflect social conceptions of intelligence. All the disorders described in this chapter hinge on assessment of intellectual functioning or IQ. Yet, IQ remains a hotly debated construct that is still poorly understood. This InfoTrac article provides an overview of the changing conceptions of intelligence. After reading this article, address the following points: (a) what is intelligence?, (b) what are some of the new views of intelligence?, (c) what are the implications of the author's position about intelligence for understanding the disorders described in this chapter? Limit your answer to 3-5 double-spaced pages.

Exercise 2: The Real Story About Facilitated Communication as a Treatment for Autism

Key Term: *Facilitated Communication*

Facilitated communication is offered as a new and viable treatment for persons with autism. This treatment purports that children with autism can understand and communicate, but lack the means to do so without a facilitator. Your task is to critically evaluate such claims in light of the available evidence. What is facilitated communication? And, what does the research say about its efficacy for autism? Does this treatment work?, and should parents and caregivers seek out such therapy for their children? Review the InfoTrac article on this topic, and prepare a critical review and response. Limit your answer to 3-5 double-spaced pages.

Exercise 3: The Nature of Williams Syndrome: Should it be Part of the DSM-IV-TR?

Key Term: *Williams Syndrome*

Williams syndrome is a rare but increasingly well understood genetic disorder usually seen in infancy and childhood. This disorder is similar in many respects to the childhood developmental disorders covered in the textbook, but it is not included anywhere in the DSM-IV-TR, or the textbook. Your task here is to assume the role of textbook author with the job of writing a concise summary section outlining the clinical features, prevalence, causes, and treatment of Williams syndrome. Conclude by making an argument to the publisher and textbook authors for inclusion of your wonderfully written section in the next edition of the textbook. Limit your answer to 3-5 double-spaced pages.

Exercise 4 (Future Trend): Does Watching TV Cause ADHD?

Many of us heard the mantra "Too much TV is bad for you" and now it is being argued that TV viewing, at a young age, can compromise cognitive development and even be a risk factor for mental illness, and particularly ADHD. This is a controversial topic that will likely spark debate and discussion in class. The links below provide useful starting points.

http://www.smh.com.au/articles/2004/04/05/1081017107931.html
http://www.limitv.org/tvaddadhd.htm
http://www.autismtoday.com/articles/ADD-ADHD-Linked-to-TV%20.htm

CLASSROOM ACTIVITIES, DEMONSTRATIONS, AND LECTURE TOPICS

1. **Activity: Lecture Discussion about Savants.** Although the text encourages students to move away from stereotypical ideas about children with autism all being savants, you want to nonetheless introduce the topic. People with savant syndromes are fascinating to students and warrant some discussion. You should tie this information to the wonders of the brain and how much we have to learn about its capabilities. Some examples of savant behavior are provided below and can be drawn from the following source:

   Source Information. Roach, M. (1989). Extraordinary people: Understanding "idiot savants." New York: Harper and Row. Martin Bolt draws the following examples from Roach's book:

   a. George and his identical twin brother, Charles, can give you the day of the week for any date over a span of 80,000 years. Ask them to identify the years in the next two centuries in which Easter will fall on March 23 and they will give correct answers with lightning speed. The twin brothers can describe the weather on any day of their adult life. At the same time, they are unable to add or count to 30, and they cannot figure change from a $10 bill for a $6 purchase.
   b. Kenneth can accurately cite the population of every American city over 5000, the distance from each city or town to the largest city in its state, the names, number of rooms, and locations of 2000 leading hotels in the United States, and statistics concerning 3000 mountains and rivers. Kenneth has a mental age of 11 years.
   c. Ellen constructs complicated chords to accompany music she hears on the radio. She was able to repeat the soundtrack of the musical "Evita" after hearing it only once, transposing orchestra and chorus to her piano by using complex, precise chords, including intense dissonances, to reproduce mob and crowd noises. Ellen is blind and has an intelligence quotient of less than 50.

2. **Activity: Would You Want to Know?** Genetic research raises several interesting ethical questions, particularly with regard to the disorders discussed in this chapter. Ask students to consider whether they would want to know as parents whether their unborn child would have Down's syndrome or perhaps even Autism (if such a test were available). Also ask students to consider the ethical implications involved if and when routine genetic testing for development disorders comes of age. Would such testing be advantageous or potentially harmful?

3. **Activity: The Movie "Rainman."** In the film *Rainman*, Dustin Hoffman plays the role of Raymond; a man with apparent autism. Many students will likely be familiar with the film, but what they may not know or appreciate is whether Hoffman's character accurately depicts autistic disorder. Most experts agree that Hoffman's character does not accurately represent autism, and the textbook similarly reinforces this point. After discussing autistic disorder, show the film and ask students to identify whether Raymond displays the three main features of autistic disorder, and whether the film fits the facts

with regard to autistic behavior. You may also open the discussion to issues related to media depiction of persons with profound developmental disabilities.

4. **Activity: Guest Lecture by a Special Education Instructor.** Ask a special education instructor to visit the class to talk about the intervention methods s/he uses to assist persons with developmental disabilities. You may also supplement this with a speaker from your college or university student disabilities services.

5. **Video Activity: Autism and Mainstreaming.** Show the segment titled "Autism," from Abnormal Psychology: Inside/Out Vol. 3. In this segment, Dr. Durand discusses the nature of autism, its characteristics and symptoms. There is live footage of a public school in New York where the teachers and children with autism are in a mainstreamed setting with other students. Aside from the real footage, this segment highlights the ongoing controversy regarding whether such children should be mainstreamed into regular classes or placed in special education classes. You may use this segment as a springboard to discuss student reactions to the idea of mainstreaming, particularly in light of the assets and liabilities of this approach. Stress that there are no right or wrong answers.

SUPPLEMENTARY READING MATERIAL FOR CHAPTER FOURTEEN

(🔍 = These sources can be found on "*Infotrac, the online library*" provided by Wadsworth and Brooks/Cole Publishing.)

Barkley, R. A. (1997). ADHD and the nature of self-control. New York: Guilford.

Cohen, S. (1998). Targeting autism: What we know, don't know, and can do to help young children with autism and related disorders. Berkeley, CA: University of California Press.

Fouse, B. A. (1997). Treasure chest of behavioral strategies for individuals with autism. Arlington, TX: Future Horizons.

Frith, U. (Ed.) (1991). Autism and Asperger's syndrome. New York: Cambridge University Press.

🔍 Gaub, M., & Carlson, C. L. (1997). Gender differences in ADHD: A meta-analysis and critical review. Journal of the American Academy of Child and Adolescent Psychiatry, 36, 1036(10).

Jordan, D. R. (1992). Attention deficit disorder: ADHD and ADD syndromes. Austin, TX: PRO-ED.

Klin, A., Volkmar, F. R., & Sparrow, S. S. (Eds.) (2000). Asperger syndrome. New York: Guilford.

Kozloff, M. A. (1998). Reaching the autistic child: A parent training program. Cambridge, MA: Brookline Books.

Kurlan, R. (Ed.) (1993). Handbook of Tourette's syndrome and related tic and behavioral disorders. New York: Dekker.

Mayes, S. D., Calhoun, S. L., & Crites, D. L. (2001). Does DSM-IV Asperger's disorder exist? Journal of Abnormal Child Psychology, 29, 263.

Pliszka, S. R., Carlson, C. L., & Swanson, J. M. (1999). ADHD with comorbid disorders: Clinical assessment and management. New York: Guilford.

Rutter, M. (2000). Genetic studies of autism: From the 1970s into the millennium. Journal of Abnormal Child Psychology, 28, 3.

Seifert, C. D. (1990). Theories of autism. Lanham, MD: University Press of America.

Shapiro, E. S. (1996). Academic skills problems. New York: Guilford.

Siegel, B. (1996). The world of the autistic child: Understanding and treating autistic spectrum disorders. Oxford: Oxford University Press.

Silverman, H. H. (1992). Stuttering and other fluency disorders. Englewood Cliffs, NJ: Prentice Hall.

Tanguay, P. E. (2000). Pervasive developmental disorders: A 10-year review. Journal of the American Academy of Child and Adolescent Psychiatry, 39, 1079.

Teeter, P. A. (2000). Interventions for ADHD: Treatment in developmental context. New York: Guilford.

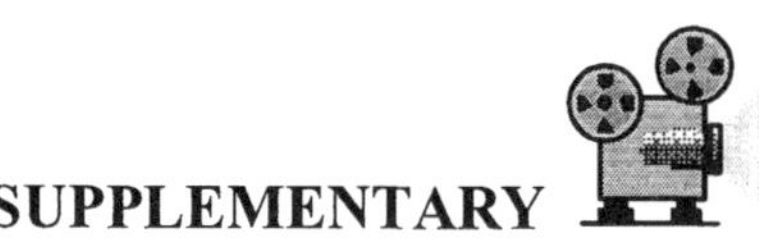

SUPPLEMENTARY VIDEO RESOURCES FOR CHAPTER FOURTEEN

Abnormal psychology inside/out, vol 3. (*available through your International Thomson Learning representative).* The segment titled, "Attention Deficit Hyperactivity Disorder," presents Jim Swanson of the University of California-Irvine interviewing the parent of an 11 year old child with ADHD. This segment covers the DSM-IV characteristics of attention deficit hyperactivity disorder, and shows how this child behaved at 5 and 6 prior to behavioral treatment combined with medication. Dr. Swanson discusses the theories of neuropsychological causes of ADHD and the role of dopamine as well.

A second segment titled, "Autism," presents an interview with V. Mark Durand of SUNY-Albany. Dr. Durand discusses the nature of autism, its characteristics and symptoms.

There is live footage of a public school in New York where the teachers and children with autism are in a mainstreamed setting with other students. It gives students a chance to see what this disorder looks like, and gives a chance to talk with their teachers. The footage also shows the clinical, school, and home settings of the child, giving a full picture of how this child's behavior changed pre to post-therapy.

ADHD: What do we know? (Insight Media: 2162 Broadway, New York, NY 10024/ (800)-233-9910). This video outlines the etiology and prevalence of ADHD and describes its manifestations, comorbidity, and long-term outcome. (35 min)

Autism: A world apart. (Fanlight Productions, 1-800-937-4113). This film depicts the stories of three families and what it is like to love and care for children with autism. (29 min)

Behavior disorders of childhood. (Insight Media: 2162 Broadway, New York, NY 10024/ (800)-233-9910). This video visits families of youngsters with attention deficit hyperactivity disorder, conduct disorder, separation anxiety disorder, and autism. It also features experts in child development and psychology who discuss how to differentiate abnormal behavior from normal developmental patterns. (60 min)

Behind the glass door: Hannah's story. (Fanlight Productions, 1-800-937-4113). Following the struggle of the Shepard family over a period of five years, this powerful and evocative video documents the slow, painful process of reaching one autistic child. It offers tremendous insight into the stress families and educators face as they tackle this mysterious disorder, while giving hope and inspiration to those who are determined to bring their children out from behind the glass door of autism. (52 min)

CNN today: Abnormal psychology, vol. 1. (*available through your International Thomson Learning representative)*. The segment titled, "Developmental Disorders: Learning Disabilities" presents the case of a boy with ADHD, and discusses the importance of early detection of all learning disabilities. (4 min, 37 sec)

A second segment titled, "ADHD Overdiagnosed," presents the results of a research study which found that approximately 3-5% of school children have ADHD, yet 3-17% of children are medicated for ADHD. This discrepancy is discussed in terms of over diagnosing ADHD in children. (3 min, 21 sec)

Dyslexia. (Fanlight Productions, 1-800-937-4113). This film is part of the "The Doctor Is In" series and examines the experiences of people with learning disabilities as well as the potential value to society of their alternative ways of learning. (30 min)

Forrest Gump. (Hollywood Film; Fantasy). This film traces the life of a character named Forrest Gump, with an IQ of 75. The film is useful to examine stereotypes about mental retardation.

One of us. (Fanlight Productions, 1-800-937-4113). This film depicts four stories about integrating people with developmental disabilities into mainstream society. (27 min)

Rainman. (Hollywood Film; Drama). This film depicts Dustin Hoffman as Raymond, an autistic savant. On the one hand, the film nicely illustrates some of the more salient features of autistic behavior. On the other, it also misrepresents the nature of autistic disorder.

Raymonds portrait. (Fanlight Productions, 1-800-937-4113). Raymond Hu is an accomplished artist who was born with Down Syndrome. This moving documentary looks at what can happen when a child is encouraged to develop to his full potential. (27 min)

Understanding Asperger's. (Insight Media: 2162 Broadway, New York, NY 10024/ (800)-233-9910). Designed for educators and therapists, this video outlines the major characteristics of this disorder and illustrates them with footage of children with Asperger's. (30 min)

What's eating Gilbert Grape. (Hollywood Film; Drama). This film portrays a mentally retarded 17 year old boy and how he and his family attempt to cope with his problems.

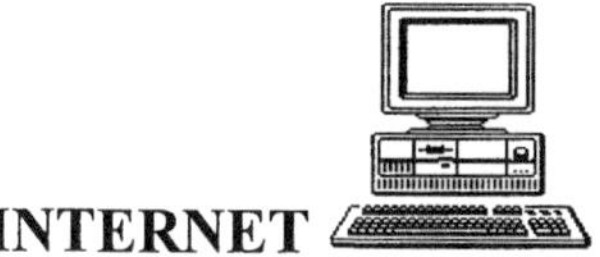

INTERNET RESOURCES FOR CHAPTER FOURTEEN

The American Academy of Child and Adolescent Psychiatry Homepage
http://www.aacap.org/
Provides information for children and their families (including research, education, and treatment) on many childhood disorders.

Asperger's Disorder
http://www.mentalhealth.com/dis/p20-ch07.html
This site contains a wealth of scholarly information and links related to Asperger's disorder.

Ask NOAH About Autism
http://www.noah-health.org/english/illness/genetic_diseases/autism.html#PERVASIVE
This is an excellent mega site on information related to child developmental disorders and includes many useful links to teaching and scholarly resources.

Attention Deficit Disorder
http://www.mentalhealth.com/dis/p20-ch01.html
This site contains a wealth of scholarly information and links related to ADHD.

Attention Deficit Hyperactivity Disorder (NIMH)
http://www.nimh.nih.gov/HealthInformation/adhdmenu.cfm
This NIMH web site provides a wealth of information and resources related to ADHD.

Autistic Disorder
http://www.mentalhealth.com/dis/p20-ch06.html
This site contains a wealth of scholarly information and links related to autistic disorder.

Autism Center
http://www.patientcenters.com/autism/

This web page, in addition to providing links to other related sources on the web, gives information on the symptoms of autism, guidelines for families and caregivers, and relevant books and resources.

Autism at NIMH
http://www.nimh.nih.gov/HealthInformation/autismmenu.cfm

This NIMH web site is exclusively devoted to the nature and treatment of autism.

CH.A.D.D. (Children and Adults with Attention Deficit Disorders)
http://www.chadd.org/

CH.A.D.D. is a non-profit organization devoted to educating the public about attention deficit and hyperactivity disorders. This site includes information on the symptoms of ADDHD, treatments, and as well as CH.A.D.D. chapters throughout the country.

Down Syndrome WWW Page
http://www.nas.com/downsyn/

This WWW page was established in 1995 and provides information on healthcare guidelines for patients, education resources, events & conferences, and Down Syndrome organizations worldwide.

Dyslexia Online
http://www.dyslexiaonline.com/

A website maintained by Dr. Harold Levinson devoted to "resolving the traditional misconceptions of dyslexia and related attention deficit and anxiety disorders."

Early Childhood Links
http://www.dec-sped.org/

This web site provides links related to early intervention information for developmental disorders.

Learning Disabilities Association of America
http://www.ldanatl.org/

This web site provides information and news updates on learning disabilities. This site is aimed at parents, teachers, and other professionals.

New York Autism Network
http://www.albany.edu/psy/autism/autism.html

This site provides a wealth of information related to research and treatment of autism.

NLDline
http://www.NLDline.com

This is a non-verbal learning disabilities website with a huge array of information about learning disabilities common in people with pervasive developmental disorders.

WARNING SIGNS OF ATTENTION DEFICIT/HYPERACTIVITY DISORDER

- Often fidgeting with hands or feet, or squirming while seated
- Having difficulty remaining seated when required to do so
- Being easily distracted by extraneous stimuli
- Having difficulty awaiting turn in games or group activities
- Often blurting out answers before questions are completed
- Having difficulty in following instructions
- Having difficulty sustaining attention in tasks or play activities
- Often shifting from one uncompleted task to another
- Having difficulty playing quietly
- Often talking excessively
- Often interrupting or intruding on others
- Often not listening to what is being said
- Often forgetting things necessary for tasks or activities
- Often engaging in physically dangerous activities without considering possible consequences

WARNING SIGNS OF LEARNING DISABILITIES (PRESCHOOL)

Does the child have trouble with or delayed development in:

- Learning the alphabet
- Rhyming words
- Connecting sounds and letters
- Counting and learning numbers
- Being understood when he or she speaks to a stranger
- Using scissors, crayons, and paints
- Reacting too much or too little to touch
- Using words or, later, stringing words together into phrases
- Pronouncing words
- Walking forward or up and down stairs
- Remembering the names of colors
- Dressing self without assistance

WARNING SIGNS OF LEARNING DISABILITIES (ELEMENTARY SCHOOL)

Does the child have trouble with:

- Learning new vocabulary
- Speaking in full sentences
- Understanding the rules of conversation
- Retelling stories
- Remembering newly learned information
- Playing with peers
- Moving from one activity to another
- Expressing thoughts orally or in writing
- Holding a pencil
- Handwriting
- Computing math problems at his or her grade level
- Following directions
- Self-esteem
- Remembering routines
- Learning new skills
- Understanding what he or she reads
- Succeeding in one or more subject areas
- Drawing or copying shapes
- Understanding what information presented in class is important
- Modulating voice (may speak to loudly or in a monotone)
- Keeping notebook neat and assignments organized
- Remembering and sticking to deadlines
- Understanding how to play age-appropriate board games

WARNING SIGNS OF LEARNING DISABILITIES (ADULTHOOD)

Does the adult have trouble with:

- Remembering newly learned information
- Staying organized
- Understanding what he or she reads
- Getting along with peers or coworkers
- Finding or keeping a job
- Sense of direction
- Understanding jokes that are subtle or sarcastic
- Making appropriate remarks
- Expressing thoughts orally or in writing
- Following directions
- Basic skills (such as reading, writing, spelling, and math)
- Self-esteem
- Using proper grammar in spoken or written communication
- Remembering and sticking to deadlines

WARNING SIGNS OF AUTISM

- Difficulty in mixing with other children
- Insistence on sameness; resists changes in routine
- Inappropriate laughing and giggling
- No real fear of dangers
- Little or no eye contact
- Sustained odd play
- Apparent insensitivity to pain
- Echolalia (repeating words or phrases in place of normal language)
- Prefers to be alone; aloof manner
- May not want cuddling or act cuddly
- Spins objects
- Not responsive to verbal cues; acts as though deaf
- Inappropriate attachment to objects
- Difficulty in expressing needs; uses gestures or pointing instead of words
- Noticeable physical overactivity or extreme underactivity
- Tantrums - displays extreme distress for no apparent reason
- Unresponsive to normal teaching methods
- Uneven gross/fine motor skills (e.g., may not want to kick ball but can stack blocks)

"EARLY" WARNING SIGNS OF AUTISM

If your child displays any of these signs, bring it to the attention of your doctor:

- No babbling by 12 months
- No pointing, waving and other gesturing by 12 months
- No single words by 16 months
- No two-word spontaneous (not echoed) phrases by 24 months
- Any loss of language or social skills at any age
- Inability to make or hold eye contact
- Inability to respond to the child's name being called
- Inability to look where you point
- Lack of interest in pretend play by 18 months
- Arches back to avoid touch
- Rocks or bangs head
- Makes little attempt to communicate

WARNING SIGNS OF ASPERGER'S SYNDROME

Often individuals with Asperger's syndrome have many of the behaviors listed below:

Language:

- Lucid speech before age 4; grammar and vocabulary are usually very good
- Speech is sometimes stilted and repetitive
- Voice tends to be flat and emotionless
- Conversations revolve around self

Cognition:

- Obsessed with complex topics, such as patterns, weather, music, history, etc.
- Often described as eccentric
- I.Q.'s fall along the full spectrum, but many are in the above normal range in verbal ability and in the below average range in performance abilities
- Many have dyslexia, writing problems, and difficulty with mathematics
- Lack common sense
- Concrete thinking (versus abstract)

Behavior:

- Movements tend to be clumsy and awkward
- Odd forms of self-stimulatory behavior
- Sensory problems appear not to be as dramatic as those with other forms of autism
- Socially aware but displays inappropriate reciprocal interaction

DSM-IV-TR Criteria for Attention Deficit Hyperactivity Disorder Criterion A

A. Either (1) or (2):

1. inattention: six (or more) of the following symptoms of inattention have persisted for at least 6 months to a degree that is maladaptive and inconsistent with developmental level:
   a. often fails to give close attention to details or makes careless mistakes in schoolwork, work, or other activities
   b. often has difficulty sustaining attention in tasks or play activities
   c. often does not seem to listen when spoken to directly
   d. often does not follow through on instructions and fails to finish school work, chores, or duties in the workplace (not due to oppositional behavior or failure to understand instructions)
   e. often has difficulty organizing tasks and activities
   f. often avoids, dislikes, or is reluctant to engage in tasks that require sustained mental effort (such as schoolwork or homework)
   g. often loses things necessary for tasks or activities (e.g., toys, school assignments, pencils, books, or tools)
   h. is often easily distracted by extraneous stimuli
   i. is often forgetful in daily activities
2. hyperactivity-impulsivity: six (or more) of the following symptoms of hyperactivity-impulsivity have persisted for at least 6 months to a degree that is maladaptive and inconsistent with developmental level:

Hyperactivity

a. often fidgets with hands or feet or squirms in seat
b. often leaves seat in classroom or in other situations in which remaining seated is expected
c. often runs about or climbs excessively in situations in which it is inappropriate (in adolescents or adults, may be limited to subjective feelings of restlessness)
d. often has difficulty playing or engaging in leisure activities quietly
e. is often "on the go" or often acts as if "driven by a motor"
f. often talks excessively

Impulsivity

g. often blurts out answers before questions have been completed
h. often has difficulty awaiting turn often interrupts
i. intrudes on others (e.g., butts into conversations or games)

DSM-IV-TR Criteria for Attention Deficit Hyperactivity Disorder Criteria B, C, D, and E

B. Some hyperactive-impulsive or inattentive symptoms that caused impairment were present before age 7 years.

C. Some impairment from the symptoms is present in two or more settings (e.g., at school [or work] and at home).

D. There must be clear evidence of clinically significant impairment in social, academic, or occupational functioning.

E. The symptoms do not occur exclusively during the course of a Pervasive Developmental Disorder, Schizophrenia, or other Psychotic Disorder and are not better accounted for by another mental disorder (e.g., Mood Disorder, Anxiety Disorder, Dissociative Disorders, or a Personality Disorder).

Code based on type:

Attention-Deficit/Hyperactivity Disorder, Combined Type: if both Criteria A1 and A2 are met for the past 6 months

Attention-Deficit/Hyperactivity Disorder, Predominantly Inattentive Type: if Criterion A1 is met but Criterion A2 is not met for the past 6 months

Attention-Deficit/Hyperactivity Disorder, Predominantly Hyperactive-Impulsive Type: if Criterion A2 is met but Criterion A1 is not met for the past 6 months

Coding note: For individuals (especially adolescents and adults) who currently have symptoms that no longer meet full criteria, "In Partial Remission" should be specified.

DSM-IV-TR Criteria for Mathematics Disorder

A. Mathematical ability, as measured by individually administered standardized tests, is substantially below that expected given the person's chronological age, measured intelligence, and age-appropriate education.

B. The disturbance in Criterion A significantly interferes with academic achievement or activities of daily living that require mathematical ability.

C. If a sensory deficit is present, the difficulties in mathematical ability are in excess of those usually associated with it.

Coding note: If a general medical (e.g., neurological) condition or sensory deficit is present, code the condition on Axis III.

DSM-IV-TR Criteria for Reading Disorder

A. Reading achievement, as measured by individually administered standardized tests of reading accuracy or comprehension, is substantially below that expected given the person's chronological age, measured intelligence, and age-appropriate education.

B. The disturbance in Criterion A significantly interferes with academic achievement or activities of daily living that require reading skills.

C. If a sensory deficit is present, the reading difficulties are in excess of those usually associated with it.

Coding note: If a general medical (e.g., neurological) condition or sensory deficit is present, code the condition on Axis III.

DSM-IV-TR Criteria for Disorder of Written Expression

A. Writing skills, as measured by individually administered standardized tests (or functional assessments of writing skills), are substantially below those expected given the person's chronological age, measured intelligence, and age-appropriate education.

B. The disturbance in Criterion A significantly interferes with academic achievement or activities of daily living that require the composition of written texts (e.g., writing grammatically correct sentences and organized paragraphs).

C. If a sensory deficit is present, the difficulties in writing skills are in excess of those usually associated with it.

Coding note: If a general medical (e.g., neurological) condition or sensory deficit is present, code the condition on Axis III.

DSM-IV-TR Criteria for Stuttering

A. Disturbance in the normal fluency and time patterning of speech (inappropriate for the individual's age), characterized by frequent occurrences of one or more of the following:

1. sound and syllable repetitions
2. sound prolongations
3. interjections
4. broken words (e.g., pauses within a word)
5. audible or silent blocking (filled or unfilled pauses in speech)
6. circumlocutions (word substitutions to avoid problematic words)
7. words produced with an excess of physical tension
8. monosyllabic whole-word repetitions (e.g., "I-I-I-I see him")

B. The disturbance in fluency interferes with academic or occupational achievement or with social communication.

C. If a speech-motor or sensory deficit is present, the speech difficulties are in excess of those usually associated with these problems.

Coding note: If a speech-motor or sensory deficit or a neurological condition is present, code the condition on Axis III.

DSM-IV-TR Criteria for Expressive Language Disorder

A. The scores obtained from standardized individually administered measures of expressive language development are substantially below those obtained from standardized measures of both nonverbal intellectual capacity and receptive language development. The disturbance may be manifest clinically by symptoms that include having a markedly limited vocabulary, making errors in tense, or having difficulty recalling words or producing sentences with developmentally appropriate length or complexity.

B. The difficulties with expressive language interfere with academic or occupational achievement or with social communication.

C. Criteria are not met for Mixed Receptive-Expressive Language Disorder or a Pervasive Developmental Disorders.

D. If Mental Retardation, a speech-motor or sensory deficit, or environmental deprivation is present, the language difficulties are in excess of those usually associated with these problems.

Coding note: If a speech-motor or sensory deficit or a neurological conditic is present, code the condition on Axis III.

DSM-IV-TR Criteria for Selective Mutism

A. Consistent failure to speak in specific social situations (in which there is an expectation for speaking, e.g., at school) despite speaking in other situations.

B. The disturbance interferes with educational or occupational achievement or with social communication.

C. The duration of the disturbance is at least 1 month (not limited to the first month of school).

D. The failure to speak is not due to a lack of knowledge of, or comfort with, the spoken language required in the social situation.

E. The disturbance is not better accounted for by a Communication Disorder (e.g., Stuttering) and does not occur exclusively during the course of a Pervasive Developmental Disorder, Schizophrenia, or other Psychotic Disorder.

DSM-IV-TR Criteria for Chronic Motor or Vocal Tic Disorder

A. Single or multiple motor or vocal tics (i.e., sudden, rapid, recurrent, nonrhythmic, stereotyped motor movements or vocalizations), but not both, have been present at some time during the illness.

B. The tics occur many times a day nearly every day or intermittently throughout period of more than 1 year, and during this period there was never a tic-free perio of more than 3 consecutive months.

C. The onset is before age 18 years.

D. The disturbance is not due to the direct physiological effects of a substance (e.g., stimulants) or a general medical condition (e.g., Huntington's disease or postviral encephalitis).

E. Criteria have never been met for Tourette's Disorder.

DSM-IV-TR Criteria for Tourette's Disorder

A. Both multiple motor and one or more vocal tics have been present at some time during the illness, although not necessarily concurrently. (A tic is a sudden, rapid, recurrent, nonrhythmic, stereotyped motor movement or vocalization.)

B. The tics occur many times a day (usually in bouts) nearly every day or intermittently throughout a period of more than 1 year, and during this period there was never a tic-free period of more than 3 consecutive months.

C. The onset is before age 18 years.

D. The disturbance is not due to the direct physiological effects of a substance (e.g., stimulants) or a general medical condition (e.g., Huntington's disease or postviral encephalitis).

Transparency 14-11

DSM-IV-TR Criteria for Autistic Disorder

A. A total of six (or more) items from (1), (2), and (3), with at least two from (1), and one each from (2) and (3):

1. qualitative impairment in social interaction, as manifested by at least two of the following:
   a. marked impairment in the use of multiple nonverbal behaviors such as eye-to-eye gaze, facial expression, body postures, and gestures to regulate social interaction
   b. failure to develop peer relationships appropriate to developmental level
   c. a lack of spontaneous seeking to share enjoyment, interests, or achievements with other people (e.g., by a lack of showing, bringing, or pointing out objects of interest)
   d. lack of social or emotional reciprocity
2. qualitative impairments in communication as manifested by at least one of the following:
   a. delay in, or total lack of, the development of spoken language (not accompanied by an attempt to compensate through alternative modes of communication such as gesture or mime)
   b. in individuals with adequate speech, marked impairment in the ability to initiate or sustain a conversation with others
   c. stereotyped and repetitive use of language or idiosyncratic language
   d. lack of varied, spontaneous make-believe play or social imitative play appropriate to developmental level
3. restricted repetitive and stereotyped patterns of behavior, interests, and activities, as manifested by at least one of the following:
   a. encompassing preoccupation with one or more stereotyped and restricted patterns of interest that is abnormal either in intensity or focus
   b. apparently inflexible adherence to specific, nonfunctional routines or rituals
   c. stereotyped and repetitive motor mannerisms (e.g., hand or finger flapping or twisting, or complex whole-body movements)
   d. persistent preoccupation with parts of objects

B. Delays or abnormal functioning in at least one of the following areas, with onset prior to age 3 years: (1) social interaction, (2) language as used in social communication, or (3) symbolic or imaginative play.

C. The disturbance is not better accounted for by Rett's Disorder or Childhood Disintegrative Disorder.

DSM-IV-TR Criteria for Asperger's Disorder

A. Qualitative impairment in social interaction, as manifested by at least two of the following:

1. marked impairment in the use of multiple nonverbal behaviors such as eye-to-eye gaze, facial expression, body postures, and gestures to regulate social interaction
2. failure to develop peer relationships appropriate to developmental level
3. a lack of spontaneous seeking to share enjoyment, interests, or achievements with other people (e.g., by a lack of showing, bringing, or pointing out objects of interest to other people)
4. lack of social or emotional reciprocity

B. Restricted repetitive and stereotyped patterns of behavior, interests, and activities, as manifested by at least one of the following:

1. encompassing preoccupation with one or more stereotyped and restricted patterns of interest that is abnormal either in intensity or focus
2. apparently inflexible adherence to specific, nonfunctional routines or rituals
3. stereotyped and repetitive motor mannerisms (e.g., hand or finger flapping or twisting, or complex whole-body movements)
4. persistent preoccupation with parts of objects

C. The disturbance causes clinically significant impairment in social, occupational, or other important areas of functioning.

D. There is no clinically significant general delay in language (e.g., single words used by age 2 years, communicative phrases used by age 3 years).

E. There is no clinically significant delay in cognitive development or in the development of age-appropriate self-help skills, adaptive behavior (other than in social interaction), and curiosity about the environment in childhood.

F. Criteria are not met for another specific Pervasive Developmental Disorder or Schizophrenia.

Transparency 14-13

DSM-IV-TR Criteria for Rett's Disorder

A. All of the following:
   1. apparently normal prenatal and perinatal development
   2. apparently normal psychomotor development through the first 5 months after birth
   3. normal head circumference at birth

B. Onset of all of the following after the period of normal development:
   1. deceleration of head growth between ages 5 and 48 months
   2. loss of previously acquired purposeful hand skills between ages 5 and 30 months with the subsequent development of stereotyped hand movements (e.g., hand-wringing or hand washing)
   3. loss of social engagement early in the course (although often social interaction develops later)
   4. appearance of poorly coordinated gait or trunk movements
   5. severely impaired expressive and receptive language development with severe psychomotor retardation

DSM-IV-TR Criteria for Childhood Disintegrative Disorder

A. Apparently normal development for at least the first 2 years after birth as manifested by the presence of age-appropriate verbal and nonverbal communication, social relationships, play, and adaptive behavior.

B. Clinically significant loss of previously acquired skills (before age 10 years) in at least two of the following areas:

1. expressive or receptive language
2. social skills or adaptive behavior
3. bowel or bladder control
4. play
5. motor skills

C. Abnormalities of functioning in at least two of the following areas:

1. qualitative impairment in social interaction (e.g., impairment in nonverbal behaviors, failure to develop peer relationships, lack of social or emotional reciprocity)
2. qualitative impairments in communication (e.g., delay or lack of spoken language, inability to initiate or sustain a conversation, stereotyped and repetitive use of language, lack of varied make-believe play)
3. restricted, repetitive, and stereotyped patterns of behavior, interests, and activities, including motor stereotypies and mannerisms

D. The disturbance is not better accounted for by another specific Pervasive Developmental Disorder or by Schizophrenia.

DSM-IV-TR Criteria for Mental Retardation

A. Significantly subaverage intellectual functioning: an IQ of approximately 70 o below on an individually administered IQ test (for infants, a clinical judgment of significantly subaverage intellectual functioning).

B. Concurrent deficits or impairments in present adaptive functioning (i.e., the person's effectiveness in meeting the standards expected for his or her age by his o her cultural group) in at least two of the following areas: communication, self-care home living, social/interpersonal skills, use of community resources, self-direction functional academic skills, work, leisure, health, and safety.

C. The onset is before age 18 years.

Code based on degree of severity reflecting level of intellectual impairment:

Mild Mental Retardation: IQ level 50-55 to approximately 70
Moderate Mental Retardation: IQ level 35-40 to 50-55
Severe Mental Retardation: IQ level 20-25 to 35-40
Profound Mental Retardation: IQ level below 20 or 25
Mental Retardation, Severity Unspecified: when there is strong presumption of Mental Retardation but the person's intelligence is untestabl by standard tests

CHAPTER FIFTEEN

COGNITIVE DISORDERS

LEARNING OBJECTIVES

1. Define the term cognitive disorder and explain why the term organic mental disorder is not consistent with current views.
2. Discuss the three main divisions of cognitive disorders.
3. Describe the symptoms of delirium, including what is known about its prevalence, causes, and treatment.
4. Describe the symptoms of dementia, including what is known about its prevalence, causes, and treatment.
5. Describe the clinical manifestations of Alzheimer's disease and presenile dementia.
6. Describe neurobiological research on Alzheimer's disease, particularly with regard to the role of amyloid deposits.
7. Describe how conditions other than Alzheimer's disease can lead to dementia, particularly Parkinson's disease and Huntington's disease.
8. Discuss the role of psychologists with regard to assisting those who care for persons with dementia.
9. Describe the clinical manifestations of amnestic disorder, including prevention efforts.

OUTLINE

I. Perspectives on Cognitive Disorders
   A. This chapter concerns itself with **cognitive disorders** that affect cognitive processes such as learning, memory, and consciousness, most of which develop much later in life. Three main classes of cognitive disorders are delineated:
      1. The first, **delirium** is often a temporary condition involving confusion and disorientation.
      2. The second, **dementia** is a progressive and degenerative condition marked by gradual and broad cognitive deterioration.
      3. Finally, **amnestic disorders** refer to memory dysfunctions caused by a medical condition or a drug or toxin.

   B. The DSM-IV-TR label "cognitive disorders" reflects a shift in the way these disorders are viewed.
      1. Previous versions of the DSM defined cognitive disorders as **organic mental disorders**, with the term "organic" used to indicate that brain damage or dysfunction was believed to be involved. Most DSM disorders, however, involve some level of brain dysfunction, and most disorders are organic in this sense. The term organic was dropped.
      2. The term **cognitive disorders** captures the central feature of such disorders, namely, impairments in memory, attention, perception, and thinking. Consequences of cognitive disorders often involve profound changes in

behavior and personality, including anxiety, depression, paranoia, agitation, aggression, including problems relating with family and other persons. Such disorders appear in the DSM because of profound changes seen in behavior and personality.

II. Delirium

A. **Delirium** is characterized by impaired consciousness and cognition that develops somewhat rapidly over the course of several hours or days. Such persons appear confused, disoriented, out of touch with their surroundings, have difficulty focusing and sustaining attention, and show marked impairments in memory and language. The textbook illustrates delirium with the case of Mr. J.

B. About 10% to 30% of persons in acute care facilities, such as emergency rooms, are believed to suffer from delirium. It is most prevalent among older adults, people undergoing medical procedures, cancer patients, and persons with AIDS.

1. 44% of persons with dementia suffer at least one episode of delirium.
2. Delirium subsides quickly, with full recovery expected within several weeks; though some continue to have problems and may lapse into coma or die.

C. **Medical conditions** linked with delirium include drug intoxication, poisons, withdrawal from drugs (e.g., alcohol, sedative, hypnotic, or anxiolytic drugs), infections, head injury, and several forms of brain trauma. The DSM-IV-TR recognizes several causes of delirium among its subtypes.

1. **Delirium due to a general medical condition** includes a disturbance of consciousness and a change in cognitive abilities (e.g., language, memory) occurring over a short period of time and resulting from a general medical condition.
2. Other subtypes include **substance-induced delirium**, **delirium due to multiple etiologies**, and **delirium not otherwise specified**. The latter two categories indicate the complex nature of delirium.
3. Delirium is common in the elderly as a consequence of improper use of medications, and can also be experienced by children who have high fevers or who are taking certain kinds of medications.
4. **Age itself** is an important factor in delirium, with older adults being more susceptible to developing delirium as a result of mild infection or medication changes compared to younger persons.
5. Sleep deprivation, immobility, and excessive stress can also cause delirium.

D. **Treatment for delirium** usually involves attention to precipitating medical problems. For example, delirium brought on by withdrawal from alcohol or other drugs is usually treated with benzodiazepines.

1. The antipsychotic drug Haloperidol is prescribed for persons in acute delirium.
2. **Psychosocial interventions** include reassurance in dealing with agitation, anxiety, and hallucinations related to delirium. Such interventions are aimed at helping the person cope and manage the disruptions caused by delirium until medical causes are identified and addressed.

E. **Prevention** is most successful in persons who are susceptible to delirium, and may include efforts geared toward proper medical care for illnesses and therapeutic drug monitoring.

III. Dementia

A. **Dementia** is a cognitive disorder that includes a gradual deterioration of brain functioning that affects judgment, memory, language, and other advanced cognitive processes. The textbook illustrates dementia with the case of Diana.

1. Dementia may be caused by several medical conditions, and by the abuse of drugs or alcohol.
2. Some forms of this disorder, such as Alzheimer's disease, are not reversible.
3. Like delirium, dementia has many causes, including stroke, infectious diseases such as syphilis and HIV, severe head injury, toxic or poisonous substances, and diseases such as Parkinson's, Huntington's, and the most common cause, Alzheimer's disease.
4. Dementia may be reversible or irreversible, but usually develops slowly.

B. The gradual progression of dementia may include a range of symptoms.

1. **In the initial stages**, memory impairment typically manifests as an inability to register ongoing events (e.g., forgetting how to talk, difficulty remembering recent events, but able to remember past events). In addition, deficits are present in visuospatial skills such as returning home.
    a. **Agnosia**, an inability to recognize and name objects, is the most common symptom.
    b. **Facial agnosia**, an inability to recognize familiar faces, may also occur and is extremely distressing to family members.
    c. Emotional changes may happen as well, including **delusions, depression**, **agitation**, **aggression**, and **apathy**.
2. **Cognitive functioning** continues to deteriorate until the person requires almost total support to carry out day-to-day activities.
3. Death results from inactivity combined with onset of other illnesses such as pneumonia.

C. **Dementia can occur at any age** but is more common among the elderly. The prevalence of dementia is a bit over 1% in persons between 65-74 years of age and increases to 4% in persons 75-84 years old, and is over 10% in those 85 years and older.

1. It is estimated that as many as 47% of adults over the age of 85 may have dementia of the Alzheimer's type; a condition that rarely occurs in people under 45 years of age.
2. As survival rates influence prevalence data, incidence figures may be more reliable. One study notes the incidence of dementia as 2.3% for people 75-79 years of age, 4.6% for people 80-84 years of age, and 8.5% for those 85 and older. Rates of new cases appear to double with every 5 years of age.

3. Incidence rates of dementia are comparable for men and women and are equivalent across educational level and social class.
4. Generally, studies suggest that dementia is common among older adults and risk for dementia increases rapidly after the age of 75.

D. DSM-IV-TR delineates **five classes of dementia** based on etiology and include: (1) **dementia of the Alzheimer's type**, (2) **vascular dementia**, (3) **dementia due to other general medical conditions**, (4) **substance-induced persisting dementia**, and (5) **dementia due to multiple etiologies**. A sixth **dementia not otherwise specified** is included when etiology cannot be determined.
   1. The textbook focuses on dementia of the Alzheimer's type because of the high prevalence rate of this condition and the amount of research on its etiology and treatment.

E. **Dementia of the Alzheimer's Type** was first described by a German psychiatrist Alois Alzheimer in 1906.
   1. DSM-IV-TR diagnostic criteria for dementia of the Alzheimer's type include:
      a. Multiple **cognitive deficits** that develop gradually and steadily.
      b. Predominant **impairment in memory, orientation, judgment, and reasoning**. This feature includes an inability to integrate new information and the failure to learn new associations; forgetting important events or losing objects; narrowed interest in routine activities; loss of interest in others.
      c. Progression of the disorder can include agitation, confusion, depression, anxiety, or combativeness. Such difficulties are more pronounced late in the day; a phenomenon referred to as **sundowner syndrome**.
      d. Cognitive disturbances can include **aphasia** (i.e., difficulty with language), **apraxia** (i.e., impaired motor functioning), **agnosia** (i.e., failure to recognize objects), or difficulties with planning, organizing, sequencing, or abstracting information.
      e. Such impairments have a significant negative impact on social and occupational functioning and represent a significant decline from previous abilities.
   2. A definitive diagnosis of Alzheimer's disease can be made only after an **autopsy** determines that certain characteristic types of damage are present in the brain. Clinicians can accurately identify this condition 85% of the time via a mental status exam.
   3. **Cognitive deterioration** of the Alzheimer's type is slow during the early and later stages but more rapid during the middle stages, with average survival time being about 8 years.
      a. Some forms of the disease can occur during the 40s or 50s (i.e., referred to as **presenile dementia**), but the disorder usually appears during the 60s or 70s.

b. Approximately 50% of cases of dementia are ultimately found to be the result of Alzheimer's disease, which is believed to affect 4 million Americans and many millions more worldwide.
c. Alzheimer's disease may be more prevalent in people who are poorly educated. Higher educational attainment may create a **mental reserve** (i.e., a learned set of skills) that helps one cope longer with cognitive deterioration that marks the beginnings of dementia.
d. The **cognitive reserve hypothesis** suggests that more synapses are built up with education and thus delay the full signs of dementia longer.
e. Alzheimer's disease may be more prevalent among women, even when considering that women typically live longer than men.
f. Prevalence of Alzheimer's disease also varies by race, with Japanese, Nigerian, certain Native American, and Amish persons being less likely to develop the disorder.

F. **Vascular Dementia** is a progressive brain disorder that is the second leading cause of dementia next to Alzheimer's disease. Vascular dementia is caused by blockage or damage to the blood vessels that provide the brain with oxygen and other nutrients. For example, damaged areas or multiple infarctions may be caused by a stroke.

1. Neurological signs that indicate brain tissue damage are characteristic of this population, and patterns of impairment vary from person to person.
2. The **DSM-IV-TR criteria for vascular dementia** includes memory and other cognitive disturbances that are identical to dementia of the Alzheimer's type; however, neurological signs of brain tissue damage (e.g., abnormal walking or weakness in the limbs) occur in persons with vascular dementia, but not in the early stages of Alzheimer's disease.
3. Few studies of vascular dementia exist, and the incidence is believed to be about 4.7% or men and 3.8% of women. Men are more likely than women to develop vascular dementia, perhaps due to the higher risk of cardiovascular disease in men.
4. Onset of vascular dementia is more sudden than Alzheimer's disease, often because of stroke. The outcome of vascular disease and Alzheimer's disease is similar, requiring formal nursing care until they succumb to an infectious disease such as pneumonia.

G. **Dementia due to Other Medical Conditions** includes **dementia due to HIV disease, dementia due to head trauma, dementia due to Parkinson's disease, dementia due to Huntington's disease, dementia due to Pick's disease**, and **dementia due to Creutzfeldt-Jakob disease**.

1. Other medical conditions that may lead to dementia include **hydrocephalus** (i.e., excessive water in the cranium, due to brain shrinkage), **hypothyroidism** (i.e., an underactive thyroid gland), **brain tumor**, and **vitamin B12 deficiency**.

2. The **human immunodeficiency virus-type-1 (HIV-1)** causes AIDS and also causes dementia. HIV itself seems to be responsible for the neurological impairment.
    a. Symptoms of HIV dementia are cognitive slowness, impaired attention, and forgetfulness, a tendency to be clumsy, repetitive movements such as tremors and leg weakness, apathy, and social withdrawal.
    b. Cognitive impairments tend to occur during the later stages of HIV infection and are observed in 29% to 87% of people with AIDS.
    c. Dementia resulting from HIV is sometimes referred to as **subcortical dementia** because it affects primarily the inner areas of the brain. Subcortical dementia does not involve aphasia, but often involves severe depression and anxiety, including impairment in motor skills.
3. **Head trauma** is typically caused by accidents and can lead to cognitive impairments in children and adults, with memory loss being the most common symptom.
4. **Parkinson's disease** is a degenerative brain disorder that affects about 1 out of 1,000 people worldwide. Motor problems are characteristic of this disorder, and include stooped posture, slow body movements (i.e., **bradykinesia**), tremors, and jerkiness in walking. Speech tends to be very soft and monotone.
    a. Damage to **dopamine** pathways are believed to be responsible for motor problems, such as tremors and muscle weakness.
    b. Risk for dementia in Parkinson's disease is twice that found in the general population, and the pattern of impairments is similar to subcortical dementia.
5. **Huntington's disease** is a genetic disorder that initially affects motor movements, typically in the form of **chorea** (i.e., involuntary limb movements). About 20% to 80% of persons with this disease go on to display dementia, and it tends to follow the subcortical pattern.
    a. Huntington's disease is inherited as an **autosomal** dominant disorder, meaning that 50% of the offspring of an adult with Huntington's will develop the disease. The deficit appears to chromosome 4 and one gene.
5. **Pick's disease** is a rare neurological condition that produces a cortical dementia similar to that of Alzheimer's disease. The course of this disease is about 5 to 10 years and its cause is unknown.
    a. Pick's disease, like Huntington's disease, occurs early in life (around 40s or 50s) and is an example of presenile dementia for that reason.
6. **Creutzfeldt-Jakob disease** affects 1 out of 1,000,000 persons and has been linked to mad cow disease.

H. **Substance-induced-persisting dementia** results from drug use in combination with poor diet and results in dementia in some cases. About 7% of alcohol dependent persons meet criteria for dementia.

1. DSM-IV-TR identifies **alcohol**, **inhalants**, and **sedative**, **hypnotic**, and **anxiolytic drugs** that are known to lead to dementia. The resulting brain damage can be permanent and can cause the same symptoms seen in dementia of the Alzheimer's type.
2. Diagnostic criteria for this form of dementia are essential the same as for the other forms of dementia and include memory impairment and one of the following cognitive disturbances: aphasia, apraxia, agnosia, or disturbance in executive functioning.

I. The following causes of dementia have been identified:

1. Several **genetic and biological influences** on dementia have been reported, but premature conclusions are often made.
    a. For example, several researchers have explored a link between **aluminum** and Alzheimer's disease. However, another study indicates that aluminum seen in neuritic plaques is simply a lab contaminant.
    b. In addition, a negative correlation between smoking and Alzheimer's disease may not imply a protective effect but instead reflect differential survival rates.
    c. Brains of Alzheimer's patients atrophy to a greater extent than would be expected through normal aging. The brains of all persons with Alzheimer's disease also show large numbers of tangled strand-like filaments (referred to as **neurofibrillary tangles**), and the cause of this feature is unknown. Accumulation of neurofibrillary tangles and amyloid plaques are believed to produce the characteristic cognitive disorders.
    d. Accumulation of gummy protein deposits (called **amyloid plaques** or referred to as **senile** or **neuritic plaques**) occur in the brains of Alzheimer's patients more so than in older adults who do not show symptoms of dementia. This buildup of amyloid protein appears to involve **precursor protein (APP)**, whose production is controlled by a gene on **chromosome 21**; the same site as Down syndrome.
    e. Amyloid build-up may also result from **apolipoprotein E** (ApoE) which helps transport cholesterols, including amyloid protein, through the bloodstream. Three forms of this transporter protein include **apoE-2**, **apoE-3**, and **apoE-4**. The gene for apoE-4 on chromosome 19 is present in 80% of those with Alzheimer's disease who have a family history of the disease. Having two genes for ApoE-4 increases the risk for Alzheimer's disease, including an earlier onset. Amyloid protein may also cause brain cells to self-destruct and die through a natural process called **apoptosis**.
    f. Genetic research suggests that multiple genes are involved in Alzheimer's disease, particularly genes on chromosomes 21, 19, 14, 12, and 1. **Chromosome 14** is associated with early onset Alzheimer's, whereas **chromosome 19** is associated with a late onset form of this disease.

g. Some of these genes have been identified as being either **deterministic** genes or **susceptibility** genes. Having one of the deterministic genes means having nearly 100% chance of developing Alzheimer's. Having susceptibility genes, increases risk of developing Alzheimer's only slightly.
h. **Head trauma** is an external factor that can produce dementia, with repeated blows to the head increasing the chances of developing **dementia pugilistica**; a condition named after boxers who suffer this type of dementia. Boxers who carry that apoE-4 gene may be at greater risk for developing dementia due to head trauma.

2. **Psychological and Social Influences** do not cause dementia, but may influence its onset and course.
   a. **Lifestyle factors,** such as continued drug use, may produce dementia. Other examples include factors that influence cardiovascular disease and risk for vascular dementia such as **diet, exercise, and stress**.
   b. **Cultural factors** also impinge on this process. For example, hypertension and strokes are prevalent among African-Americans and certain Asian Americans and so too is vascular dementia. Dementia caused by head trauma and malnutrition are common in pre-industrial rural societies.
   c. **Psychosocial factors**, such as educational attainment, can influence the onset and course of dementia, including coping skills, social resources, and familial support.

J. **Treatment of dementia** is not as promising when compared to other cognitive disorders. A key factor working against the treatment of dementia is the extensive brain damage caused by the disorder. Although some damage can be compensated for via brain **plasticity**, there is a limit to how many neurons can be destroyed before functioning is disturbed. As a result, the goals of treatment are focused on prevention, stopping the progression of the disease, and helping people cope with advancing deterioration.

1. Dementia due to known infectious diseases, nutritional deficiencies, and depression can be **treated medically** if caught early.
2. Yet, there is no known treatment for most of the different types of dementia that are responsible for the vast majority of cases (e.g., stroke, HIV, Parkinson's disease, Huntington's disease).
   a. Such persons may be helped with new treatments that involve substances that attempt to preserve or even restore neurons, known as **glial cell-derived neurotrophic factor or GDNE**.
   b. Efforts are also underway examining the benefits of transplanting fetal brain tissue into the brains of people with dementia, and preliminary results appear promising.
   c. Drugs can help prevent strokes and are increasingly developed and tested for persons with dementia of the Alzheimer's type. **Tacrine hydrochloride (Cognex)** and **donepezil (Aricept)** are FDA approved drugs for Alzheimer's disease that prevent the breakdown of

acetylcholine which is often deficient in persons with Alzheimer's. Such drugs appear to improve the cognitive functioning of Alzheimer's patients, but only temporarily and continued decline cannot be prevented with such drugs.

d. High doses of **vitamin E** appears to delay the progression of Alzheimer's disease, and beneficial effects of estrogen replacement therapy and **aspirin** and other **nonsteroidal anti-inflammatory drugs** have also been observed.

e. The best available medications provide some recovery of function, but do not stop progressive deterioration.

3. **Psychosocial treatments** focus on enhancing the lives of people with dementia and their families and include **teaching skills** to compensate for lost abilities.

a. Such interventions may include prosthetic devices to assist with memory (e.g., index cards, note pads). Examples include **memory wallets** to improve conversations, reorientation, and prevention of socially stigmatizing behaviors. As an alternative to restraint for those who wander and get lost, **navigational cues** may be used.

b. In addition, caregiver treatment may include supportive counseling, assertiveness training, and reduction of stress and elder abuse. The main emphasis of psychosocial interventions appears to be on the caregivers of those with dementia.

K. **Prevention** of dementia in older adults includes the following:

1. **Estrogen-replacement therapy** appears related to decreased risk of dementia of the Alzheimer's type among women.
2. Proper treatment of systolic hypertension, stroke, and cardiovascular disease may also cut the risk of dementia, including the use of anti-inflammatory medications.
3. Increased safety behaviors to reduce head trauma and exposure to neurotoxins are also part of prevention efforts.

IV. Amnestic Disorder

A. **Amnestic disorder** is characterized by circumscribed loss of memory and an inability to transfer information into long-term memory. This is often due to medical conditions, head trauma, or long-term drug use. The textbook illustrates amnestic disorder with the case of S. T., who suffers from Wernicke-Korsakoff syndrome.

B. The DSM-IV-TR criteria for amnestic disorder cover the inability to learn new information or to recall previously learned information, with memory disturbance causing significant impairment in social or occupational functioning.

1. One type of amnestic disorder is **Wernicke-Korsakoff syndrome**, which is caused by thalamic damage resulting from stroke or more commonly chronic heavy alcohol use. Efforts to prevent damage caused by Wernicke-Korsakoff syndrome have focused on supplements to restore a deficiency in **thiamine** (i.e., vitamin B-1) due to alcohol abuse.

2. To date little research has addressed long-term assistance in treating people with amnesic disorders.

OVERALL SUMMARY

This chapter outlines the primary features of cognitive disorders, which involve delirium, dementia, and amnesia. In so doing, forms of each of these cognitive disorders are described, with an emphasis on Alzheimer's disease. Coverage also includes discussion of known biological, environmental, and psychosocial factors that cause, maintain, or are related to the prevention and alleviation of cognitive disorders.

KEY TERMS

Agnosia (p. 524)
Alzheimer's disease (p. 527)
Amnestic disorder (p. 538)
Aphasia (p. 526)
Creutzfeldt-Jakob disease (p. 531)
Delirium (p. 521)
Dementia (p. 523)
Dementia of the Alzheimer's type (p. 526)
Deterministic (p. 533)
Facial agnosia (p. 524)
Head trauma (p. 530)
HIV-1 disease (p. 529)
Huntington's disease (p. 530)
Parkinson's disease (p. 530)
Pick's disease (p. 531)
Susceptibility (p. 533)
Vascular dementia (p. 528)

INFOTRAC KEY TERM EXERCISES

Each exercise is linked to key terms from the Wadsworth InfoTrac on-line searchable database. Key terms must be entered exactly as written.

Exercise 1: Agnosias: A Review of Diagnostic, Assessment, and Treatment Approaches
Article: A114168255
Citation: (Clinical management of agnosia). Martha S. Burns. Topics in Stroke Rehabilitation, Wntr 2004 v11 i1 p1(9)

Agnosia is a neurological recognition deficit that affects a single modality (e.g., visual, auditory). Rapid advances are being made in the diagnosis and clinical management of agnosias. This InfoTrac article outlines the history, diagnosis and assessment, and clinical interventions for various forms of agnosia. After reading this article, briefly describe (a) the various forms of agnosia, (b) relevant research outlining underlying brain abnormalities that give rise to them, and

(c) assessment and treatment approaches used for persons suffering from agnosia. Limit your answer to 3-5 double-spaced pages.

Exercise2: Stroke and Depression: What is the Relation?
Key Term: *Stroke, depression*

The effects of a stroke vary from patient to patient, and much of this variability has been attributed to the area of the brain where the rupture occurs. Yet, stroke is often associated with other emotional effects, namely depression. What is the relation between stroke and depression, including suicide? Is depression related to stroke a consequence of damage to specific regions of the brain, or is it a consequence of other factors? Review the InfoTrac article on the relation between stroke and depression in the context of addressing the general questions posed above. In so doing, attempt to identify what factors contribute to depression in stroke survivors and what can be done about it. Limit your answer to 3-5 double-spaced pages.

Exercise 3: Elder Abuse in Older Persons Who Cannot Take Care of Themselves
Key Term: *Elder Abuse*

Caregivers of older persons with delirium, dementia, or amnestic disorders often suffer along with their loved ones. Increasingly it appears that some caregivers may be inflicting deliberate suffering on those older persons under their care. This phenomenon is commonly referred to as elder abuse. What is the prevalence of elder abuse, what are the risk factors for such abuse (i.e., perpetrator and victim characteristics), and what is psychology's role in preventing such abuse from occurring. Review the InfoTrac article on elder abuse with the above questions in mind, and evaluate whether psychology is truly doing enough to address what appears to be a growing problem in the United States. Limit your answer to 3-5 double-spaced pages.

Exercise 4 (Future Trend): Stem Cell Research: An Eventual Cure for Cognitive Disorders?

Embryonic stem cell research has been described as a one of the major new developments in medical science over the past decade or so. This promising area of science is also leading scientists to investigate the possibility of cell-based therapies to treat disease, which is often referred to as regenerative or reparative medicine. Though still in its early stages, this line of research offers the potential to cure the incurable cognitive disorders described in this chapter. As an instructor, you may wish to describe the nature of stem cell research in detail, including the potential ethical and moral issues that are involved, while relating this approach to the specific cognitive disorders outlined in this chapter. The links below provide additional relevant information about stem cell research.

http://stemcells.nih.gov/index.asp
http://www.stemcellresearchnews.com/
http://www.ninds.nih.gov/parkinsonsweb/events_2002.htm
http://www.aaas.org/spp/sfrl/projects/stem/main.htm
http://www.religioustolerance.org/res_stem.htm
http://www.time.com/time/magazine/article/0,9171,1101040531-641157,00.html
http://serendip.brynmawr.edu/bb/neuro/neuro04/web2/abruce.html

CLASSROOM ACTIVITIES, DEMONSTRATIONS, AND LECTURE TOPICS

1. **Activity: Distinguishing Episodic, Semantic, and Procedural Memories.** Episodic (autobiographical) memories, and semantic memories (memories for learned facts) are typically affected in both amnestics and demented patients. However, procedural memories (memory for the ability to perform skills, such as riding a bike) are often spared in these patients. Make copies of HANDOUT 15.1 and give it to your students. Remind students that episodic and semantic memories fall under the category of *declarative memories* (i.e., memories that a person can state in words) whereas *procedural* memories are motor skill memories.

2. **Activity: Demonstrate the Mini-Mental Status Examination.** This is an evaluation scale developed by Evelyn Lee Teng and others (1987) and is often used to diagnose dementia. Allow students to examine this test in order to review the various impairments associated with Alzheimer's disease and other dementias. Many questions found on this examination will seem quite simple to students, but remind them that individuals suffering from dementia, particularly in the later stages, are often challenged by such problems.

   Source Information. Teng, E. L., Chui, H. C., Schneider, L. S., & Metzger, L. E. (1987). Mini-mental status examination. Journal of Consulting and Clinical Psychology, 55, 96-100.

3. **Activity: How is Your Memory?** It is easy for students to be lulled into thinking that memory problems are unique to persons with the disorders covered in this chapter. Indeed, memory problems are quite common and are quite often related to inattention. Ask students in the class to answer the following simple questions, originally posed by Kenneth Higbee, and then read the correct answers and ask for a show of hands as to how many in the class got each question wrong. This activity may be used as a springboard to a discussion of attention and memory, including the role of increasing attention in assisting persons with various cognitive disorders.
   a. Which color is on top of a stoplight? (*answer*: red)
   b. Whose image is on a penny? (*answer*: Lincoln); Is he wearing a tie? (*answer*: yes, a bow tie)
   c. What five words besides "In God We Trust" appear on most U.S. coins? (*answer*: United States of American and Liberty)
   d. When water goes down the drain, does it swirl clockwise or counterclockwise? (*answer*: counterclockwise in the Northern Hemisphere; clockwise in the Southern Hemisphere)
   e. What letters, if any, are missing on a telephone dial? (*answer*: Q, Z)

4. **Activity: The Role of Schemas and Memory.** Schemas are mental frameworks used to interpret/filter information and influence the retrieval of information stored in long-term memory. Some of the disorders covered in this chapter illustrate problems with this process to an extreme degree. To demonstrate this effect in your "normal" students, use the following exercise developed by Drew Appleby. Tell students that you are going to show them a list of 12 words and that they should try to remember them. Then, slowly

display on index cards or transparencies the following words one at a time as you read them aloud: REST, TIRED, AWAKE, DREAM, SNORE, BED, EAT, SLUMBER, SOUND, COMFORT, WAKE, NIGHT.

After completing the list, distract the class for 30 seconds or so, and then give the students 2 minutes to write down as many words as they can recall. Ask for a show of hands from all those who recalled the word AARDVARK. Most students will look at you as though you were crazy. Then ask for a show of hands for those who remembered the word SLEEP. Appleby reports that 80 to 95 percent of students typically recall the word SLEEP, and most students will be shocked to learn that SLEEP was not on the list (you can show them that this was, in fact, the case). This exercise nicely illustrates how schemas do influence recall, and how their "sleep schema" was invoked by the words in this list leading most to make errors in recall. You may want to discuss the issue of whether people can mistakenly remember information because it is consistent with their schemas, and whether it may also be possible that persons can mistakenly forget information that is inconsistent with their schemas and the implications (if any) for understanding cognitive disorders.

Source Information. Appleby, D. (1987). Producing a déjà vu experience. In V. P. Makosky, L. G. Whittemore, & A. M. Rogers (Eds.), Activities handbook for the teaching of psychology, vol. 2 (pp. 78-79). Washington, DC: American Psychological Association.

5. **Video Activity: Amnestic Disorder.** Show the segment on "Amnestic Disorders," from Abnormal Psychology: Inside/Out, Video 2. In this segment, a patient (Mike) is interviewed about his brain injury following a car accident and his inability to learn or remember new information. Ask the students to place themselves in Mike's shoes and to consider how their lives would be different if they had similar problems. Discuss what might have been done to prevent some of the negative life consequences of his injury, particularly with regard to the role of psychologists.

HANDOUT 15.1

Distinguishing Episodic, Semantic, and Procedural Memories

Below you will find a list of situations. Read each one carefully and decide if it is an example of episodic, semantic, or procedural memory.

E = Episodic (Autobiographical memory; memory for events that happened directly to you)
S = Semantic (Memory for facts or knowledge not directly related to you)
P = Procedural (Memory for motor skills)

1.	Riding a bike.	E	S	P
2.	Describing your trip to Las Vegas on New Year's Eve.	E	S	P
3.	Naming the capital of Michigan.	E	S	P
4.	Stating what you were doing when the Challenger space shuttle exploded.	E	S	P
5.	Driving a car home from school.	E	S	P
6.	Being able to read and play music.	E	S	P
7.	Describing what you had for breakfast this morning.	E	S	P
8.	Stating the 12 cranial nerves (in order).	E	S	P
9.	Recalling events from your 10th birthday.	E	S	P
10.	Playing tennis or golf.	E	S	P

SUPPLEMENTARY READING MATERIAL FOR CHAPTER FIFTEEN

(I = These sources can be found on "*Infotrac, the online library*" provided by Wadsworth and Brooks/Cole Publishing.)

Caplan, L. R., Dyken, M. L., & Easton, J. D. (1994). American Heart Association family guide to stroke treatment, recovery, and prevention. New York: Time Books.

Cummings, J. L. (Ed.) (1990). Subcortical dementia. New York: Oxford University Press.

Davies, P. (1994). Starting again: Early rehabilitation after traumatic brain injury or other severe brain lesion. New York: Springer.

Edwards, A. J. (1994). When memory fails: Helping the Alzheimer's and dementia patient. New York: Plenum.

Eide, M. (1987). Alzheimer's disease. Phoenix, AZ: Oryx Press.

Fisher, J. E., & Carstensen, L. L. (1990). Behavior management of the dementias. Clinical Psychology Review, 10, 611-629.

Jackson, J. E., Katzman, R., & Lessin, P. J. (Eds.) (1992). Alzheimer's disease: Long term care. San Diego: San Diego State University Press.

McGowin, D. F. (1993). Living in the labyrinth: A personal journey through the maze of Alzheimer's. New York: Delacorte.

Sacks, O. (1985). The man who mistook his wife for a hat and other clinical tales. New York: Summit.

Storandt, M., & VandenBos, G. R. (Eds.) (1994). Neuropsychological assessment of dementia and depression in older adults : A clinician's guide. New York: American Psychological Association.

Weiner, M. F. (Ed.) (1996). The dementias: Diagnosis, management, and research, 2nd ed. Washington, DC: American Psychiatric Press.

Wright, L. K. (1993). Alzheimer's disease and marriage: An intimate account. Newbury Park, CA: Sage.

SUPPLEMENTAL 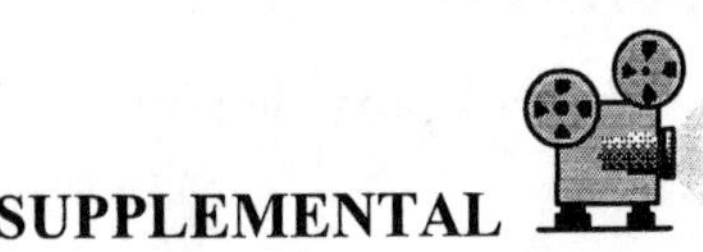 VIDEO RESOURCES FOR CHAPTER FIFTEEN

Abnormal psychology inside/out, vol. 1, video 2. (*available through your International Thomson Learning representative*). An interview with a patient named Mike is presented. Mike suffered a brain injury after racing his car and cannot learn or remember new information. However, he has retained over-learned memories, such as how to build an engine. He carries a notebook with information with him at all times with activities he must do every half hour. Consequences of the brain injury include development of a temper control problem, depression, loss of his job, wife and home. (14 min)

Agitation...it's a sign. (Fanlight Productions, 1-800-937-4113). A variety of caregivers share their experiences and thoughts on providing for residents with Alzheimer's while providing vivid examples of the techniques and concepts that have worked in their facilities. (14 min)

Communicating with older adults and people with dementia. (Insight Media: 2162 Broadway, New York, NY 10024/ (800)-233-9910). Good communication begins with listening skills and common courtesy. This program discusses how to augment communication skills when dealing with a client suffering from a hearing deficit or dementia. It features the commentary of an Alzheimer's specialist who discusses the five A's: agnosia, amnesia, aphasia, apraxia, and attention deficit. (55 min)

Caring...sharing: The Alzheimer's caregiver. (Fanlight Productions, 1-800-937-4113). Explores the frustrations, fears, loneliness, anger and guilt – as well as moments of joy – experienced by those who care for loved ones with Alzheimer's Disease. (38 min)

He's doing this to spite me. (Fanlight Productions, 1-800-937-4113). In this frank video, three caregivers openly share their experiences of conflict and frustration in interactions with their loved one who has dementia. These scenes are integrated with comments and guidance from professionals in dementia care. The result is a program which teaches both family and professional caregivers how to reframe the dynamic into one which is more comfortable and productive for both caregiver and patient. (22 min)

Philadelphia. (Hollywood Film; Drama). This film, starring Tom Hanks, depicts a young man who suffers from AIDS and the effects of the illness on his neurological functioning.

Regarding Henry. (Hollywood Film; Drama). This film depicts a man who experienced a stroke and the impact it has on his family and how they learned to cope.

Wandering: Is it a problem? (Fanlight Productions, 1-800-937-4113). A variety of caregivers share their experiences and thoughts on providing for residents with Alzheimer's while providing vivid examples of the techniques and concepts that have worked in their facilities. (14 min)

INTERNET 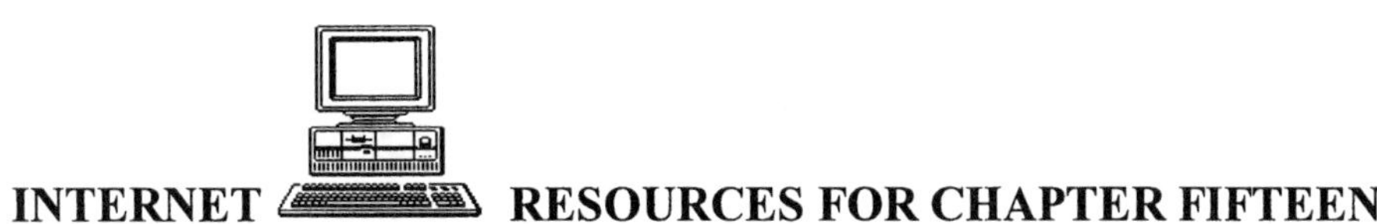 RESOURCES FOR CHAPTER FIFTEEN

Alzheimer's Association
http://www.alz.org/

The Alzheimer's Association web site contains information on local chapters, coping strategies for caregivers, and scientific progress towards effective treatment and understanding of this disorder.

Delirium
http://www.mentalhealth.com/p20-grp.html

This web page provides diagnostic and clinically-relevant research information and links about delirium.

Dementia
http://www.mentalhealth.com/p20-grp.html

This web page provides diagnostic and clinically-relevant research information and links about dementia.

Dementia of the Alzheimer's Type
http://www.mentalhealth.com/p20-grp.html

This web page provides diagnostic and clinically-relevant research information and links about dementia of the Alzheimer's Type.

Dementia Web
http://dementia.ion.ucl.ac.uk/

Good site with a lot of information/links on a wide variety of topics/research. Includes a support database.

WARNING SIGNS OF ALZHEIMER'S DISEASE

- Memory loss that affects job skills
- Difficulty performing familiar tasks
- Problems with language
- Disorientation of time and place
- Poor or decreased judgment
- Problems with abstract thinking
- Misplacing things
- Changes in mood or behavior
- Changes in personality
- Loss of initiative

DSM-IV-TR Criteria for Delirium Due to... [Indicate the General Medical Condition]

A. Disturbance of consciousness (i.e., reduced clarity of awareness of the environment) with reduced ability to focus, sustain, or shift attention.

B. A change in cognition (such as memory deficit, disorientation, language disturbance) or the development of a perceptual disturbance that is not better accounted for by a preexisting, established, or evolving dementia.

C. The disturbance develops over a short period of time (usually hours to days) and tends to fluctuate during the course of the day.

D. There is evidence from the history, physical examination, or laboratory findings that the disturbance is caused by the direct physiological consequences of a general medical condition.

Coding note: If delirium is superimposed on a preexisting Dementia of the Alzheimer's Type or Vascular Dementia, indicate the delirium by coding the appropriate subtype of the dementia, e.g., 290.3 Dementia of the Alzheimer's Type, With Late Onset, With Delirium.

Coding note: Include the name of the general medical condition on Axis I, e.g., 293.0 Delirium Due to Hepatic Encephalopathy; also code the general medical condition on Axis III.

DSM-IV-TR Criteria for Substance Intoxication Delirium

A. Disturbance of consciousness (i.e., reduced clarity of awareness of the environment) with reduced ability to focus, sustain, or shift attention.

B. A change in cognition (such as memory deficit, disorientation, language disturbance) or the development of a perceptual disturbance that is not better accounted for by a preexisting, established, or evolving dementia.

C. The disturbance develops over a short period of time (usually hours to days) and tends to fluctuate during the course of the day.

D. There is evidence from the history, physical examination, or laboratory findings of either (1) or (2):

1. the symptoms in Criteria A and B developed during Substance Intoxication
2. medication use is etiologically related to the disturbance*

Note: This diagnosis should be made instead of a diagnosis of Substance Intoxication only when the cognitive symptoms are in excess of those usually associated with the intoxication syndrome and when the symptoms are sufficiently severe to warrant independent clinical attention.

*Note: The diagnosis should be recorded as Substance-Induced Delirium if related to medication use. Refer to Appendix G for E-codes indicating specific medications.

Code [Specific Substance] Intoxication Delirium:

Alcohol, Amphetamine [or Amphetamine-Like Substance], Cannabis, Cocaine, Hallucinogen, Inhalant, Opioid, Phencyclidine [or Phencyclidine-Like Substance], Sedative, Hypnotic, or Anxiolytic, Other [or Unknown] Substance (e.g., cimetidine, digitalis, benzotropine)

DSM-IV-TR Criteria for Substance Withdrawal Delirium

A. Disturbance of consciousness (i.e., reduced clarity of awareness of the environment) with reduced ability to focus, sustain, or shift attention.

B. A change in cognition (such as memory deficit, disorientation, language disturbance) or the development of a perceptual disturbance that is not better accounted for by a preexisting, established, or evolving dementia.

C. The disturbance develops over a short period of time (usually hours to days) and tends to fluctuate during the course of the day.

D. There is evidence from the history, physical examination, or laboratory findings that the symptoms in Criteria A and B developed during, or shortly after, a withdrawal syndrome.

Note: This diagnosis should be made instead of a diagnosis of Substance Withdrawal only when the cognitive symptoms are in excess of those usually associated with the withdrawal syndrome and when the symptoms are sufficiently severe to warrant independent clinical attention.

Code [Specific Substance] Withdrawal Delirium:

Alcohol, Sedative, Hypnotic, or Anxiolytic, Other [or Unknown] Substance

DSM-IV-TR Criteria for Delirium Due to Multiple Etiologies

A. Disturbance of consciousness (i.e., reduced clarity of awareness of the environment) with reduced ability to focus, sustain, or shift attention.

B. A change in cognition (such as memory deficit, disorientation, language disturbance) or the development of a perceptual disturbance that is not better accounted for by a preexisting, established, or evolving dementia.

C. The disturbance develops over a short period of time (usually hours to days) and tends to fluctuate during the course of the day.

D. There is evidence from the history, physical examination, or laboratory findings that the delirium has more than one etiology (e.g., more than one etiological general medical condition, a general medical condition plus Substance Intoxication or medication side effect).

Coding note: Use multiple codes reflecting specific delirium and specific etiologies, (e.g., 293.0 Delirium Due to Viral Encephalitis; 291.0 Alcohol Withdrawal Delirium).

DSM-IV-TR-TR Criteria for Dementia of the Alzheimer's Type

A. The development of multiple cognitive deficits manifested by both (1) memory impairment (impaired ability to learn new information or to recall previously learned information) (2) one (or more) of the following cognitive disturbances:

1. aphasia (language disturbance)
2. apraxia (impaired ability to carry out motor activities despite intact motor function)
3. agnosia (failure to recognize or identify objects despite intact sensory function)
4. disturbance in executive functioning (i.e., planning, organizing, sequencing, abstracting)

B. The cognitive deficits in Criteria A1 and A2 each cause significant impairment in social or occupational functioning and represent a significant decline from a previous level of functioning.

C. The course is characterized by gradual onset and continuing cognitive decline.

D. The cognitive deficits in Criteria A1 and A2 are not due to any of the following:

1. other central nervous system conditions that cause progressive deficits in memory and cognition (e.g., cerebrovascular disease, Parkinson's disease, Huntington's disease, subdural hematoma, normal-pressure hydrocephalus, brain tumor)
2. systemic conditions that are known to cause dementia (e.g., hypothyroidism, vitamin B or folic acid deficiency, niacin deficiency, hypercalcemia, neurosyphilis, HIV infection)
3. substance-induced conditions

E. The deficits do not occur exclusively during the course of a delirium.

F. The disturbance is not better accounted for by another Axis I disorder (e.g., Major Depressive Episode, Schizophrenia).

Code based on presence or absence of a clinically significant behavioral disturbance:
Without Behavioral Disturbance or With Behavioral Disturbance.

Specify subtype:

With **Early Onset** or With **Late Onset**.

DSM-IV-TR Criteria for Substance-Induced Persisting Dementia

A. The development of multiple cognitive deficits manifested by both

1. memory impairment (impaired ability to learn new information or to recall previously learned information)
2. one (or more) of the following cognitive disturbances:
   a. aphasia (language disturbance)
   b. apraxia (impaired ability to carry out motor activities despite intact motor function)
   c. agnosia (failure to recognize or identify objects despite intact sensory function)
   d. disturbance in executive functioning (i.e., planning, organizing, sequencing, abstracting)

B. The cognitive deficits in Criteria A1 and A2 each cause significant impairment in social or occupational functioning and represent a significant decline from a previous level of functioning.

C. The deficits do not occur exclusively during the course of a delirium and persist beyond the usual duration of Substance Intoxication or Withdrawal.

D. There is evidence from the history, physical examination, or laboratory findings that the deficits are etiologically related to the persisting effects of substance use (e.g., a drug of abuse, a medication).

Code [Specific Substance]-Induced Persisting Dementia:

Alcohol, Inhalant, Sedative, Hypnotic, or Anxiolytic, Other [or Unknown] Substance

DSM-IV-TR Criteria for Vascular Dementia

A. The development of multiple cognitive deficits manifested by both
   1. memory impairment (impaired ability to learn new information or to recall previously learned information)
   2. one (or more) of the following cognitive disturbances:
      a. aphasia (language disturbance)
      b. apraxia (impaired ability to carry out motor activities despite intact motor function)
      c. agnosia (failure to recognize or identify objects despite intact sensory function)
      d. disturbance in executive functioning (i.e., planning, organizing, sequencing, abstracting)

B. The cognitive deficits in Criteria A1 and A2 each cause significant impairment in social or occupational functioning and represent a significant decline from a previous level of functioning.

C. Focal neurological signs and symptoms (e.g., exaggeration of deep tendon reflexes, extensor plantar response, pseudobulbar palsy, gait abnormalities, weakness of an extremity) or laboratory evidence indicative of cerebrovascular disease (e.g., multiple infarctions involving cortex and underlying white matter) that are judged to be etiologically related to the disturbance.

D. The deficits do not occur exclusively during the course of a Delirium.

Code based on predominant features:

With Delirium: if delirium is superimposed on the dementia
With Delusions: if delusions are the predominant feature
With Depressed Mood: if depressed mood (including presentations that meet full symptom criteria for a Major Depressive Episode) is the predominant feature. A separate diagnosis of Mood Disorder Due to a General Medical Condition is not given.
Uncomplicated: if none of the above predominates in the current clinical presentation

Specify if: **With Behavioral Disturbance**
Coding note: Also code cerebrovascular condition on Axis III.

DSM-IV-TR-TR Criteria for Dementia Due to Other General Medical Conditions

A. The development of multiple cognitive deficits manifested by both

1. memory impairment (impaired ability to learn new information or to recall previously learned information)
2. one (or more) of the following cognitive disturbances:
   a. aphasia (language disturbance)
   b. apraxia (impaired ability to carry out motor activities despite intact motor function)
   c. agnosia (failure to recognize or identify objects despite intact sensory function)
   d. disturbance in executive functioning (i.e., planning, organizing, sequencing abstracting)

B. The cognitive deficits in Criteria A1 and A2 each cause significant impairment in social or occupational functioning and represent a significant decline from a previous level of functioning.

C. There is evidence from the history, physical examination, or laboratory findings that the disturbance is the direct physiological consequence of one of the general medical conditions listed below.

D. The deficits do not occur exclusively during the course of a Delirium.

Code based on presence or absence of a clinically significant behavioral disturbance.
Without Behavioral Disturbance: if the cognitive disturbance is not accompanied by any clinically significant behavioral disturbance.
With Behavioral Disturbance: if the cognitive disturbance is accompanied by a clinically significant behavioral disturbance (e.g., wandering, agitation).

- Dementia Due to HIV Disease
- Dementia Due to Head Trauma
- Dementia Due to Parkinson's Disease
- Dementia Due to Huntington's Disease
- Dementia Due to Pick's Disease
- Dementia Due to Creutzfeldt-Jakob Disease

Coding note: Also code the general medical condition on Axis III.

DSM-IV-TR Criteria for Dementia Due to Multiple Etiologies

A. The development of multiple cognitive deficits manifested by both
   1. memory impairment (impaired ability to learn new information or to recall previously learned information)
   2. one (or more) of the following cognitive disturbances:
      a. aphasia (language disturbance)
      b. apraxia (impaired ability to carry out motor activities despite intact motor function)
      c. agnosia (failure to recognize or identify objects despite intact sensory function)
      d. disturbance in executive functioning (i.e., planning, organizing, sequencing, abstracting)

B. The cognitive deficits in Criteria A1 and A2 each cause significant impairment in social or occupational functioning and represent a significant decline from a previous level of functioning.

C. There is evidence from the history, physical examination, or laboratory findings that the disturbance has more than one etiology (e.g., head trauma plus chronic alcohol use, Dementia of the Alzheimer's Type with the subsequent development of Vascular Dementia).

D. The deficits do not occur exclusively during the course of a Delirium.

Coding note: Use multiple codes based on specific dementias and specific etiologies, (e.g., Dementia of the Alzheimer's Type, With Late Onset, Uncomplicated; Vascular Dementia, Uncomplicated).

DSM-IV-TR Criteria for Substance-Induced Persisting Amnestic Disorder

A. The development of memory impairment as manifested by impairment in the ability to learn new information or the inability to recall previously learned information.

B. The memory disturbance causes significant impairment in social or occupational functioning and represents a significant decline from a previous level of functioning.

C. The memory disturbance does not occur exclusively during the course of a Delirium or a Dementia and persists beyond the usual duration of Substance Delirium or Withdrawal.

D. There is evidence from the history, physical examination, or laboratory findings that the memory disturbance is etiologically related to the persisting effects of substance use (e.g., a drug of abuse, a medication).

Code [Specific Substance]-Induced Persisting Amnestic Disorder:
Alcohol, Sedative, Hypnotic, or Anxiolytic, Other [or Unknown] Substance

DSM-IV-TR Criteria for Amnestic Disorder Due to...[Indicate the General Medical Condition]

A. The development of memory impairment as manifested by impairment in the ability to learn new information or the inability to recall previously learned information.

B. The memory disturbance causes significant impairment in social or occupational functioning and represents a significant decline from a previous level of functioning.

C. The memory disturbance does not occur exclusively during the course of a Delirium or a Dementia.

D. There is evidence from the history, physical examination, or laboratory findings that the disturbance is the direct physiological consequence of a general medical condition (including physical trauma).

Specify if:

Transient: if memory impairment lasts for 1 month or less
Chronic: if memory impairment lasts for more than 1 month

Coding note: Include the name of the general medical condition on Axis I, e.g., 294.0 Amnestic Disorder Due to Head Trauma; also code the general medical condition on Axis III

CHAPTER SIXTEEN

MENTAL HEALTH SERVICES: LEGAL AND ETHICAL ISSUES

LEARNING OBJECTIVES

1. Define and differentiate the concept of mental illness from a psychological disorder.
2. Compare and contrast civil commitment and criminal commitment by outlining the historical evolution of such concepts, including the criteria that now generally apply for each.
3. Describe how the law relates to the mentally ill, including various standards of the insanity defense (e.g., not guilty by reason of insanity, guilty but mentally ill) and the issue of competency to stand trial.
4. Discuss the relation between violence/dangerousness and mental illness, and similarly the relation between mental illness, deinstitutionalization, and homelessness.
5. Define and discuss the concept of patient rights, including the right to treatment, the right to refuse treatment, the right to the least restrictive alternative, and other rights in the context of mental health law and ethics.
6. Describe the parameters of informed consent and how it relates to research participation, including its relation to ethics to psychological treatment more generally.
7. Discuss standards of psychological practice, and distinguish between efficacy vs. effectiveness research, including its relation to validity, managed care, and delivery of psychological services more generally.

OUTLINE

I. Civil Commitment

A. The **legal system** exercises significant influence over the mental health system, and professional behavior is dictated by laws and ethical principles. Each state has civil commitment laws that detail when a person can be legally declared to have a mental illness and be placed in a hospital for treatment. The following two trends in mental health law are evident in the recent history of the United States: liberal and neoconservative eras.

1. The **liberal era**, from 1960 to 1980, was characterized by a commitment to individual rights and fairness. During this period, the rights of people with mental illness dominated.
2. The **neoconservative era**, from 1980 to present, was a reaction against the liberal reforms of the 1960s and 1970s and was characterized by an emphasis on law and order. During this era, the rights of people with mental illness were limited to provide greater protection of society.

B. **Civil commitment** laws in the United States date back to the late 19th century. Before that time, people with mental illness were cared for by family members, the community at large, or were left to care for themselves. The advent of large public hospitals ushered in an alarming trend; namely, commitment of people for reasons that were unrelated to mental illness (e.g., holding different political views).

C. **Criteria for civil commitment** have evolved.

1. Historically, states permitted civil commitment when *either* of the following conditions were met.
    a. The person was shown to have a **mental illness** and a need for treatment.
    b. The person was deemed **dangerous** to self or others.
    c. The person was unable to care for him or herself, a situation referred to as a **grave disability**.
2. The **government** justifies its right to act against the wishes of the individual under two types of authority.
    a. Under **police power** authority, the government takes responsibility for protecting public health, safety, and welfare and can create laws and regulations to ensure such protection.
    b. Under **parens patriae**, the state applies power when citizens are not likely to act in their own best interest (e.g., to assume custody of children who have no living parents). This power is also used to commit individuals with severe mental illness to mental health facilities when it is believed they might be harmed for not being able to secure basic life necessities, or because they fail to recognize the need for treatment. Under this power the state acts as a surrogate parent.
3. The **civil commitment process** unfolds when the person does not voluntarily seek help, but others feel that treatment is necessary.
    a. Specifics of this process vary by state, but it usually begins with a petition by a relative or mental health professional to a judge. This process is similar to legal proceedings and the person under question has all the rights and protections provided by the law. Such persons must be notified that civil commitment proceedings are taking place, must be present during the trial, must have representation by an attorney, and can request witnesses and independent evaluation.
    b. In emergency situations involving clear immediate danger, a short-term commitment can be made without formal proceedings required of civil commitment. Certification of dangerousness is usually made by family members or the police.

D. The **concept of mental illness** figures prominently in civil commitment and how this concept is defined is important. **Mental illness** is a legal concept, meaning severe emotional or thought disturbances that negatively affect an individual's health and safety. Each state has its own definition of mental illness, and the *term mental illness is not synonymous with psychological disorder*. Many states exclude mental retardation or substance-related disorders from the definition of mental illness.

1. **Assessment of dangerousness** is a critical and controversial feature of the civil commitment process. An important issue is whether persons with mental illness are more dangerous or prone to violent behavior then the general population.
    a. Research on this issue is mixed. One explanation for this is that different definitions of mental illness are used. In general, however, persons with hallucinations and delusions are at increased risk for violence but are more likely to have a higher number of arrests.
    b. Research also suggests that mental health professionals can identify groups of people who are at greater risk than the general population for being violent (e.g., having a previous history of violence) and can so advise the court. What cannot be done is to predict with certainty whether a particular person will or will not become violent.

E. **Problems with the process of civil commitment**, particularly with regard to ambiguity and subjectivity, have resulted in several legal developments with economic and social consequences.

1. The Supreme Court stated in 1957, in the case of **O'Connor v. Donaldson**, that a state cannot constitutionally confine a non-dangerous individual who is capable of surviving safely in freedom by himself or with the help of willing and responsible family and friends. Similarly, in 1979, in the case of **Addington v. Texas**, the Supreme Court stated that more than just a promise of improving one's quality of life is required to commit someone involuntarily. Needing treatment or having a grave disability was not sufficient to involuntarily commit someone with a mental illness. The effect of this later decision was to limit substantially the government's ability to commit persons unless they were dangerous.
2. **Tighter restrictions on involuntary commitment** in the 1970s and 1980s led many who would have been committed to mental health facilities for treatment to be instead handled by the criminal justice system. Severely mentally ill persons were living in the community without needed mental health services and their behavior often resulted in problems with the police. **Criminalization** of the mentally ill became a concern as the justice system was not prepared to care for such individuals. The following trends also emerged during this time:
    a. The number of **homeless** persons increased dramatically. Presently, about 250,000 to 3 million persons in the United States are homeless, 25% of these have a previous history of hospitalization for mental health problems, and 30% are considered severely mentally ill. For a time, homelessness was blamed on strict civil commitment criteria, limits on stays at hospitals, and deinstitutionalization.
    b. **Deinstitutionalization** aimed to close large state psychiatric hospitals and to create a network of community mental health centers where the released persons could be treated. The goal of providing alternative community care has not been attained. Instead **transinstitutionalization** (i.e., the movement of people with severe mental illness from large psychiatric hospitals to nursing homes or

other group residences, including jails and prisons) occurred. Deinstitutionalization is largely considered a failure.
c. The perception that civil commitment restrictions and deinstitutionalization caused homelessness led to changes in commitment procedures.

F. **Changes with regard to commitment procedures** resulted from a culmination of factors (e.g., lack of success with deinstitutionalization, the rise of homelessness, and criminalization of people with severe mental illness). The textbook illustrates the clash of concerns with individual freedoms of people with mental illness and society's responsibility to treat them with the case of Joyce Brown.
1. Rulings such as **O'Connor v. Donaldson** and **Addington v. Texas** argued that mental illness and dangerousness should be criteria for involuntary commitment. However, concerns about homelessness and criminalization led to calls for a return to broader civil commitment procedures that would permit commitment in cases of dangerousness, but also for individuals who were not dangerous but in need of treatment and for those with grave disability.
2. The **National Alliance for the Mentally Ill (NAMI)** argued for legal reform to make involuntary commitment easier, and several states in the late 1970s and early 1980s changed their civil commitment laws in an attempt to address such concerns. Hospitals began to fill due to longer stays, repeated admissions, and acceptance of only involuntary admissions.

II. Criminal Commitment

A. **Criminal commitment** is the process by which people are detained in a mental health facility for assessment of fitness to stand trial because they have been accused of committing a crime or if they have been found not guilty of a crime by reason of insanity.

B. With respect to the **insanity defense**, the law recognizes that people are not responsible for their behavior under certain circumstances and that punishment would therefore be unfair. Current views of criminal commitment have been shaped by a case recorded over 150 years ago in England involving Daniel M'Naghten.
1. The **M'Naghten rule** reflects the decision of the English court that a person is not responsible for their criminal behavior if they do not know what they are doing, or if they do not know that what they are doing is wrong. The insanity defense originated with this ruling, and this ruling was used for more than 100 years to determine culpability when a person's mental state was in question.
2. In more recent times, **other standards** have been introduced to modify the M'Naghten rule because some viewed reliance of a person's knowledge of right versus wrong as too limiting. Modifications were designed to account for one's entire range of functioning when determining responsibility for behavior.
   a. The **Durham rule**, initiated in 1954 in the case of **Durham v. United States**, broadened the criteria for responsibility from knowledge of

right versus wrong to include the presence of a mental disease or defect. This was discarded, however, because mental health professionals lacked the expertise to reliably assess whether one's mental illness caused criminal behavior. Though the Durham rule is no longer used, its effect was to cause reexamination of the criteria used in the insanity defense.

b. **American Law Institute (ALI)** criteria were established in 1962. ALI reaffirmed the importance of distinguishing behavior of people with and without mental illness. ALI concluded that people are not considered responsible for their criminal behavior if, because of their mental illness, they could not recognize the inappropriateness of their criminal behavior or control it. The ALI test stipulates that a person must either be unable to distinguish right from wrong (as set forth by M'Naghten) or be incapable of self-control to be shielded from legal consequences. Also included in these writings were provisions for **diminished capacity**, or the idea that one's ability to understand the nature of his/her behavior and criminal intent (mens rea) could be lessened by mental illness. Criminal intent requires proof of the physical act (**actus rea**) and the mental state (**mens rea**) of the person committing the act.

3. Court rulings though the 1960s and 1970s on criminal responsibility parallel that of civil commitment. The focus was on the needs of people with mental illness who also broke the law and to provide mental health treatment instead of punishment. Use of insanity or diminished capacity in criminal cases alarmed the public.
   a. The case that prompted the strongest outrage against the insanity defense and calls for its abolition was that of **John W. Hinckley, Jr.** who attempted to assassinate President Ronald Regan. Hinckley was judged not guilty by reason of insanity (NGRI) using the ALI standard.
   b. After this verdict, more than 50% of U.S. states considered abolishing the insanity defense. Most of the public believes that the insanity defense is a legal loophole and that it is used too often. This was partly due to high-profile criminal cases where diminished capacity was used as a successful defense. As a result, an unfavorable public perception of the insanity defense may have been created.
   c. The public overestimates how often the insanity defense is used, how often the defense is successful, how often those acquitted with the insanity defense are freed, and length of confinement. *The insanity defense is used in less than 1% of criminal cases*, and persons judged NGRI spend more time in a hospital than they would have in jail.
4. Major changes were made in criteria for the insanity defense after the John Hinckley verdict.
   a. Congress passed the **Insanity Defense Reform Act** in 1984, which made use of the insanity defense more difficult by moving toward M'Naghten-like definitions.

b. Another attempt to reform the insanity plea has been to replace **"not guilty by reason of insanity"** to **"guilty but mentally ill"** (GBMI). Persons found GBMI are not sent to prison initially but are evaluated, and later if they recover from the mental illness they are sent to prison. The latter verdict allows for treatment and subsequent punishment.
c. The second version of GBMI is even harsher for the mentally ill offender. Convicted individuals are imprisoned, and the prison authorities may provide mental health services if they are available. The GBMI verdict in such cases is simply a declaration by the jury that the person was mentally ill at the time the crime was committed and does not result in differential treatment for the perpetrator.
d. Research shows that persons who receive the GBMI verdict are more likely to be imprisoned and to receive longer sentences than people pleading NGBI and are no more likely to receive treatment than other prisoners who have mental illnesses.

C. The judicial system and the mental health system have two different goals: the judicial system is adversarial, and the mental health system attempts to resolve psychological problems, without placing blame on the individual. New "problem-solving" courts have been created to resolve the conflict involved when these two systems collide. These courts are based on the concept of **therapeutic jurisprudence**, that is, using what we know about behavior change to help people in trouble with the law. This type of criminal justice system may be an effective alternative for people with severe mental illness.

D. **Competence to stand trial** requires that a person understand the charges against them and be able to assist with their own defense, as outlined in the Supreme Court in **Dusky v. United States**. A person may thus be judged insane at the time of a criminal act but still be competent to stand trial.

1. A person determined **incompetent** to stand trial typically loses the authority to make decisions and faces commitment. The amount of time a person can be committed to determine competency cannot be indefinite, and after a reasonable amount of time, the person must be found competent, set free, or committed under civil law. Determining competency usually requires the removal of decision-making authority from the individual and results in commitment.
2. The burden of proof in competence proceedings is on the defendant.

E. The professional issue of **duty to warn** in the case of a dangerous client was highlighted in the case of **Tarasoff v. Regents of the University of California**. In this case, the court ruled that therapists must warn persons at risk of harm by their clients. Other cases have since further defined the role of the therapist to warn others. For example, threats must be specific in nature (Thompson v. County of Alameda).

F. Courts often rely on **expert witnesses** or those with specialized knowledge to assist them in making decisions. Public perception of expert witnesses is characterized by ambivalence, see the expert as valuable in educating the jury on the one hand, and on the other the expert as a hired gun whose opinions suite the side that pays their bills.

1. Research suggests that mental health professionals can make reliable predictions of **dangerousness** over a short-term (i.e., 2 to 20 days after the evaluation), but not over long periods of time.
2. Research also suggests that mental health professionals can assist in making reliable DSM diagnoses. However, statements about whether someone has a mental illness reflects determinations made by the court, not the mental health professional.
3. Areas in which mental health professionals do appear to have expertise are the assessment of **malingering** (i.e., faking or grossly exaggerating symptoms) and **competence** (i.e., ability to understand and assist with one's own defense). However, personal and professional opinions about certain issues that go beyond the competence of an expert witness can influence what information is presented and how it is relayed to a court (e.g., not believing in involuntary commitment).

III. Patients' Rights and Clinical Practice Guidelines

A. A fundamental right of those in mental health facilities is the **right to treatment**. Starting in the 1970s, a series of class action lawsuits helped establish the rights of people with mental illness and mental retardation.

1. A landmark case, **Wyatt v. Stickney**, helped set standards for minimum staff-to-patient ratios, structural requirements (e.g., number of showers per resident), and that facilities make positive efforts to attain treatment goals for their patients. In addition, this case expanded upon the concept of **least restrictive alternative**, indicating that people should be provided with treatment in the least confining and limiting environment. Yet, a gap was left as to what constituted proper treatment.
2. In 1986, Congress passed the **Protection and Advocacy for Mentally Ill Individuals Act**, which established a series of protection and advocacy agencies in each state to investigate allegations of abuse and neglect and to act as legal advocates.

B. A more controversial patient right is the **right to refuse treatment**, particularly with respect to psychotropic (antipsychotic) medications. This often pits mental health concerns against individual rights. In addition, the issue has arisen as to whether one can be forced to become competent.

1. A Supreme Court ruling, **Riggins v. Nevada**, stated that because of the potential negative side effects (e.g., tardive dyskinesia), people cannot be forced to take antipsychotic medication.

C. **Research participants** have the following rights: the right to be **informed** about the purpose of the research study, the right to **privacy**, the right to be treated with

respect and **dignity**, the right to be **protected from physical and mental harm**, the right to choose **to participate** or **to refuse to participate** without prejudice or reprisals, the right to **anonymity** in reporting results, and the right to **safeguarding their records**. Such rights are particularly important for people with psychological disorders who may not be able to understand them fully.

1. One of the most important concepts in research is information about the risks and benefits of a study. Simple consent is not enough, it must be **informed consent** (i.e., formal agreement by the subject to participate after being fully apprised of all important aspects of the study, including possibility of harm. The textbook illustrates informed consent with the case of Greg Aller who was involved in a UCLA study involving antipsychotic medication.

D. Evidence based practice and clinical practice guidelines

1. The **Food and Drug Administration (FDA)** routinely regulates drugs and it is unclear whether a similar form of protections will be applied to psychosocial interventions. Yet, recognition of wide differences in treating the same disorder and the increasing demand of managed-care companies for knowledge of appropriate and effective treatments has led to the creation in 1989 of a new branch of the federal government called the **Agency for Health Care Policy and Research (AHCPR)**.
2. The AHCPR's aim is to establish uniformity in the delivery of effective health and mental health care and to communicate to practitioners throughout the country the latest developments in treating certain disorders effectively.
   a. AHCPR has published **clinical practice guidelines** for specific disorders (e.g., sickle cell disease, unstable angina, depression in primary care), and also facilitates guideline construction by other agencies.
   b. Through the AHCPR, the government hopes to reduce costs related to unnecessary or ineffective treatments and to facilitate **dissemination** based on the latest research evidence.
3. The **American Psychological Association** composed a template, or set of principles, in 1995 (i.e., *Division 12 Task Force for the Promotion and Dissemination of Psychological Procedures*) for constructing and evaluating guidelines for clinical interventions for both psychological disorders and psychosocial aspects of physical disorders. The guidelines are aimed to facilitate decision making on the part of practitioners, and to restrain unnecessary cost cutting by health care plans via prohibition of certain treatments or treatment durations. The **APA task force's clinical practice guidelines** for specific disorders were constructed based on two simultaneous considerations.
   a. The first, the **clinical efficacy** axis, involves a thorough consideration of the scientific evidence to determine whether the intervention in question is effective. That is, is the treatment effective when compared to an alternative treatment or to no treatment in a controlled clinical research context? Answering this question requires that experiments show that the intervention in question is better than no

therapy, better than a nonspecific therapy, or better than an alternative therapy, with the latter providing the highest level of evidence for the treatment's effectiveness. This axis is concerned largely with **internal validity**. Such efforts may rely on amass data from practitioners via **quantified clinical observations** or **clinical replication series**.

b. The second axis, or **clinical utility**, is concerned with the **effectiveness** of the intervention in the practice setting, regardless of the research evidence on its efficacy. That is, will an intervention with proven efficacy in a research setting also be effective in less controlled practice settings when applied by frontline practitioners? This axis is concerned with **external validity**. Here practitioners will be concerned with feasibility and acceptability of the intervention, including generalizability from research to routine practice contexts.

OVERALL SUMMARY

This chapter outlines the primary legal and ethical issues associated with the study, assessment, and treatment of abnormal behavior. In addition, changing societal views about those with mental illness are discussed. Specific issues such as civil and criminal commitment, dangerousness, homelessness, deinstitutionalization, insanity defense, competency to stand trial, duty to warn, expert witnesses, and patient and research participant rights are discussed. Contemporary issues in mental health are also covered, with an emphasis on practice guidelines for efficacy and effectiveness of psychosocial interventions.

KEY TERMS

Civil commitment laws (p. 545)
Clinical efficacy (p. 559)
Clinical utility (p. 559)
Competence (p. 555)
Criminal commitment (p. 551)
Dangerousness (p. 547)
Deinstitutionalization (p. 548)
Diminished capacity (p. 552)
Duty to warn (p. 555)
Expert witnesses (p. 555)
Informed consent (p. 557)
Malingering (p. 556)
Mental illness (p. 547)
Transinstitutionalization (p. 549)

INFOTRAC KEY TERM EXERCISES

Each exercise is linked to key terms from the Wadsworth InfoTrac on-line searchable database. Key terms must be entered exactly as written.

Exercise 1: What to do About Mentally Ill Criminal Offenders
Article: A54099150
Citation: (A critical assessment of disposition options for mentally ill offenders). Donald M. Linhorst; P. Ann Dirks-Linhorst.
Social Service Review, March 1999 v73 i1 p65(1)

This InfoTrac article evaluates three disposition options for mentally ill offenders: (a) abolishing the insanity defense, (b) substituting a guilty but mentally ill verdict, or (c) retaining the insanity defense with a conditional release. What are the foundations of each position and the research on implementation and policy outcomes? How did the state of Missouri handle such issues and has it been successful in doing so? Argue for or against the authors' recommendation that retaining the insanity defense with conditional release and community monitoring is the most viable option. Limit your answer to 3-5 double-spaced pages.

Exercise 2: Sex Offenders: Blurred Boundaries Between Civil and Criminal Commitment
Key Term: *Criminal Commitment*

Sexual offenders, particularly pedophiles and incest perpetrators, represent unique cases where clinical disorders (i.e., pedophilia, incest) are also criminal offenses, punishable by law. In such cases, the boundaries between civil and criminal commitment are often blurred. What are the issues with regard to civil and criminal commitment of sex offenders of the types described above? What does the law say regarding civil commitment of such offenders, particularly after such persons have served their full prison terms? Does the state have the right to involuntarily commit such individuals, even after they have served their sentences, under the powers of parens patriae? Review the InfoTrac articles on this complex topic, and outline the background and rulings with regard to the issues. How do you think society and the courts should balance civil vs. criminal commitment standards in such cases? Take a position and defend it as best you can. Limit your answer to 3-5 double-spaced pages.

Exercise 3: Assessment of Decision-Making Capacity in Older Persons
Key Term: *Assessment of Decision-Making Capacity*

Legal, medical, and psychological decisions often rely on the ability of the person involved to understand, and hence, to be able to make reasonable decisions on their behalf. That is, it is assumed in most cases that such persons have some decision-making capacity. Though the chapter discusses this issue in the context of mental health law (e.g., competence) and ethics (e.g., informed consent), a broader issue concerns how one would go about assessing whether and to what extent such decision-making capacity exists in a person. Your task here is to review the InfoTrac article (only one) on this complex topic written by Barry Edelstein, and to outline the issues involved in assessing competence, particularly with regard to older persons. What methods are employed and what do psychologists look for in assessing decision-making capacity, and hence competence? Based on such considerations, evaluate the extent to which such issues apply to the assessment of competence in a legal sense. Limit your answer to 3-5 double-spaced pages.

Exercise 4 (Future Trend): Practice Guidelines and Standards, Oh My!

Mental health practitioners are increasingly being forced to practice consistent with the tenets of the scientist practitioner model. Managed care, with its focus on accountability, cost containment, quality and efficient delivery of services, has been a driving force behind such changes. Practice guidelines and standards are part of this process, and though controversial, are meant to serve as guidelines for best practices consistent with best available scientific evidence. One could even think of practice guidelines as being somewhat analogous to the FDA model of treatment development. The links below provide resources for a more detailed about practice guidelines and standards of care, including some of the controversies surrounding them.

http://www.guideline.gov/
http://www.psych.org/psych_pract/treatg/pg/prac_guide.cfm
http://kspope.com/ethcodes/index.php
http://www.apa.org/pi/oema/guide.html
http://www.cpa.ca/guide10.html

CLASSROOM ACTIVITIES, DEMONSTRATIONS, AND LECTURE TOPICS

1. **Activity: Lecture About Forensic Psychology.** The specialized field of forensic psychology is relatively new, and yet many students are quite interested in it based upon news and media depictions of mentally ill persons, criminal profiling, mass murders, and the like. You may want to review the literature on the role psychologists have in the legal profession. The following review article is a good place to start:

   Source Information. Wrightsman, L. S. (2001). Forensic psychology. Belmont, CA: Wadsworth/Thomson Learning.

2. **Activity: Defining Mental Illness.** The text discusses how the laws defining mental illness vary from state to state. Ask your students to research your state laws regarding the definition of mental illness as well as the topic of persecution of those with mental illness. You may also ask them to research how ethical concerns are handled in your state. For example, what course of action must a consumer take to file a charge against a psychologist who has violated ethical or legal practices? Have your students write a brief paper indicating who they spoke with to receive information and what they learned about this process.

3. **Activity: Discuss the Nature of Manualized Psychotherapy.** Practice guidelines are increasingly pointing toward flexible use of psychotherapy manuals in routine clinical practice. Yet, there are many misunderstandings and myths surrounding manualized treatments, most of them negative. Try to get a copy of an empirically supported psychosocial treatment manual and present some of it to the class, including why such

manuals are used in efficacy trials, and the assets and liabilities of such manuals in routine clinical practice.

4. **Activity: Invited Lecture by Expert Witness or Forensic Psychologist.** Students will often be curious as to the role of psychologists in their capacity as expert witnesses, including the routine work of forensic psychologists. Try inviting someone who has extensive experience in these areas to come and speak to the class. Prior to the invited lecture, ask students to prepare 1 or 2 anonymous questions that they are curious about and provide them to the guest lecturer beforehand.

5. **Video Activity: Perceptions of the Mentally Ill.** Show the CNN today video segment titled "Mental Health Services: Britain Bedlam." This relatively brief segment depicts images from Bethlehem (i.e., Bedlam) hospital then and now, and goes on to discuss de-institutionalization of the mentally ill, and how societal attitudes about persons with mental illness have changed over the years. You may use this video as a prompt to ask students whether societal attitudes have really changed. For example, ask your students for a show of hands to the following question: How many of you would mind having a community residence for chronically mentally ill persons in your neighborhood, or perhaps right next door to your house? Alternatively, ask your students for a show of hands to the following question: how many of you would feel comfortable telling a friend or family member that you had mono, or that they were going to see a doctor for the flu? Many hands will go up. Now ask those who put up their hands whether they would be equally comfortable telling the same persons that they are going to see a psychologist, or that they suffer from bi-polar disorder, alcoholism, or anorexia? Discuss with the students their perceptions of whether societal attitudes about the mentally ill have really changed, and if so, where do they see the changes?

SUPPLEMENTARY READING MATERIAL FOR CHAPTER SIXTEEN

(= These sources can be found on *"Infotrac, the online library"* provided by Wadsworth and Brooks/Cole Publishing.)

Accordino, M. P., Porter, D. F., & Morse, T. (2001). Deinstitutionalization of persons with severe mental illness: Context and consequences. The Journal of Rehabilitation, 67, 16.

American Psychological Association (1992). Ethical principles of psychologists and code of conduct. Washington, DC: Author.

Annas, G. J. (1989). The rights of patients: The basic ACLU guide to patient rights (2nd ed.). Carbondale, IL: Southern Illinois University Press.

Bersoff, D. N. (1995). Ethical conflicts in psychology. Washington, DC: American Psychological Association.

Chambless, D. L., & Ollendick, T. H. (2000). Empirically supported psychological interventions: Controversies and evidence. Annual Review of Psychology, 685.

Crespi, T. D. (1989). Child and adolescent psychopathology and involuntary hospitalization: A handbook for mental health professionals. Springfield, IL: Thomas.

Edelstein, B. (2000). Challenges in the assessment of decision-making capacity. Journal of Aging Studies, 14, 423.

Falk, A. J. (1999). Sex offenders, mental illness and criminal responsibility: The constitutional boundaries of civil commitment. American Journal of Law & Medicine, 25, 117(1).

La Fond, J. Q., & Durham, M. L. (1992). Back to the asylum: The future of mental health law and policy in the United States. New York: Oxford University Press.

Lilienfeld, S. O. (1995). Seeing both sides: Classic controversies in abnormal psychology. Pacific Grove, CA: Brooks/Cole.

Mindell, J. A. (1993). Issues in clinical psychology. Madison, WI: Wm. C. Brown.

Spiegel, A. D., & Spiegel, M. B. (1998). The insanity plea in early nineteenth century America. Journal of Community Health, 23, 227(21).

Spring, R. L. (1989). Patients, psychiatrists, and lawyers: Law and the mental health system. Cincinatti, OH: Anderson.

Steadman, H. J., McGreevy, M. A., & Morrisey, J. P. (1993). Before and after Hinckley: Evaluating insanity defense reform. New York: Guilford.

Winick, B. J. (1997). The right to refuse mental health treatment. Washington, DC: American Psychological Association.

SUPPLEMENTARY 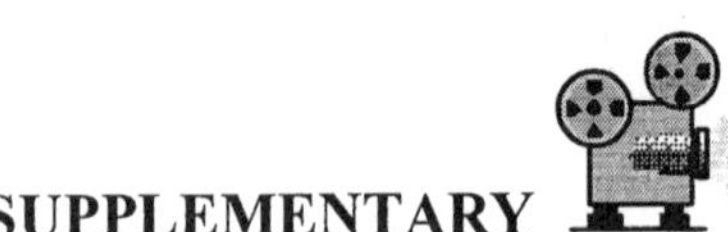 VIDEO RESOURCES FOR CHAPTER SIXTEEN

A defendant's state of mind: The insanity defense. (Insight Media: 2162 Broadway, New York, NY 10024/ (800)-233-9910). This panel discussion probes issues related to the insanity defense, asking whether or not it is used in too many cases. It focuses on the cases of Colin Ferguson, Jeffrey Dahmer, Susan Smith, and John Salvi. It also considers how juries react to sensational trials. (48 min)

A fine madness. (Hollywood Film; Drama). This film stars Sean Connery as Samson, an eccentric poet who is hospitalized and later lobotomized because of this sexual exploits and his failure to conform to societal expectations. This film nicely depicts important issues about the rights of persons with mental illness.

Anatomy of a murder. (Hollywood Film; Drama). This film depicts a courtroom case involving rape and promiscuity and an interesting analysis of the irresistible impulse defense.

CNN today: Abnormal psychology, vol. 1. (*available through your International Thomson Learning representative).* The segment titled "Mental Health Services: Britain Bedlam" shows pictures of Bedlam then and now, discusses the de-institutionalization of the mentally ill, and how societal attitudes about persons with mental illness have changed over the years. (3 min, 30 sec)

Criminally insane. (Insight Media: 2162 Broadway, New York, NY 10024/ (800)-233-9910). Taking viewers on an unprecedented tour of the Clifton T. Perkins hospital in Jessup, Maryland, this video explores the world of a maximum-security institution for the criminally insane. It explains that while virtually all of the patients at Perkins have committed extremely violent crimes, all of them have been found not guilty by reason of insanity. (60 min)

Dark side of the moon. (Fanlight Productions, 1-800-937-4113). Documents the struggles and successes of three formerly homeless men with mental illnesses. (25 min)

Ethics for the mental health professional. (Insight Media: 2162 Broadway, New York, NY 10024/ (800)-233-9910). This video teaches the basics of ethical behavior for psychologists, social workers, and counselors. It discusses licensing law and violations of ethical guidelines, and shows how to terminate treatment, make referrals, and maintain records. It also considers malpractice. (160 min)

Inside the criminal mind 1. (Insight Media: 2162 Broadway, New York, NY 10024/ (800)-233-9910). An exploration of the workings of the deviant psyche, this video enables viewers to witness therapy sessions with incarcerated men and women. (60 min)

King of hearts. (Hollywood film; Drama). This film nicely illustrates societal attitudes about mental illness.

Nuts. (Hollywood Film; Drama). This film, starring Barbara Streisand and Richard Dreyfuss, portrarys a woman's fight to defend her claims of sanity, and illustrates issues related to the process of commitment.

Pleading insane. (Insight Media: 2162 Broadway, New York, NY 10024/ (800)-233-9910). Tracing the history of the insanity plea from the Hatfield case in 19th-century England, this video shows how the defense has evolved and discusses some of the issues it raises. It profiles several well-known cases, focusing on the Hinckley verdict. (50 min)

Rampage. (Hollywood Film; Drama/Thriller). This is a William Friedkin film depicting a sociopath who is arrested and tried for murder. The film raises important issues about capital punishment, the not guilty by reason of insanity plea, and the role of the expert witness in the courtroom.

Testifying about child sexual abuse: A courtroom guide. (Insight Media: 2162 Broadway, New York, NY 10024/ (800)-233-9910). Professionals evaluating children for alleged sexual abuse must be aware that they may ultimately be called upon to present their findings in a court of law. This video helps viewers understand their role in legal proceedings, prepare and deliver testimony effectively, and minimize the stress involved for children. (35 min)

The mind of a serial killer. (Insight Media: 2162 Broadway, New York, NY 10024/ (800)-233-9910). This video presents an inside look at the FBI's use of psychological profiling. It shows how the FBI unit made famous in The Silence of the Lambs used a detailed psychological profile to help a New York state police department catch a serial killer. (60 min)

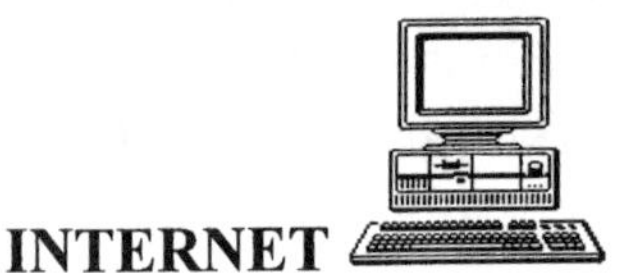

INTERNET RESOURCES FOR CHAPTER SIXTEEN

A Brief Summary of the Insanity Defense
http://ua1vm.ua.edu/~jhooper/insanity.html

This web site entitled "Forensic Psychiatry Resource Page" is maintained by Dr. J. Hooper at the University of Alabama Department of Psychiatry & Neurology. This page is an elaborate outline of the history of the insanity defense.

American Psychological Association (APA) Ethics Office
http://www.apa.org/ethics/

This is the official APA ethics web site, with links to the ethical principles and code of conduct and related topics about ethical violations.

Dodging the Insanity Defense With Diminished Capacity
http://www.diminishedcapacity.com/

This is an interesting web site with a wealth of information regarding the nature and use of the insanity defense, most of it somewhat critical.

Empirically Supported Treatment (EST) Archive
http://www.wpic.pitt.edu/research/sscp/empirically_supported_treatments.htm

This web site, sponsored by the Society for a Science of Clinical Psychology (SSCP), offers links to current articles on empirically supported psychotherapies, including available manualized treatments for a range of DSM disorders.

Federal Bureau of Investigation
http://www.fbi.gov/

The FBI's web site; includes the "Ten Most Wanted" list of fugitives.

Forensic Science Resources
http://www.tncrimlaw.com/forensic/f_psych.html
This web site provides several links to topics related to mental health and the law.

Law for Psychiatrists
http://ua1vm.ua.edu/~jhooper/law-psy.html
This web site entitled "Forensic Psychiatry Resource Page" is maintained by Dr. J. Hooper. This page describes information on legal issues, including the insanity defense, for psychiatrists.

Mental Health Info Source
http://www.mhsource.com/
This web site provides a wealth of information about psychological disorders and their treatment, including information on practice guidelines and managed care.

National Alliance for the Mentally Ill (NAMI)
http://www.nami.org
This web site provides information and status reports about state and federal laws that affect people with mental illness, including their families.

National Guideline Clearinghouse
http://www.guideline.gov/
The National Guideline Clearinghouse TM (NGC) is a public resource for evidence-based clinical practice guidelines.

Psychiatry for Attorneys
http://ua1vm.ua.edu/~jhooper/psy-law.html
This web site entitled "Forensic Psychiatry Resource Page" is maintained by Dr. J. Hooper at the University of Alabama Department of Psychiatry & Neurology. This page describes an overview of psychiatric principles for attorneys.

Violence and Mental Illness
http://www.hc-sc.gc.ca/hppb/mentalhealth/pubs/mental_illness/
This Canadian site presents a comprehensive review and data regarding the relation between violence and mental illness.

WARNING SIGNS OF TEEN VIOLENCE

The following signs indicate the potential for violent behavior. Note that having a mental illness is not a warning sign of violent behavior!

- Loss of temper on a daily basis
- Frequent physical fighting
- Significant vandalism or property damage
- Serious drug or alcohol use, or an increase in such use
- Increase in risk-taking behavior
- Detailed plans to commit acts of violence
- Announcing threats or plans for hurting others
- Enjoying hurting animals
- Carrying a weapon
- A history of violent or aggressive behavior
- Gang membership or strong desire to be in a gang
- Access to or fascination with weapons, especially guns
- Threatening others regularly
- Trouble controlling feelings like anger
- Withdrawal from friends and usual activities
- Feeling rejected or alone
- Having been a victim of bullying
- Poor school performance
- History of discipline problems or frequent run-ins with authority
- Feeling constantly disrespected
- Failing to acknowledge the feelings or rights of others

<table>
<tr><th>21Barlow and Durand: Abnormal Psychology, An Integrative Approach, 4/e</th><th>Davison, Neale, and Kring: Abnormal Psychology with Cases, 9/e</th></tr>
<tr><td>Chapter 1: Abnormal Behavior in Historical Context

• Understanding Psychopathology (2-5)
• The Science of Psychopathology (5-8)
• Historical Conceptions of Abnormal Behavior (8-11)
• The Biological Tradition (11-14)
• The Psychological Tradition (14-16)

• Psychoanalytical Theory (16-21)
• Humanistic Theory (21-22)

• The Behavioral Model (22-25)
• The Present: The Scientific Method and An Integrative Approach (25-26)</td><td>Chapter 1: Historical and Scientific Considerations and Chapter 2: Current Paradigms in Psychopathology and Therapy

What is Abnormal Behavior? (3-5)
• Science: A Human Enterprise (15-17)
• History of Psychopathology (6-11)

• The Biological Paradigm (21-25)

• The Psychoanalytic Paradigm (26-36)
• Humanitarian and Existential Paradigms (37-43)
• Learning Paradigms (43-51)
• The Cognitive Paradigm (52-56)</td></tr>
<tr><td>Chapter 2: An Integrative Approach to Psychopathology

• One Dimensional or Multidimensional Models (31-34)
• Genetic Contributions to Psychopathology (34-40)
• Neuroscience and Its Contribution to Psychopathology (41-53)
• Behavioral and Cognitive Science (54-57)
• Emotions (57-60)
• Cultural, Social, and Interpersonal Factors (60-63)
• Life-Span Development (64)</td><td>Chapter 2: Current Paradigms in Psychopathology and Therapy

• Consequences of Adopting a Paradigm (58)

• Diathesis-Stress: An Integrative Paradigm (58)

• Different Perspectives on a Clinical Problem (60)
• Ecclecticism in Psychotherapy (61)</td></tr>
</table>

21Barlow and Durand: Abnormal Psychology, An Integrative Approach, 4/e	Davison, Neale, and Kring: Abnormal Psychology with Cases, 9/e
Chapter 3: Clinical Assessment and Diagnosis • Assessing Psychological Disorders (69-74) • Behavioral Assessment (74-77) • Psychological Testing (77-82) • Neuropsychological Testing (82-84) • Psychophysiological Assessment (84-85) • Diagnosing Psychological Disorders (86-96)	**Chapter 3: Classification and Diagnosis and Chapter 4: Clinical Assessment Procedures** • Issues in the Classification of Abnormal Behavior (72-78) • The Diagnostic System of the American Psychiatric Association (DSM-IV-TR) (65-71) • Psychological Assessment (82-96) • Biological Assessment (97-104) • Reliability and Validity in Assessment (80-81) • Cultural Diversity and Clinical Assessment (105-106) • The Consistency and Variablity of Behavior (107-108)
Chapter 4: Research Methods • Important Concepts (100-103) • Studying Individual Cases (103-104) • Research by Correlation (104-106) • Research by Experiment (106-108) • Single Case Experimental Designs (108-111) • Studying Genetics (111-113) • Studying Behavior Over Time (113-114) • Studying Behavior Across Cultures (114-115) • The Power of a Program of Research (115-116) • Replication (116-117) • Research Ethics (117)	**Chapter 5: Research Methods in the Study of Abnormal Behavior** • Science and Scientific Methods (111-113) • The Research Methods of Abnormal Psychology (114-130) • The Case Study (115-116) • The Correlational Method (118-120) • The Experiment (121-126) • Single Subject Experimental Research (127)

21Barlow and Durand: Abnormal Psychology, An Integrative Approach, 4/e	Davison, Neale, and Kring: Abnormal Psychology with Cases, 9/e
Chapter 5: Anxiety Disorders • Anxiety, Fear, and Panic (121-123) • Causes (123-126) • Comorbidity of Anxiety Disorders (126) • Generalized Anxiety Disorder (127-131) • Panic Disorder with and without Agoraphobia (132-141) • Nocturnal Panic (135) • Specific Phobia (141-148) • Separation Anxiety Disorder (143-144) • Social Phobia (148-152) • Post Traumatic Stress Disorder (152-158) • Obsessive Compulsive Disorder (159-162)	**Chapter 6: Anxiety Disorders** • Generalized Anxiety Disorder (152-155) • Panic Disorder (145-151) • Phobias (134-144) • Posttraumatic Stress Disorder (163-170) • Obsessive Compulsive Disorder (156-162)
Chapter 6: Somatoform and Dissociative Disorders • Hypochondriasis (169-173) • Somatization Disorder (173-177) • Conversion Disorders (177-182) • Pain Disorder (182) • Body Dysmorphic Disorder (182-186) • Depersonalization Disorder (187-188) • Dissociative Amnesia (188-189) • Dissociative Fugue (189-190) • Dissociative Trance Disorder (190) • Dissociative Identity Disorder (191-198)	**Chapter 7: Somatoform and Dissociative Disorders** • Pain Disorder, Body Dysmorphic Disorder, and Hypochondriasis (173) • Conversion Disorder (174) • Depersonalization Disorder (187) • Dissociative Amnesia (186) • Dissociative Fugue (186) • Dissociative Identity Disorder (187)

21Barlow and Durand: *Abnormal Psychology, An Integrative Approach*, 4/e	**Davison, Neale, and Kring: *Abnormal Psychology with Cases*, 9/e**
Chapter 7: Mood Disorders and Suicide	**Chapter 10: Mood Disorders**
• Understanding and Defining Mood Disorders (205-206) • An Overview of Depression and Mania (206) • The Structure of Mood Disorders (206-208)	• General Characteristics of Mood Disorders (268-272)
• Depressive Disorders (208-212)	• Depression (268)
• Bipolar Disorders (212-215)	• Mania (268)
• Additional Defining Criteria (215-216) • Differences in the Course of Mood Disorders (216-218) • Prevalence of Mood Disorders (219-223) • The Overlap of Anxiety and Depression (223-224)	• Psychological Theories of Mood Disorders (273-282) • Biological Theories of Mood Disorders (283-287)
• Causes of Mood Disorders (225-236)	
• Treatment of Mood Disorders (236-242) • Preventing Relapse (242-245)	• Therapies for Mood Disorders (287-299)
• Suicide (246-250)	• Suicide (304-316)
Chapter 8: Eating and Sleep Disorders	**Chapter 9: Eating Disorders**
• Major Types of Eating Disorders (257-258)	
• Bulimia Nervosa (258-261)	• Bulimia Nervosa (248)
• Anorexia Nervosa (261-264)	• Anorexia Nervosa (246-247)
• Binge-Eating Disorder (264-265)	• Binge-Eating Disorder (250)
• Cross-Cultural Considerations (265-267) • Developmental Considerations (267)	
• Causes (267-273)	• Etiology of Eating Disorders (251-260)
• Treatment of Eating Disorders (273-279)	• Treatment of Eating Disorders (261-265)
• Obesity (279-282) • Sleep Disorders: The Major Dyssomnias (282-291) • Treatment of Sleep Disorders (292-296)	

21Barlow and Durand: Abnormal Psychology, An Integrative Approach, 4/e	Davison, Neale, and Kring: Abnormal Psychology with Cases, 9/e
Chapter 9: Physical Disorders and Health Psychology • Psychological and Social Factors That Influence Behavior (303-305) • The Nature of Stress (305-309) • Stress and the Immune Response (309-311) • Psychosocial Effects on Physical Disorders (312-323) • Psychosocial Treatment of Pain Disorders (324-328) • Modifying Behaviors to Promote Health (328-331)	**Chapter 8: Psychophysiological Disorders and Health Psychology** • Stress and Health (199-205) • Theories of the Stress-Illness Link (206-209) • Socioeconomic Status, Ethnicity, and Health (229-230) • Therapies for Psychophysiological Disorders (231-243)

21Barlow and Durand: Abnormal Psychology, An Integrative Approach, 4/e	**Davison, Neale, and Kring: Abnormal Psychology with Cases, 9/e**
Chapter 10: Sexual and Gender Identity Disorders	**Chapter 14: Sexual and Gender Identity Disorders**
• What is Normal Sexuality? (337-339) • Gender Differences (339-340) • Cultural Differences (340-342)	
• Gender Identity Disorders (342-346)	• Gender Identity Disorder (435-440)
• Overview of Sexual Dysfunctions (346-353) • Assessing Sexual Behavior (353-355) • Causes of Sexual Dysfunction (356-360) • Interaction of Psychological and Physical Factors (360)	• Descriptions and Etiology of Sexual Dysfunctions (462-465) • General Theories of Sexual Dysfunctions (466-468)
• Treatment of Sexual Dysfunction (360-364) • Paraphilia: Clinical Descriptions (364-369) • Causes of Paraphilia (369-371) • Assessing and Treating Paraphilia (371-373)	Therapies for Sexual Dysfunctions (469-472) • The Paraphilias (441-453) • Etiology of the Paraphilias (449-450) • Therapies for the Paraphilias (451-453)
Chapter 11: Substance-Related and Impulse-Control Disorders	**Chapter 12: Substance-Related Disorders**
• Perspectives on Substance-Related Disorders (379-380) • Levels of Involvement (380-384) • Diagnostic Issues (384) • Depressants (385-389)	• Alcohol Abuse and Dependence (359-364)
• Sedative, Hypnotic, or Anxiolytic Substance Use Disorders (389-390) • Stimulants (390-396) • Opiods (396-398)	• Sedatives and Stimulants (372-377)
• Hallucinogens (398-401) • Causes of Substance-Related Disorders (401-406)	LSD and Other Hallucinogens (378-381) Etiology of Substance Abuse and Dependence (382-387)
• Treatments (407-411) • Relapse Prevention (411) • Prevention (412) • Impulse-Control Disorders (412-414)	• Treatments (388-403) • Prevention of Substance Abuse (404-406)

21Barlow and Durand: Abnormal Psychology, An Integrative Approach, 4/e	Davison, Neale, and Kring: Abnormal Psychology with Cases, 9/e
Chapter 12: Personality Disorders • An Overview of Personality Disorders (421-422) • Categorical and Dimensional Models (422-424) • Statistics and Development (424) • Gender Differences (424-426) • Comorbidity (426) • Personality Disorder Under Study (415-416) • Paranoid Personality Disorder (427-429) • Schizoid Personality Disorder (429-430) • Schizotypal Personality Disorder (430-432) • Antisocial Personality Disorder (432-440) • Borderline Personality Disorder (440-443) • Histrionic Personality Disorder (443-444) • Narcissistic Personality Disorder (444-446) • Avoidant Personality Disorder (446-447) • Dependent Personality Disorder (447-448) • Obsessive Compulsive Personality Disorder (448-449)	**Chapter 13: Personality Disorders** • Classifying Personality Disorders: Clusters, Categories and Problems (410-411) • Paranoid Personality Disorder (411) • Schizoid Personality Disorder (412) • Schizotypal Personality Disorder (412) • Antisocial Personality Disorder (418-423) • Borderline Personality Disorder (413-415) • Histrionic Personality Disorder (416) • Narcissistic Personality Disorder (417) • Avoidant Personality (424) • Dependent Personality Disorder (425) • Obsessive-Compulsive Personality Disorder (425-426)

21Barlow and Durand: *Abnormal Psychology, An Integrative Approach, 4/e*	Davison, Neale, and Kring: *Abnormal Psychology with Cases, 9/e*
Chapter 13: Schizophrenia and Other Psychotic Diseases • Perspectives on Schizophrenia (455-456) • Identifying Symptoms (456-457) • Clinical Description, Symptoms, and Subtypes (458-464) • Other Psychotic Disorders (464-467) • Prevalence of Schizophrenia (467-468) • Development (468) • Cultural Factors (469) • Causes (469-476) • Psychological and Social Influences (476-477) • Treatment of Schizophrenia (478-482) • Prevention (482-483)	**Chapter 11: Schizophrenia** • Clinical Symptoms of Schizophrenia (319-323) • History of the Concept of Schizophrenia (324-327) • Etiology of Schizophrenia (328-340) • Therapies for Schizophrenia (341-354)
Chapter 14: Developmental Disorders • What Is Normal? What is Abnormal? (490) • Attention Deficit / Hyperactivity Disorder (490-495) • Learning Disorders (495-499) • Pervasive Developmental Disorders (499-503) • Asperger's Disorder (503-505) • Treatment of Pervasive Developmental Disorders (505-507) • Mental Retardation (507-515) • Prevention of Developmental Disorders (515)	**Chapter 15: Disorders of Childhood** • Classification of Childhood Disorders (476-477) • Attention Deficit/Hyperactivity Disorder (478-483) • Learning Disabilities (492-497) • Autistic Disorder (506-517) • Mental Retardation (498-505)

<table>
<tr><th>21Barlow and Durand: Abnormal Psychology, An Integrative Approach, 4/e</th><th>Davison, Neale, and Kring: Abnormal Psychology with Cases, 9/e</th></tr>
<tr><td>Chapter 15: Cognitive Disorders

• Delirium (521-523)
• Dementia (523-526)
• Dementia of the Alzheimer's Type (526-528)
• Vascular Dementia (528-529)
• Dementia Due to Other General Medical Conditions (529-531)
• Substance-Induced Persisting Dementia (531-532)
• Biological Influences (532-534)
• Psychological and Social Influences (534-535)
• Treatment (535-537)
• Prevention (537-538)
• Amnestic Disorder (538-539)</td><td>Chapter 16: Aging and Psychological Disorders

• Delirium (531-533)
• Dementia (524-530)
• Old Age and Psychological Disorders (534-552)

• Treatment and Care of Older Adults (553-558)</td></tr>
<tr><td>Chapter 16: Mental Health Services: Legal and Ethical Issues

• Civil Commitment (545-551)
• Criminal Commitment (551-556)
• Patient's Rights (556-557)
• Research Participants Rights (557-558)
• Clinical Practice Guidelines (558-560)</td><td>Chapter 18: Legal and Ethical Issues

• Civil Commitment (621-636)
• Criminal Commitment (608-620)
• Ethical Dilemmas in Therapy and Research (637-646)</td></tr>
</table>